Nursing Acutely Ill Adults

This comprehensive and clinically focused textbook is designed for student and qualified nurses concerned with caring effectively for deteriorating and acutely ill adults outside of specialist intensive care units.

Divided into six parts, the book begins with chapters on assessment and the deteriorating patient, including monitoring vital signs and interpreting blood results. This is followed by two parts focusing on breathing and cardiovascular problems respectively. Part 4 explores issues around disability and impairment, including chapters on neurology, pain management, psychological needs and thermoregulation. The penultimate part looks at maintaining the internal environment, with chapters on issues such as nutrition, fluid management and infection control. The text ends with a discussion of legal issues and accountability.

Nursing Acutely Ill Adults includes a full range of pedagogical features, including sections on: identifying fundamental knowledge; highlighting implications for practice; suggesting further reading and resources; describing case scenarios, which help readers relate theory to practice; and providing 'time out' exercises. It is the ideal textbook for students taking modules in caring for critically ill adults, and qualified nurses working with these patients.

Philip Woodrow is the Practice Development Nurse for Critical Care in East Kent Hospitals University NHS Foundation Trust, UK. He teaches a number of critical care courses, and maintains clinical practice across the Trust's three intensive care units.

In acknowledging that nurses are an important safety net in hospitals, this text sets out to provide information for nurses on how to recognise, understand and respond to problems in the acutely unwell ward patient. Even a cursory glance over the contents list gives an indication of the breadth of this book. Chapters cover a wide range of topics including vital signs, intrapleural chest drainage, acute kidney injury, tissue donation and accountability. This text can be used to dip in and out of whilst working on the ward, or to sit down and read systematically: there is something here for everyone. So whether you're an 'old hand' in ward nursing or a novice nurse just about to embark on your hospital career, this text is recommended reading.

Maureen Coombs, Victoria University of Wellington, NZ

Nursing Acutely Ill Adults

Philip Woodrow

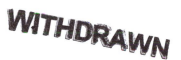
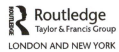
Routledge
Taylor & Francis Group

LONDON AND NEW YORK

First published 2016
by Routledge
2 Park Square, Milton Park, Abingdon, Oxon OX14 4RN

and by Routledge
711 Third Avenue, New York, NY 10017

Routledge is an imprint of the Taylor & Francis Group, an informa business

British Library Cataloguing-in-Publication Data
A catalogue record for this book is available from the British Library

Library of Congress Cataloging in Publication Data
Woodrow, Philip, 1957– , author.
Nursing acutely ill adults/written by Philip Woodrow.
p. cm.
Includes bibliographical references and index.
I. Title.
[DNLM: 1. Critical Care Nursing – methods. 2. Critical Illness – nursing. 3. Critical Care – methods. WY 154]
RT120.I5
616.02′8 – dc23
2015004456

ISBN: 978-1-138-01887-7 (hbk)
ISBN: 978-1-138-01888-4 (pbk)
ISBN: 978-1-315-77945-4 (ebk)

Typeset in Times
by Florence Production Ltd, Stoodleigh, Devon, UK
Printed by Ashford Colourr Press Ltd.

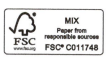

Contents

Part 3: Cardiovascular

Part 4: Disability

Part 5: Environment (internal)

Part 6: Professional contexts

Figures

Tables

Preface

This book is written for nurses caring for acutely ill adults in general hospital wards. It is based on the 'Caring for the Acutely Ill Patient' course, which I facilitate for East Kent Hospitals University NHS Trust, and uses the A-B-C-D-E assessment recommended by the Resuscitation Council.

Acute illness is a large topic, and so selection has been necessary to make the book affordable, manageable and readable. I have therefore largely avoided duplication of material in my *Intensive Care Nursing* book, viewing these two books essentially as companion texts, and making some cross references to the other text.

While issues about acutely ill and deteriorating patients are largely global, structures of healthcare can differ significantly between countries. This book is written primarily from a UK perspective, and should be interpreted in local contexts for readers elsewhere. Similarly, although many aspects may also be applicable for sick children, readers caring for children should check paediatric sources. Similarly, readers working in specialist areas will need to extend their specialist knowledge beyond aspects covered in this book.

Inevitably many texts and guidelines are likely to be published and updated during the shelf-life of this book, so readers should check the internet and other sources for any superseding versions. Many guidelines have been cited in this book, but readers can find useful information on websites such as those for the

- National Institute for Clinical Excellence
- National Patient Safety Agency
- Department of Health
- Scottish Intercollegiate Guidelines Network

as well as special interest groups (such as the British Thoracic Society). Similar bodies exist in many countries.

No book is perfect, but my hope is that this book provides an overview of acute illness and the deteriorating patient, to enable readers to deliver improved care and to inspire readers to develop their own knowledge further as part of their continuing professional development. Many chapters are prefixed by FUNDAMENTAL KNOWLEDGE, a list of aspects that readers should revise if unsure about; as most items in FUNDAMENTAL KNOWLEDGE are anatomical, an anatomy and physiology resource will be useful. Each chapter ends with suggested further reading and a clinical scenario or set of exercises to help readers consolidate the chapter. Some chapters also include TIME OUT exercises to encourage reflection. As most readers are likely to dip in and out of the book, rather than read it cover-to-cover, the text includes cross-references to other chapters.

Thank you to everyone who has helped in the production of this book: the team at Routledge, illustrator Jane Fallows, copy-editor Carolyn Holleyman, Proofreader Kilmeny MacBride, the production team at Florence Production and to the many people 'behind the scenes' who have helped make this book what it is.

Philip Woodrow

Abbreviations

A-B-C-D-E	airway – breathing – circulation – disability – exposure (or environment), the nationally recommended first-responder initial assessment
ACS	acute coronary syndrome
AECOPD	acute exacerbation of chronic obstructive pulmonary disease
AKI	acute kidney injury
AMI	acute myocardial infarction
aPPT	activated Partial Thromboplastin Time
ATN	acute tubular necrosis
ATP	adenosine triphosphate, produced in cells and used by cells for energy
AVPU	Alert – Verbal – Pain – Unresponsive
BACCN	British Association of Critical Care Nurses
bpm	breaths per minute (in context of breathing) or beats per minute (in context of pulse)
C diff	*Clostridium difficile*
CAD	coronary artery disease
CCO	Critical Care Outreach
CK	creatine kinase (cardiac biomarker)
CKD	chronic kidney disease
CLOD	Clinical Lead for Organ Donation (the doctor identified within the Trust to promote donation services)
CNST	Clinical Negligence Scheme for Trusts
COPD	chronic obstructive pulmonary disease
CPAP	continuous positive airway pressure
CRE	carbapenem-resistant *Enterobacteriacae*
CRP	C-reactive protein
CRT	capillary refill time
CSL	compound sodium lactate ('Hartmann's solution')
cTnI, cTnT	cardiac-specific troponin I, troponin T (cardiac biomarkers)
CVC	central venous catheter

DES	drug eluding stent
DKA	diabetic ketoacidosis
DOH	Department of Health
DVT	deep vein thrombosis
EF	ejection fraction
EMLA	eutectic mixture of local anaesthetics
EMRSa	epidemic meticillin resistant *Staphylococcus aureus*
EN	enternal nutrition
ESBL	extended spectrum beta-lactamase (increases resistance)
ESRF	end-stage renal failure
FBC	full blood count
FG	french gauge (sizing of cannula/catheter)
FRIII	fixed rate intravenous insulin infusion
GCS	Glasgow Coma Scale
GFR	glomerular filtration rate
GRE	glycopeptide resistant *Enterococci*
GTN	glyceryl trinitate
HAS	human albumin solution
HCAI	healthcare-associated infection (also called hospital-acquired infection)
HHS	hyperosmolar hyperglycaemic state
HONKS	hyperosmolar non-ketotic state (now called hyperosmolar hyperglycaemic state)
I:E	inspiratory to expiratory ratio (normally 1:2)
ICD	implantable cardiac defibrillator
ICS	Intensive Care Society
INR	international normalised ratio, a measurement of clotting time (see Chapter 3)
IVI	intravenous infusion
kDa	kilodaltons; molecular weight
LDL	low density lipoprotein
LFTs	liver function tests
MAP	mean arterial pressure
MC+S	microscopy, culture and sensitivity (the standard microbiology test)
MI	myocardial infarction
MRSa	meticillin resistant *Staphylococcus aureus* (meticillin was previously called methicillin)
NAFLD	non-alcoholic fatty liver disease
NASH	non-alcoholic straeto-hepatitis
NEWS	National Early Warning Score
ng	nanograms (millionths of grams)
NHSLA	NHS Litigation Authority
NICE	National Institute for Clinical Excellence
NIV	noninvasive ventilation
NPSA	National Patient Safety Agency (now disbanded)
NSAID	non-steroidal anti-inflammatory drugs (many of the medium strength pain-killers)

NSTEMI	Non ST elevation myocardial infarction
PE	pulmonary embolism
PEA	pulseless electrical activity
PERTL	pupils equal, react to light
PICC	peripherally inserted central catheter
PN	parenteral nutrition
pPCI	primary percutaneous coronary intervention
PPIs	protein pump inhibitors
PT	Prothrombin Time
RCN	Royal College of Nursing
rt-PA	recombinant tissue plasminogen activator
SBAR	Situation Background Assessment Response
SBP	systolic blood pressure
SIADH	syndrome of inappropriate antidiuretic hormone
SIRS	systemic inflammatory response syndrome
SNOD	Senior Nurse for Organ Donation
SSI	signs and symptoms of infection (see Table 13.1)
STEMI	ST elevation myocardial infarction
TBI	traumatic brain injury
TC	total cholesterol
TEDS	thromboembolytic deterrent stockings
TIA	transient ischaemic attack
TPN	total parenteral nutrition
U+Es	urea + electrolytes (biochemistry blood test)
UA	unstable angina
ViEWS	VitalPac Early Warning Score
VRE	vancomycin resistant *Enterococci* (now called glycopeptide resistant *Enterococci* – GRE)
VTE	venous thromboembolism
WCC	white cell count

Part 1

Assessment

Chapter 1

The deteriorating patient

Contents

Introduction

Significant avoidable morbidity and mortality occurs in acute hospitals (NICE, 2007; NPSA, 2007a; Yoon *et al.*, 2014). In recent years, average acuity of patients in acute hospitals has increased (Needleman, 2013), placing all acute hospital patients at potential risk of deterioration. This book aims to help readers recognise the deteriorating patient, and identify what interventions may help avoid or reduce avoidable mortality.

Healthcare has faced many challenges and changes over the last quarter century. While 25 years may seem a long perspective, many buildings in which acute hospitals function are older, and many structures of, and expectations from, healthcare delivery predate these changes.

Arguably, the most significant change in acute care coincided with the new millennium: in 2000 the Department of Health (DOH) published *Comprehensive Critical Care*. Among the report's many recommendations, all of which were accepted in full, was the expectation to replace 'the existing division into high dependency and intensive care based on beds

... by a classification that focuses on the level of care that individual patients need, regardless of location' (paragraph 16). From a patient-centred perspective, this appears desirable. However, most general wards were not designed, equipped or staffed to provide high dependency or intensive care, and most ward staff had little or no experience of those specialities. The expectations of *Comprehensive Critical Care* therefore placed significant pressures on acute hospitals and their staff.

The challenges would have been significant had expectations been matched by increased funding, staffing and resources. But publication of *Comprehensive Critical Care* coincided with multiple other internal and external pressures, including

- year-on-year budget restrictions encouraging cost-saving reductions in numbers of staff (Francis, 2013; Aiken *et al.*, 2014);
- national and international directives and legislation, such as the European Union working time directives;
- society moving from a duty-based ethic to a rights-based one;
- promotion of evidence-based practice (Stevens, 2013).

Recent years have seen much turbulence within healthcare, potentially destabilising practice and confidence. An example of this turbulence is the number of relatively recently created national organisations which, having highlighted many of the issues discussed in this book, have now been disbanded, such as the NHS Modernisation Agency, and the National Patient Safety Agency (transferred to the NHS Commissioning Board Special Health Authority).

Staffing levels

Maintaining safety is fundamental to healthcare (Nightingale, 1859/1980; Roper *et al.*, 1996). Staffing costs, and especially nursing staff, form the largest part of the NHS budget, so financial prioritisation has sometimes encouraged reduction of staffing levels (Francis, 2013). But this may be a false economy: lower staffing levels increase

- mortality (Aiken *et al.*, 2014; Needleman *et al.*, 2011);
- pressure ulcer rates (Twigg *et al.*, 2010);
- incidence of falls (RCN, 2012);
- medication errors (Twigg *et al.*, 2010);
- readmission rates (McHugh and Chenjuan, 2013);

and many other causes of morbidity and mortality. Many nurses feel unable to provide safe care due to excessive work pressures. The Royal College of Nursing (RCN, 2012), and many other organisations have proposed that the UK should, like some other countries, adopt minimum staffing levels. In the wake of Francis (2013), NHS England (2014) published guidance for nurse staffing levels, and now requires Trusts to publish data on the internet.

Levels of care

Comprehensive Critical Care defined four levels of care for hospitalised patients (see Table 1.1), level 2 patients being what were previously called 'high dependency'. This book focuses of level 2 patients, although aspects are also relevant to patients needing other levels of care. Level 1 was later (AUKUH, 2007) subdivided into 1a (sicker) and 1b (less sick), although this division tends to be used more for administration than ward-level care.

The 2007 document further specified level 2 as patients

- with single organ system monitoring and support (not advanced respiratory support);
- needing preoperative optimisation: invasive monitoring and treatment to improve organ function;
- needing extended post-operative care: including short term (less than 24 hours), routine post-operative ventilation with no other organ dysfunction (e.g. fast track cardiac surgery patients);
- needing greater degree of observation and monitoring;
- moving to step-down care;
- major uncorrected physiological abnormalities.

Previously, the Intensive Care Society (ICS, 2002) had listed examples of level 2 patients as those

- needing more than 50% oxygen;
- with haemodynamic instability due to hypovolaemia/haemorrhage/sepsis;
- with acute impairment of renal, electrolyte or metabolic function;
- having undergone major elective surgery;

Table 1.1 Levels of Care (DOH, 2000; ICS, 2009)

Level 0:
Patients whose needs can be met through normal ward care in an acute hospital

Level 1:
Patients at risk of their condition deteriorating, or those recently relocated from higher levels of care, whose needs can be met on an acute ward with additional advice and support from the critical care team

Level 2:
Patients requiring more detailed observation or intervention including support for a single failing organ system or post-operative care and those 'stepping down' from higher levels of care

Level 3:
Patients requiring advanced respiratory support alone or basic respiratory support together with support of at least two organ systems. This level includes all complex patients requiring support for multi-organ failure

---

- with tachycardia above 120 bpm;
- with hypotension (systolic below 80 mmHg for more than one hour);
- with Glasgow Coma Scale (GCS) score below 10 and at risk of acute deterioration.

A 2009 update of this ICS document includes further examples. However, the shorter 2002 list illustrates that most general wards do have level 2 patients.

Microphysiology

Many acute pathologies will be outlined in later chapters, focusing on major organs and body systems. The human body is made up of more than 100 trillion (100,000,000,000, 000) cells (Maczulak, 2010). While visible organs may be easier to conceptualise, microscopic cells, cell function and dysfunction are fundamental to health. When sufficient cells fail, the organ/system fails. Crude mortality risk is approximately 25% per organ/system failure. Supporting healthy cell function can therefore prevent cell, and system, failure, reducing mortality risks for patients.

Cells need energy to function. Each cell makes its own energy, in the form of adenosine triphosphate (ATP), in its mitochondria. Normally, mitochondria produce energy by glycolysis – combustion of glucose in the presence of oxygen. There are three main waste products of glycolysis:

- carbon dioxide
- water
- metabolic acids.

These waste products can be toxic/problematic if not removed.

In the absence of glucose, mitochondria can produce energy from alternative sources (fat is usually the preferred source in the absence of glucose); in the absence of oxygen, mitochondria can produce energy anaerobically. But alternative energy source and/or anaerobic metabolism produce relatively little energy and more (and often different) waste products. Although most cells have some energy (ATP) stores, with the notable exception of brain cells, insufficient supply of either oxygen or glucose is likely eventually to cause cell failure, and cell death.

Acuity of illness is significantly affected by two homeostatic mechanisms:

- stress
- inflammation.

Normally, when the body is exposed to a threat, it mounts a stress and/or inflammatory response to resolve the problem. If the response is balanced, the threat will usually be resisted or resolved. If responses are insufficient, the threat causes pathophysiology (illness/death). If responses are excessive, they are likely to become pathological (see Figure 1.1).

Understanding these two microscopic processes is fundamental to understanding almost all pathologies described in later chapters.

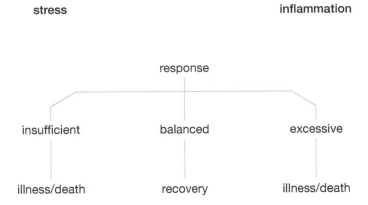

Figure 1.1 **Effects of balanced and imbalanced stress and inflammatory responses**

Adverse events

About 4% of hospitalised patients experience adverse events, about one quarter of which are preventable (Benning *et al.*, 2011). Classen *et al.* (2011) suggest that incidence is usually under-measured, and could be tenfold most estimates.

As well as morbidity and mortality, adverse incidents can have significant emotional and financial impact on all involved (patients, families, staff), and as sicker patients are likely to need longer hospitalisation and more complex and costly and complex treatments, staff workload is also likely to be increased. Humans can err, and systems can fail, so as well as reporting any harms that did occur, it is important to report 'near misses' to try and avert future patients being exposed to similar risks (WHO, 2005a).

Any treatment or aspect of care creates risks and/or problems (benefits and burdens). Professional care should therefore constantly assess risk/benefit analysis, and whenever possible discuss these openly with patients.

Fundamental care

Much recent concern about healthcare has been about failure, or perceived failure, of fundamental care, such as hygiene and nutrition. This concern has prompted such responses as the Chief Nursing Officer's advocacy of the '6 Cs' (Commissioning Board Chief Nursing Officer and DH Chief Nursing Adviser, 2012).

Some fundamental aspects are included in this book, but it is impractical to include all; some others are discussed in the companion textbook *Intensive Care Nursing;* others may be assumed, or indicated in 'fundamental knowledge', being covered in many textbooks focusing on more other aspects of nursing. If fundamental needs are not met, deterioration is more likely, and recovery less likely, to occur.

As the single largest group of staff in acute hospitals, nurses have a major role in preventing harm and helping recovery. Empowering nurses to provide safe and effective care reduces risks to patients, and improves outcome (Welch, 2000).

You are presumably reading this book because you are motivated to help your patients. The next chapter outlines vital signs which, if abnormal, are often indicators of deterioration (Welch, 2000). Empowerment can be through specific structures, such as Patient Group Directions (PGDs), enabling nurses to administer medicines which have been prescribed for a patient group rather than an individual patient, or through knowledge. This book is designed to help you recognise early warning signs of the deteriorating patient, and enable you to identify early actions that are likely to be helpful. Throughout this book you should reflect on your

- current work
- own developmental needs to meet the care of patients where you work
- your own career aims
- how you envisage you will achieve your career aim.

Such reflections on each chapter could provide valuable pages in your professional portfolio.

'Acute' versus 'chronic'

'Chronic' derives from the ancient Greek word 'chronos', meaning 'time'. Traditionally, 'chronic' referred to something present for more than 90 days, 'acute' for shorter time periods. Unfortunately, the word chronic has gained a plethora of meanings and connotations; this book generally follows this traditional, if arbitrary, division, although 'acute care', and by implications acute problems and treatments, often assumes a shorter (undefined) time period – hours or at the most days. The focus of this book is acute care, and therefore acute problems. However, patients will often be admitted with chronic co-morbidities, so aspects of chronic care and management are included where appropriate.

A note on this using book

Acute illness covers a wide range of diseases and possible interventions, nearly all of which have been studied, and written about, in depth. This book aims to provide an overview of the range of the topic. A large tome could be written on the topic, but such length would almost invariably restrict its use to selective reading for specific aspects. To achieve accessibility, this book necessarily sacrifices depth – each topic can be pursued in further detail. This book should be viewed as a resource for continuing professional development, highlighting topics which if relevant to the reader's practice, should then be pursued further.

Implications for practice

- Acute hospitals aim to cure acute disease.
- Acute illness makes patients vulnerable to further deterioration.
- Disease may manifest in macro organs, but originates at microscopic level.
- Supporting cell health and function helps prevent deterioration.

- While some deaths are unavoidable, there is an unacceptable incidence of avoidable mortality and morbidity in acute hospitals.
- If you suspect deterioration in a patient's condition, escalate your concerns ('if in doubt, shout').

Summary

Ward nurses are the only group of clinical staff who are in the patient's vicinity all the time. Nurses therefore provide an important 'safety net' for patients, being able to recognise problems early and escalate concerns promptly. Nurses therefore need to recognise the signs of acute deterioration. This chapter has introduced this core theme, and other key aspects, of this book. Many issues raised are developed in subsequent chapters.

Further reading

A recent and trusted anatomy and physiology text is a useful companion for this book. Marieb and Hoehn (2013) is the one most cited in this book, but there are many other useful ones. NICE (2007) and the companion report NPSA (2007a) highlighted problems of failure to identify deterioration. RCN (2012) comprehensively analyses nurse staffing levels.

Clinical scenario

Mr Henry Stubbings was admitted to A&E following a fall during his out-patient appointment. The wound to his leg was dressed, and he was discharged home. Four days later he was readmitted as a GP referral, due to rigors, tachycardia and hypotension. You admit him to the Clinical Decisions Unit, where his initial vital signs are

Respiratory rate	28 breaths per minute
Pulse	112 bpm (regular)
BP	98/56 (MAP 70)
Temperature	38.6°C

He is alert, and accompanied by his wife.

Generally, a healthy 74-year-old with a good quality of life, he had previously visited his GP because of periodic dizziness. The GP found his blood sugar was 9.6 mmol/litre, so had referred him to endocrinology outpatients.

1   From this information, what do you suspect is the likely cause of the fall?
2   What are your main concerns? What immediate risk factors would you need to address, and how would you address them? What further initial investigations

do you plan to undertake? What initial investigations would you expect medical staff to initiate? What questions might you ask Mr Stubbings and/or his wife to help plan his care? What other sources of information might be available to you?

3   You decide to bleep the doctor, who is busy elsewhere. Using SBAR format (or another if used in your workplace), list what you plan to say over the telephone.

Chapter 2

Vital signs

Contents

Introduction

The phrase 'vital signs' derives from the Latin word 'vita', meaning life. Vital signs are signs of life, so abnormal vital signs provide early warning of deterioration (Goldhill and McNarry, 2003). To help recognition of the deteriorating patient, various early warning scores have been developed, using what are considered to be the key vital signs. This chapter refers to the National Early Warning Score (NEWS), with its electronic variant VitalPac Early Warning Score (ViEWS) (Prytherch *et al.*, 2010; RCP, 2011; RCP, 2012a). As NEWS/ViEWS is the UK's national scoring system, other scoring systems will not be discussed, although most are broadly similar, and NEWS/ViEWS is based on the widely used Modified Early Warning Score (MEWS). Where NEWS/ViEWS parameters are available for vital signs, ideal (zero-scoring) ranges are identified as 'target'.

NEWS/ViEWS (Table 2.1) assesses

- pulse
- temperature
- systolic blood pressure
- respiration rate
- consciousness level
- oxygen saturations
- any supplemental oxygen.

But other vital signs included here may be clinically important. This chapter does not discuss oxygen therapy (NEWS/ViEWS target: any oxygen scores 2), and only briefly

Table 2.1 NEWS/ViEWS

PHYSIOLOGICAL PARAMETERS	3	2	1	0	1	2	3
Respiration Rate	≤8		9–11	12–20		21–24	≥25
Oxygen Saturations	≤91	92–93	94–95	≤96			
Any Supplemental Oxygen		Yes		No			
Temperature	≤35.0		35.1–36.0	36.1–38.0	38.1–39.0	≤39.1	
Systolic BP	≤90	91–100	101–110	111–219			≥220
Heart Rate	≤40		41–50	51–90	91–110	111–130	≥131
Level of Consciousness				A			V, P, or U

mentions temperature, as this is discussed further in Chapter 19. Many other aspects discussed are developed in subsequent chapters. The stress response, introduced in the previous chapter, is also developed.

This chapter uses two frameworks for assessment promoted by the Resuscitation Council (2010):

- A-B-C-D-E (Airway – Breathing – Circulation – Disability – Exposure/ Environment);
- look – listen – feel.

Like most early warning systems, NEWS/ViEWS recommends frequency of repeat observations. Any decision to over-ride recommended reassessment should be professionally justifiable, reasons recorded, and may be called to account.

Compensation

The body attempts to compensate for problems, so if any system disease causes hypoxia, breathing will usually increase. As human beings, compensation is a useful response to help us cope with problems. It creates a period of 'quiet deterioration' before symptoms occur, and during which people are unlikely to seek help or report problems. As healthcare professionals, compensation is problematic, as many patients will already have reached advanced stages of deterioration before seeking help; problems may be unreported and unobvious until decompensation occurs. Even 'early warning' abnormal vital signs often only appear at relatively late stages, especially in younger, otherwise healthy, adults. Any concern should therefore be escalated promptly.

Goldhill and McNarry (2003) suggest that immediate threats to life are negligible if vital signs are normal, but that two abnormal vital signs carry a 9.2% one month mortality risk, rising to 21.3% risk with three or more abnormal vital signs.

Recognising deterioration

Before *Comprehensive Critical Care*, another DOH-commissioned report (McQuillan *et al.*, 1998) identified that incidence of critical illness could have been reduced by half had there been closer monitoring of vital signs, and appropriate responses, at an earlier stage of hospital care. Similar findings were reported in two later, linked, reports (NICE, 2007; NPSA, 2007a), which highlighted three main concerns

- lack of monitoring of vital signs
- lack of reporting measured abnormal vital signs
- delay in medical staff responding to reported abnormal vital signs.

They therefore recommended that early warning scores should be used in all hospitals (NICE, 2007).

Pitfalls

Each vital sign measures an aspect of physiological function. However, body systems are part of the whole person, and dysfunction of one system can affect others. For example, breathlessness (tachypnoea) is a common response to many problems, and does not necessarily indicate respiratory disease.

Trends are more important than single or isolated figures, and therefore new concerns should be considered in the context of previous observations. If using paper charts, it is therefore useful to continue using the same chart until it is complete, and keeping recent previous charts nearby.

Many vital signs are measured with machines. Numbers displayed by machines may be subject to machine error margins – numbers displayed are not always as precise as they may appear. Machines can also be 'fooled' by artefact – for example ECG monitors sometimes double the heart rate because tall T waves are erroneously counted as QRSs. People can also make mistakes – counting respiratory rate can be significantly affected if patients are aware their rate is being counted, if they undertake some other activity during the time of it being counted, or if some abdominal movement not related to breathing is included in the count. Therefore, with any reported abnormal observations that cause concern, look at the patient, and if in doubt about the accuracy of measurements, remeasure.

A

Airway

Significant partial airway obstruction is usually audible (*listen*). A completely obstructed airway is likely to be silent, with either no signs of breathing, or severe distress (stridor). The airway may be opened by extending it, such as by tilting the head – chin lift to create a 'morning sniff' position. If obstruction from vomit or other secretions is suspected, the 'recovery' (lateral, with airway and head downward) may enable drainage. Absence of breathing, or extreme distress, suggests respiratory arrest, which should prompt an 'arrest' call (in the UK: 2222, remembering to state hospital as well as location within the hospital). Unless an obvious cause for obstruction can be removed, anaesthetic intervention (intubation) will probably be needed.

B

Breathing

The earliest warning of deterioration is usually a change in respiratory rate (Tarassenk *et al.*, 2006). Breathing gets oxygen into the body and carbon dioxide out. While gas exchange is affected by rate, respiratory assessment should also include:

- look (rate, depth, pattern, appearance)
- listen (sound of breathing, cough)
- feel (skin – e.g. clammy).

Pulse oximetry is a valuable way to assess oxygenation, the main effect of breathing.

Rate (NEWS/ViEWS target 12–20)

Respiratory *rate* normally varies to meet the body's need for oxygen and to clear carbon dioxide.

Bradypnoea (low respiratory rates) may be caused by opioid or other overdoses. Symptomatic bradypnoeas may be reversible with drugs (e.g. naloxone for opioids); if unresponsive to drugs, anaesthetists should be consulted, with a view to potential mechanical ventilation.

More often, hospitalised patients experience tachypnoea. People with chronic respiratory disease therefore usually have a chronically high respiratory rate. Any reversible causes, such as pain, should be treated. Respiratory rate normally increases on exertion, but rates above 24 are likely to precipitate crises, escalating until exhaustion and respiratory/cardiac arrest, so be urgently review by medical staff (Cretikos *et al.*, 2008).

Depth

Depth of breathing cannot be numerically quantified, but does suggest effectiveness of carbon dioxide clearance. Depth depends on

- total lung volume
- respiratory stimuli (oxygen, carbon dioxide, acid)
- inhibition.

Lung volume may be reduced by

- external pressure (e.g. obesity, faecal impaction, ascites, or other abdominal distension);
- internal collapse (e.g. pneumothorax, atelectasis);
- abnormalities occupying space (e.g. pulmonary oedema, pleural effusion, lung cancer).

Reducing these (where possible) improves respiratory function. The importance of positioning is discussed in Chapter 4.

Inhibition may be caused by pain – pain on inspiration encourages shallow breathing. Inhibition may also be caused by drugs or disease. General anaesthetics include neuromuscular blockade ('paralysing agents'), and although the drugs will have largely cleared before anaesthetists extubate patients, residual amounts can cause shallow breathing for some hours post-operatively (Yip *et al.*, 2010). Neuromuscular diseases, such as Guillain Barré Syndrome, can also impair depth of breathing – these are discussed further in *Intensive Care Nursing*, Chapter 31.

Pattern

Most people usually breathe relatively regularly; if breathing *pattern* becomes irregular, the patient is usually deteriorating. Breathing is normally also symmetrical, as both lungs expand together. The only reason for asymmetrical breathing is something preventing one lung from expanding. Unless the person has had lung reduction surgery, this is likely to be an acute problem, such as a pneumothorax. Asymmetrical breathing should therefore be urgently reported. However, resting people periodically take 'sigh breaths' – extra deep slow breaths, like a sigh; this disrupts counting rate, so count should be recommenced.

Appearance

How the person breathes affects how they *appear*. Hypoxia and/or hypercapnia can affect skin colour and texture, as well as behaviour. Insufficient oxygen can cause cyanosis, and sometimes a cold clamminess just before a crisis. Peripheral cyanosis is best seen in the nailbed; central cyanosis is best seen in the lips and tongue. In people who are normally cyanosed, increased cyanosis usually indicates deterioration. Hypercapnia can cause vasodilatation, giving an overly-pink colour to skin (see Chapter 4). Most people normally breathe through their nose; new mouth-breathing is usually a sign of deterioration.

Most adults normally breathe through their nose, resorting to mouth-breathing when there is an airway problem, such as a cold. If patients start mouth-breathing, this usually indicates deterioration.

Listen

Normal breathing is inaudible, so when *listening* if breathing is heard it is abnormal. If a cough is present, is it

- strong or weak
- can you describe its sound (e.g. dry, hoarse, hacking)
- productive or unproductive?

On admission, record if coughs are absent, as later coughing suggests a healthcare-associated infection. Auscultation using a stethoscope is discussed in Chapter 6.

Sputum

Sputum is normally produced by lungs, but it is normally mobilised to the oropharynx, where it stimulates a swallowing reflex. If excessive sputum is produced, sometimes the swallow is visible. More often, copious sputum will be expectorated. As well as providing sputum pots, tissues and rubbish bags, it is useful to examine sputum for

- amount
- colour
- consistency.

Normally, sputum is *white*, but if expectorated it is seldom normal. Abnormal sputum colours include

■ *black*, which may be from smoking (tar in cigarettes), dried blood, or other sources (e.g. coal, or something staining saliva black, such as iron therapy);

■ *pink*, from fresh blood;

■ *creamy, green* or *yellow*, from infection; reporting exact colours may help doctors identify likely microbes – for example, green sputum is almost invariably pseudomonas. If infection is suspected, a specimen should be sent for MC+S.

If expectorated, sputum is normally thick (tenacious, sticky). Frothy sputum, and especially pink frothy sputum, is usually from pulmonary oedema, usually needing urgent treatment with intravenous furosemide.

Pulse oximetry (NEWS/ViEWS target ≥96)

Oxygen is relatively insoluble, so nearly all oxygen carried by blood is in haemoglobin. Pulse oximetry measures the percentage of haemoglobin carrying oxygen. The haemoglobin molecule has four 'chains', each of which can carry one oxygen molecule (two atoms). So HbO_8 is fully (100%) saturated. Normal (non-COPD) arterial saturation is 97–98%, while normal venous saturation (see Chapter 8) is 70% (Garry *et al.*, 2010), so pulse oximetry saturations below 90% result in relatively little oxygen being available for cells (Jacques *et al.*, 2006). NEWS/ViEWS target saturation conflicts with national target saturations (see Chapter 5).

Saturation is a valuable way to assess need for oxygen therapy, and to monitor oxygen therapy. However, there are limitations:

■ hypercapnia
■ anaemia
■ carbon monoxide
■ external light
■ low readings
■ dark colours.

Hypercapnia: pulse oximetry measures oxygen, not carbon dioxide. Pulse co-oximeters, which measure both gases, have been developed, but currently they are not generally used clinically (Bolliger *et al.*, 2007).

Anaemia: oximetry measures the percentage saturation of haemoglobin, but if patients are anaemic, there is relatively little haemoglobin to be saturated.

Carbon monoxide: makes haemoglobin an even brighter red than oxygen does, causing falsely high readings (Weaver *et al.*, 2013). For in-patients, the most likely source of significant carbon monoxide is from smoking.

External light: if reddish light (such as sunlight) reaches the light receiver, a falsely high reading will be obtained. Finger probes almost invariably have covers which prevent this, but if saturation is measured on ears, and the ear is in direct bright sunlight, shade the pulse oximeter probe to see if saturations readings fall.

Low readings: unless patients are moribund, very low readings (below 88%) are usually spurious, caused by insufficient bloodflow to the site of the probe. With very low readings, look at the patient, assess their level of consciousness, and check peripheries for colour and warmth; if peripheral bloodflow is poor, move the probe to a different site, or try and increase peripheral bloodflow.

Pulse oximeters work by shining red and infrared light from a light source to a light receiver. Anything between absorbs light; darker colours absorb more light. Nail varnish is therefore often considered to lower readings (BTS, 2008). Theoretically, dark nail varnish (blue, black) should absorb more light, but evidence suggests it does not make significant difference (Rodden *et al.*, 2007; Hinkelbein and Genzwuerker, 2008). Due to the cost of some acrylic nails, removing these is not recommended; if necessary, place probes sideways across the finger. Even if nail varnish does affect readings, the effect will be constant, so the trend of improvement or deterioration will be evident. Intravenous dyes are more concerning: red dyes may cause over-readings, blue dyes under-readings, and some dyes may not affect readings. Effects will only last until dye clears from blood.

C

Cardiovascular

The cardiovascular system transports gases, nutrients, waste and other things around the body. Cardiovascular assessment should include

- pulse
- blood pressure.

Other aspects included here are

- peripheral warmth/colour
- capillary refill

and arguably aspects discussed elsewhere in this book, such as temperature and urine output.

Pulse (NEWS/ViEWS target 51–90)

Pulse rate is measured by various machines, including automated blood pressure monitors and pulse oximeters. However, while these are useful for monitoring, pulse rate should also be felt for

- regularity *and*
- strength.

Irregular pulses, if new, should be reported, and an ECG should be recorded. The most likely, but not the only, cause of irregular pulses is atrial fibrillation (see Chapter 14).

If not used to feeling pulses, feel your own and those of other healthy people. Abnormally weak or strong pulses suggest abnormal stroke volumes (see Chapter 10).

Peripheral perfusion

Looking at and feeling feet, and hands, for colour and warmth indicates perfusion, or lack of it. Mottled, cold peripheries are poorly perfused. Excessive dilatation (e.g. from sepsis) makes peripheries abnormally warm and flushed. Inspecting peripheries may also reveal oedema, ulceration or other symptoms of haemodynamic compromise.

Capillary refill

Pressing on a fingertip for five seconds compresses capillaries. In health, initial blanching should disappear within two seconds (Ahern and Philpot, 2002) of releasing pressure. Delayed capillary refill indicates poor perfusion (Lima and Bakker, 2005), usually from hypovolaemia/dehydration, but may occur with vessel disease (e.g. atherosclerosis), or arterial hypotension.

(Non-invasive) blood pressure

Blood pressure is usually measured with automated machines, although some practitioners consider sphygmomanometers and stethoscopes to be more accurate. Most cuffs display marks to show how to place them on arms, and the range of arm circumferences they can be used on (see Figure 2.1). Using cuffs which are too small causes over-readings, while

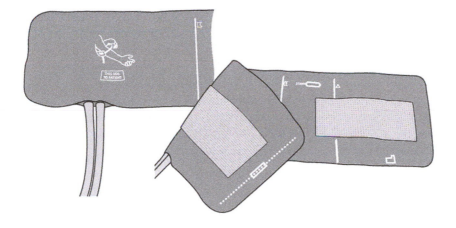

Figure 2.1 **NIBP cuff, with markings**

cuffs that are too large under-read (Lip, 2003; O'Brien *et al.*, 2013). Most adult wards only need to stock small, medium ('average') and large-sized cuffs.

Blood pressure is usually measured on the upper arm. However, contraindications to pressure on limbs includes

- patient refusal
- fractures
- renal shunts
- PICC lines
- angioedema.

If neither arm is available, measurement can be made on legs. As blood flows through the arterial system, resistance increases (Safar *et al.*, 2003), making distal systolic pressures up to one third higher (Runcimann and Ludbrook, 1996). Mean and diastolic pressures are more comparable (Moore *et al.*, 2008).

Systolic blood pressure (SBP) (NEWS/ViEWS target 111–219)

Peak, transient, pressure occurs when flow through vessels is at its greatest. Very high systolic pressure can cause bleeds, strokes or other problems. Hypotension can cause inadequate perfusion, and so cell death. Hypertension is sustained systolic pressure above 140 mmHg and diastolic above 90 mmHg (NICE, 2011a). However, most early warning scores trigger at far higher systolic pressures. Systolic blood pressure below 100 mmHg usually indicates acute hypotension; early warning scores are very sensitive for low SBP. Shock is often defined as <80 mmHg for more than one hour. However, a few people normally have very low blood pressure, and may be healthy with surprisingly low figures, while people who are normally hypertensive may suffer perfusion failure with pressures above these figures. So target blood pressure should be assessed for each patient.

Mean arterial pressure (MAP)

MAP is calculated by most automated blood pressure devices; if not available, it is normally one third of the way up between diastolic and systolic pressure:

$$\frac{(2 \times diastolic) + systolic}{3}$$

Averaging (mean) pressure across the whole pulse cycle provides a more valuable indication of whether perfusion is adequate, so with hypotension MAP is the most valuable pressure to monitor. It is also the best predictor of pre-eclampsia (Cnossen *et al.*, 2008). Normal MAP in most healthy people is 90–100 mmHg. Dellinger *et al.* (2013) suggest minimum perfusion pressure is a MAP of 65 mmHg; hypertensive people may need higher pressures (Brochard *et al.*, 2010), such as 70–80 mmHg, although Asfar *et al.* (2014) found no benefit when treating sepsis with MAP targets of 80–85 mmHg.

Diastolic pressure

The lowest arterial pressure occurs between pulses. Sustained high diastolic pressures (rule of thumb >100 mmHg) increase the risk of strokes, while very low diastolic pressures (possibly <60 mmHg, may indicate shock, probably from vasodilatation (distributive shock).

D

Disability (neurological assessment)

Neurological status may be assessed informally and formally. Informal assessments include behaviour and family reports. Formal assessment are mainly consciousness level (AVPU, Glasgow Coma Scale), and may include pupil size and reaction. Although not usually considered a neurological assessment, with acute confusion blood sugar should be checked, as confusion is often one of the first symptoms of hyper- or hypo-glycaemia (Hare *et al.*, 2008), blood sugar is easily checked, and relatively easy to treat. Assessments using technology such as intracranial pressure monitoring, are seldom used outside neurological centres, so are not discussed, but advanced neurological assessment, including Glasgow Coma Scale, is discussed in Chapter 17.

Behaviour

Often, the first detected sign of neurological deterioration may be a change in behaviour. This may be detected by nurses, other staff in the area, or relatives/friends. Nurses should therefore not only use their own observations, but note any changes reported by others – this may be as subtle as 'he seems rather tired today'. A possible, but not the only, reason for a change in behaviour is a neurological pathology. There are many possible changes in behaviour, but common examples are

- tiredness/lethargy
- aggressiveness
- confusion or altered cognition
- motor impairment (e.g. dribbling, dysphagia, dysphasia, weakness)
- hallucinations.

With any change in behaviour, the patient's neurological status should be assessed further, although the possibility of the patient just having an 'off day' should be considered.

AVPU (NEWS/ViEWS target: Alert)

- **Alert**
- **Verbal** – responds to verbal stimuli
- **Pain** – responds to painful stimuli
- **Unresponsive**

This first-aid score is incorporated into NEWS/ViEWS. Assuming there is no known chronic condition that affects response, any score below Alert should trigger further assessment, such as Glasgow Coma Scale, pupil reaction (see Chapter 17 for both) or blood sugar.

Responses to pain

Both AVPU and GCS may necessitate assessing response to pain. However, painful stimuli should only be undertaken if no higher level of consciousness is apparent. For initial AVPU assessment, vigorously shaking the patient's shoulder may be sufficient. A normal response to pain is a peripheral nervous system spinal reflex – withdrawal to pain, or guarding. Such responses therefore only confirm the peripheral nervous system is intact; unless the patient responds verbally or in some other way, they provide no information about the central nervous system. Conversely, if patients have a peripheral nervous system deficit (e.g. hemiparesis from a stroke), stimulating the peripheral nervous system may not elicit a response even though the central nervous system may be intact. So central stimuli should be used to assess the central nervous system.

Edmunds *et al.* (2011) identify three central stimuli:

- trapezium squeeze – pinching and twisting the trapezius muscle, between the head and shoulders;
- supraorbital pressure – running a finger along the bony ridge at the top of the eye;
- sternal rub – grinding the sternum with knuckles; Lower (2003) suggests this should leave an imprint of your knuckles on the patient's skin and an imprint of your nails on your fingers.

Lower (2003) and Waterhouse (2005) identify a fourth central stimulus:

- mandibular pressure (using the index and middle fingers, push upwards and inwards on the angle of the patient's jaw for a maximum of 30 seconds.

For initial assessment, where decisions about treatment or withdrawal may be based on responses, each of these may be useful. But sternal rub and manibular pressure are inappropriate for repeated assessments, and all repeated stimuli should be used cautiously. Where tissue damage is suspected, painful stimuli should not be inflicted on that area – for example, supraorbital pressure should not be used if facial bones are unstable or fractured (Edmunds *et al.*, 2011). The sternal rub and mandibular pressure can be useful for isolated assessments to determine whether or not the patient is alive, but they should not be used repeatedly (Edmunds *et al.*, 2011); their use should be confined to resuscitation situations, and they should only be used by people familiar with how to use them.

Frequency

Informal assessment, such as behaviour, should be assessed by all staff whenever they are near patients. But in general wards, there are currently other means of continuous neurological assessment. Charted observations, such as AVPU and GCS, are necessarily intermittent. Frequency of performing these observations must be a clinical decision based on risk assessment: what is the maximum time that can be left between observations that is likely to provide sufficient early warning of significant changes? Where there is no identified neurological concern, AVPU is usually scored with routine observations (e.g. every 4 to 12 hours). If there is a new concern about neurological deterioration, the time interval will probably be 10–15 minutes, with intervals being relaxed if the condition stabilises or improves. As with other nursing observations, each nurse is individually professionally accountable: observations that are either too frequent or too infrequent may reasonably be questioned.

Temperature

(NEWS/ViEWS target 36.1–38.0°C)

Raised body temperature is usually caused by increased metabolism and/or infection, but a possible (less common) cause for pyrexia is hypothalamic damage. The hypothalamus, in the brain-stem, regulates body temperature, so if damaged, thermoregulation fails, typically causing pyrexia. Damage may be permanent (e.g. stroke) or transient (e.g. oedema), and may or may not be treatable. Thermoregulation is discussed further in Chapter 19.

Stress

Stress may be caused by psychological or physiological factors – fear, pain, hypotension, pyrexia. It activates the hypothalamic-pituitary-adrenal axis: the hypothalamus (in the brain-stem) triggers the pituitary gland (control gland of the endocrine system, also in the brain-stem) to release adrenocorticotrophic hormone (ACTH). This stimulates the adrenal cortex, resulting in stress hormones: primarily

- adrenaline
- noradrenaline

but also

- cortisol
- glucagon

and others. Adrenaline (and its precursor, noradrenaline) stimulates a hyperdynamic circulation:

- tachycardia
- vasoconstriction (with tachycardia, increasing blood pressure)

which stimulates

- tachypnoea.

Cortisol increases sodium and water retention (potential oedema) and compromises the immune system. Adrenaline inhibits insulin function which, together with glycogen stores released in response to glucagon, causes hyperglycaemia. Thrombosis is more likely due to viscosity, increasing risks of thrombotic events (stroke, myocardial infarction, pulmonary embolus). These 'fight and flight' responses can be useful if facing short-term threats, but in acutely ill patients can cause an unacceptable (life-threatening) cost. Physiology and psychology therefore cannot, and should not, be separated. Providing good psychological care (information, empowerment, 'meet and greet', effective pain relief, and anything else that promotes comfort and well-being) are therefore not just beneficial from humanitarian perspectives, they also improve physiological function and reduce risks to patients.

Communicating concerns

Underuse of recommended responses places patient safety at risk (Massey *et al.*, 2010). Therefore concerns raised by early warning scores, other abnormal vital signs, and sometimes 'gut feelings', should be escalated to the appropriate people, such as medical staff and Critical Care Outreach (CCO). However, communication is often suboptimal; communication breakdown causes more than 70% of errors in healthcare (Tschannen *et al.*, 2011). Early warning scores almost invariably include recommended actions (those for NEWS/ViEWS are listed in Table 2.2). People called are likely to be busy, and unless concerns are communicated succinctly and clearly, may not elicit the desired response. Therefore when communicating concerns, especially via telephones or electronic means, plan and prioritise what will be said to include key points; further, less important, detail can be communicated when the responder arrives to review the patient.

There are various communication structures available, the most widely promoted one in UK healthcare being SBAR (www.institute.nhs.uk):

Situation
Background
Assessment
Response.

Readers should ensure familiarity with locally-used escalation tool. Escalation, and responses, should be documented.

Implications for practice

- Abnormal vital signs usually indicate problems.
- Respiratory rate is usually the earliest vital sign to change; tachypnoea usually indicates deterioration.
- If vital signs are abnormal, recheck (e.g. within 15 minutes).
- Mean arterial pressure is the best indicator of perfusion pressure – maintain above 65 mmHg.
- Changed behaviour may indicate neurological deterioration, so all staff should be encouraged to observe and report worrying changes.

- With new confusion, check blood sugar and assess neurological state further.
- If patients trigger an early warning score, nurses should initially respond by assessing the patient more fully.
- Review the trend – is the patient improving or deteriorating?
- If patients are deteriorating, escalate care.

Summary

Vital signs are signs of life. If vital signs are abnormal, mortality and morbidity risks are increased. Abnormal vital signs should therefore be reported, and if possible normalised. Early warning scores gather together key vital signs to indicate acuity and recommend initial responses. Scores are useful preliminary indicators, but should trigger further nursing assessment, and any concerns should be escalated.

Further reading

A number of useful pocket-books (such as Cooper *et al.*, 2006, Jevon and Ewens, 2012; Jevon, 2009; Adam *et al.*, 2010) discuss vital signs, and suggest responses. Readers should be familiar with local guidelines, but Dougherty and Lister (2011) provide authoritative evidence-based guidelines.

Clinical scenario

Mr Hugh Barton has been admitted following recent episodes of dizziness. He has a history of hypertension, and despite taking his daily 10 mg of atenolol this morning, blood pressure is 173/86. He feels tingling in fingers. His heart rate is 65 (regular), and his respiration rate is 22. He is alert.

1   Using an A-B-C-D-E structure, list information already known, how this may affect other aspects of assessment, and how you would identify these. What does the known information indicate? Include comments on systolic and diastolic pressures. What other haemodynamic assessments would be useful, and why?
2   His mean arterial pressure is 115. What does this indicate?
3   Calculate his NEWS/ViEWS score, and list recommended actions. Using SBAR (or locally used tools), identify what aspects you would include when initially telephoning for medical review.

Table 2.2 NEWS/ViEWS actions

ViEWS	Risk category	Observation interval	Action – first occurrence and each rise in score
0–1	Low risk	6 hours*	Ordinary vigilance
2	Low risk	6 hours	Ordinary vigilance
3–5	Medium risk	4 hours	Inform nurse in charge
<6 but with 1 or more individual triggers	High risk	1 hour	Call doctor for medical review within 1 hour
6	High risk	1 hour	**Nurse actions** • Inform nurse in charge • Reg nurse to inform doctor (FY2 or SHO) **Doctor actions** • See patient within 30 minutes • Contact Outreach team/site clinical manager
7–8	High risk	1 hour	**Nurse actions** • Reg nurse to inform doctor (FY2 or SHO) • Consider continuous patient monitoring **Doctor actions** • See patient within 30 minutes • Contact Outreach Team/Site Clinical Manager
9+	Critical risk	30 minutes	**Nurse actions** • Senior nurse to inform doctor (SpR) • Fast bleep Outreach team or site clinical manager • Commence continuous patient monitoring **Doctor actions** • See patient within 15 minutes • Fast bleep Outreach team or site clinical manager • In case of peri-arrest or medical emergency situation, call the resuscitation team using 2222 system

NEWS SCORE	FREQUENCY OF MONITORING	CLINICAL RESPONSE
0	Minimum 12 hourly	• Continue routine NEWS monitoring with every set of observations
Total: 1–4	Minimum 4–6 hourly	• Inform registered nurse who must assess the patient • Registered nurse to decide if increased frequency of monitoring and/or escalation of clinical care is required
Total: 5 or more OR 3 in one parameter	Increased frequency to a minimum of 1 hourly	• Registered nurse to urgently inform the medical team caring for the patient • Urgent assessment by a clinician with core competencies to assess acutely ill patients; • Clinical care in an environment with monitoring facilities
Total: 7 or more	Continuous monitoring of vital signs	• Registered nurse to immediately inform the medical team caring for the patient – this should be at least Specialist Registrar level • Emergency assessment by a clinical team with critical care competencies, which also includes a practitioner/s with advanced airway skills • Consider transfer of clinical care to a level 2 or 3 care facility, i.e. higher dependency or ITU

Chapter 3

Interpreting blood results

Contents

*NB biochemistry test

Fundamental knowledge

■ Vascular endothelium

Introduction

The bloodstream is the main transport mechanism for the body. In health, homeostasis normally balances gain and loss; therefore any abnormal function of organs/tissues is likely to be reflected in abnormal blood results. Although interpretation of blood results usually remains primarily the role of doctors, most nurses have access to pathology systems, and if the laboratory is especially concerned about results they telephone the ward. So nurses can readily access results, and may know the result before the doctors. Being able to interpret key results therefore enables nurses to escalate concerns. Whereas laboratories measure results against standard parameters, nurses should be able to interpret the significance in the context of their patient. Patient safety is therefore improved if nurses can identify abnormalities which are significant for their patient, and likely treatments.

There are many possible blood results, some of which are necessarily discussed in other chapters. This chapter focuses on key results in each of three areas:

■ haematology
■ liver function tests
■ biochemistry.

With each aspect, likely causes for acute abnormalities and key treatments will be identified. Reference ranges follow the national Pathology Harmony (where available; Pathology Harmony is currently work in progress). Table 3.1 provides a self-directed worksheet readers can complete while reading this chapter. Readers outside the UK may encounter different ranges, and sometimes different units of measurement.

However, with any measurement (whether vital signs, blood results or other aspects discussed in this book), there can always be 'false positives' and 'false negatives' – results that appear abnormal when there is no problem, or results that appear normal when there is a problem. It is therefore important that any measurement is interpreted in the context of the whole person. Where there is an abnormality, it can often have various causes, so although the most obvious should be investigated first, other reasonably possible causes should always be considered ('lateral thinking').

Rule of threes

Discussing blood results lends itself to grouping most aspects into threes. As interpreting blood results is likely to be relatively unfamiliar to most readers, thinking in threes will therefore be helpful for remembering most aspects discussed. This chapter will discuss three main groups of blood results:

■ haematology
■ liver function tests (LFTs)
■ biochemistry.

Each result can be

■ low
■ normal (within range)
■ high.

Causes for low results are likely to be from

■ dilution
■ loss (e.g. renal, gut)
■ failure of supply or to produce.

Causes for high results are likely to be from

■ dehydration (haemoconcentration)
■ failure to clear
■ excessive intake/production.

So, three questions that should be asked are

■ What is the source/use/loss? Where is it from? What is it used for? Where do we lose it?
■ what is its significance (for my patient)? Is it a symptom of a problem? (If so treat the cause.) Is it a problem? (If so treat the problem.) Or is it both a symptom *and* a problem? (Treat both.)
■ What is the best treatment?

Time out 3.1

As you read through this chapter, complete the relevant parts of Table 3.1. Normal ranges are cited with each item discussed, and also summarised in Table 3.3 at the end of the chapter.

1: HAEMATOLOGY

There are three types of cells in blood

■ red cells (erythrocytes)
■ white cells (leukocytes)
■ platelets (thrombocytes).

Table 3.1 Normal ranges worksheet

	Normal	Source?	Loss?	What is its significance? (what is it used for?)	What do I do about it?
Haemoglobin					
White cell count (overall)					
CRP					
Platelets					
LFTs – bilirubin					
LFTs – transaminases					
LFTs – protein					
Sodium					
Potassium					
Calcium (total)					
Glucose					
Magnesium					
Phosphate					
Creatinine					

All blood cells are initially produced in the bone marrow. A full blood count reflects these three types of cells, the main results being

- haemoglobin
- white cell count (WCC)
- platelets.

Most haematology measurements are $\times 10^9$/litre (i.e. 100,000,000 times the preceding number). In the USA most results are per cubic millimetre.

Haemoglobin (Hb)

> **Normal 140–180 (male), 115–165 (female) grams/litre (WHO, 1968)**

NB In 2012 Pathology Harmony changed the unit of measurement from grams per decilitre to grams per litre. Older resources will therefore cite in the older measurement (1 gram/decilitre = 10 grams/litre).

Haemoglobin is haem (iron) and globin (a plasma protein), and forms a substance which has high affinity for oxygen. Nearly all oxygen in blood is carried by haemoglobin (see Chapter 5). Abnormal haemoglobin levels therefore affect oxygen carriage. Ninety nine per cent of blood cells are red cells (Asharani *et al.*, 2010), and as plasma is mostly (90%) water (Marieb and Hoehn, 2013), blood is essentially red cells and water; haemoglobin therefore affects viscosity and blood flow (see Chapter 10).

When released from bone marrow, red cell lose their nucleus, so are unable to develop further. If released in an immature state, they remain immature, and so are relatively inefficient at carrying oxygen. Immature red cells are called reticulocytes. Normally, 1–2% of red cells are reticulocytes (Higgins, 2013), but excessive haemolysis (breakdown of red cells) causes earlier release of cells from bone marrow, and so raised reticulocyte counts (indicating haemolytic anaemia).

In health, erythrocytes survive about 120 days (Kindt *et al.*, 2007). As cells age, membranes become less pliable. Average erythrocyte diameter is about 8 micrometers; average capillary diameter is about 6 micrometers. Therefore, red cells change their shape ('squash up') to squeeze through capillaries. Old cells are less able to do this, so become trapped in capillaries, where they are broken down by macrophages (see below – white cells).

High haemoglobin (*polycythemia*) is rarely seen in acute care, and rarely problematic if seen. Chronic raised haemoglobin can occur in hypoxic conditions, such as living at high altitudes, or occasionally with severe chronic lung disease. If seen, the cause of polycythemia should be treated; very occasionally, venesection is needed to reduce levels.

A number of conditions can cause anaemia (see Chapter 15), but the most likely causes of rapidly reduced haemoglobin (within one day) are either blood loss or dilution from aggressive fluid therapy. If oxygen carriage is compromised, blood (as packed cells) can be transfused. However, if blood loss is suspected, its source should be investigated, and if possible resolved. Increased haemolysis often occurs with severe illness, resulting in slight anaemia. However, this appears to improve survival; Hebert *et al.* (1999) found optimal survival with haemoglobin of 70–90 grams/litre, although some (not all) subsequent studies found that older patients, and patients with cardiac disease, had optimal survival with Hb of 80–100 grams/litre. Therefore 70 or 80 grams/litre is usually the trigger for transfusion.

White cell count

Normal 4–11 × 10^9/litre

Unlike red cells, white cells retain their nuclei when released from bone marrow, so continue to develop. White cells are a key part of the immune system; different types of white cells are discussed below.

White cells normally only remain in blood for a few hours, transferring into tissues where they normally remain – hence the preferred term in this chapter of 'white cells' rather than the more commonly used 'white blood cells' (WBCs). Infection typically provokes inflammatory responses, causing pro-inflammatory mediators to attract white cells back into blood, to travel to wherever they are needed. Acutely raised white cell counts therefore usually indicate acute inflammation, which in acute healthcare is most likely to result from infection. Raised counts are not per se harmful, so the cause of the raised count, rather than the raised count itself, should be treated.

Low white cell counts (*leucopaenia*) may be caused by diseases (such as leukaemia) and treatments (such as chemotherapy). Severe infections, such as sepsis, can also cause low counts, due to rapid depletion of white cells. While leucopaenia is a symptom, it also exposes the person to increased risk of infection, so may necessitate protective isolation.

As well as overall WCC, differential measurements will be made (see Table 3.3). White cells are divided into two main groups:

- granulocytes
- agranulocytes.

Granulocytes (cells with granules in their membranes) tackle acute infections. Most granulocytes are neutrophils, which are normally the first subgroup to increase. The other types of granulocytes, basophils and eosinophils, are almost invariably few in number, and rarely raised.

Agranulocytes (without granules in cell membranes) provide underlying immunity. Most agranulocytes are lymphocytes: T and B cells that recognise and respond to antigens. A few agranulocytes and monocytes, which once in tissues develop to form the macrophages ('big eaters') that destroy unwanted substances, such as old red cells trapped in capillaries.

C-reactive protein (CRP)

> **Normal 0–10 mg/litre**
> **(Lobo *et al.*, 2003)**

Although a biochemistry test, this is placed here as CRP is almost invariably considered with WCC. It is an acute phase protein, released by the liver (Higgins, 2013) in response to inflammation. Most serious illnesses cause inflammation, so CRP is often raised in sicker patients. Like WCC, raised CRP is not per se harmful, so treatment should focus on the cause of the raised count.

Platelets

> **Normal 150–400 × 10^9/litre**

Platelets (thrombocytes) are used for clotting (some other clotting measurements are included in LFTs below). Platelets are normally kept inactive by antithrombin and other anti-clotting chemicals released by vascular endothelium, but damaged vessels release pro-clotting, rather than anti-clotting, factors, such as platelet activating factor.

Acutely raised counts are rare, and usually caused by haemoconcentration; high counts predispose towards excessive clotting formation, which can cause strokes, myocardial infarction and pulmonary emboli. Acutely low counts usually result from bleeding – platelets are used attempting to stop the bleed. Most in-hospital patients are routinely given daily subcutaneous (low molecular weight) heparin to prevent deep vein thromboses. If platelet counts are insufficient, platelets (or fresh frozen plasma if other clotting factors are needed) can be transfused. Spontaneous bleeding risk increases significantly when count falls below 30 (Higgins, 2008), so routine transfusion is not usually indicated until levels are very low, unless any procedures are likely to provoke dangerous bleeds – 'platelet cover' may be given for surgery and invasive procedures. If counts are low, medical advice should be sought about whether or not to give prescribed heparin – many teams only omit DVT prophylaxis with platelet counts below 50.

2: LIVER FUNCTION TESTS (LFTS)

The liver has hundreds of functions, so many tests can measure aspects of liver function. The main groups of tests are usually

- bilirubin
- transaminases
- proteins.

Further clotting tests are also discussed. Most waste, drugs and other substances are metabolised in the liver. Many LFTs measure results of metabolism.

Bilirubin

Normal <21 micromols/litre (μmol/litre)

When erythrocytes are metabolised, bilirubin is released. Bilirubin is metabolised by the liver into bile, which flows into the gall bladder, from where it is released in response to fat in the duodenum – bile helps emulsify (break down) fat, so it can be absorbed as a nutrient. Obstructive liver disease, such as cirrhosis, prevents bloodflow through the liver, causing serum bilirubin to rise, with potential jaundice as excess bilirubin is deposited in tissues. Lack of bile causes steatorrhoea (fatty stools that are pale and offensive, and float on water).

Bilirubin is not harmful in itself, but is a symptom of obstructive liver disease.

Transaminases (e.g. Alk Phos, ALT, AST)

Transaminases are enzymes inside hepatocytes, enabling liver cells to function. Extensive liver cell damage (e.g. from hepatitis) causes excessive release of transaminases into blood. However, as these chemicals can be released from elsewhere, two or more are usually measured to reduce the risk of false positives. Alkaline phosphatase (Alk Phos) is usually measured, together with either alanine (amino)transferase (ALT) or aspartate aminotransferase (AST). Sometimes gamma glutamyl transpeptidase (GGT) is measured. Alkaline phosphatase is present in bone (Kee, 2009), so bone degeneration during bedrest can increase serum levels.

As most drugs are metabolised by the liver, increase in transaminase levels while in hospital suggests that one or more therapeutic drugs have caused toxic liver damage.

Proteins

The liver synthesises plasma proteins from dietary protein. There are many plasma proteins, including the globin in haemoglobin. Total protein and albumin are usually measured in routine U+Es. Albumin forms more than half total plasma protein, and is important for

- osmotic pull (see Chapter 23)
- drug/chemical binding (see CALCIUM below).

Protein/albumin levels are invariably low with acute illness. This may in part be due to malnutrition, and partly to liver hypofunction, but is probably also related to illness itself (mechanisms remain unclear). Levels are sometimes viewed as a marker of severity of illness, although parallels are imprecise. Low levels can cause

- hypovolaemia
- oedema
- muscle weakness (Schalk *et al.*, 2005)

and possibly

- increased mortality (Palma *et al.*, 2007)

although this last may simply reflect the acuity of illness rather than be a direct result. Giving exogenous albumin only causes a transient rise in levels, so is only indicated if there is a specific need, such as increasing osmotic pull following ascitic drainage (see Chapter 26).

While early feeding benefits most patients, excessive dietary protein should almost always be avoided, as it causes excessive nitrogenous waste, such as urea.

Clotting

Many chemicals combine to form clots, so many tests can measure aspects of clotting, including platelet count (above). Three are included here:

- PT
- PTT
- INR.

The clotting cascade combines two pathways:

- extrinsic
- intrinsic.

Extrinsic chemicals are those released by vascular endothelium, such as platelet activating factor and thromboplastin. The extrinsic pathway can be measured by *prothrombin time* (PT or aPT; a = activated). The intrinsic pathway involves chemicals already in the bloodstream, such as factor IX. Intrinsic pathway chemicals are released from the liver, which is why people with liver disease are prone to bruising and bleeding. The intrinsic pathway can be measured by *partial thromboplastin time* (PTT or aPTT). Intrinsic and extrinsic pathways combine to form a clot, which in health stabilises in about 5 minutes. Overall clotting time is measured by the *international normalised ratio* (INR). Normal INR is 0.9–1.1, so if a patient's INR is 10, clots take about 50 minutes to stabilise.

Mildly prolonged clotting is desirable if patients are treated with anticoagulants; target INR for these patients should usually be 2.5 (Keeling *et al.*, 2011). If heparin therapy is used, this affects the intrinsic system, so should be monitored with aPTT (Reding and Cooper, 2012).

3: BIOCHEMISTRY

There are many biochemistry tests, some included in later chapters. Three groups are included here:

electrolytes:

- sodium
- potassium
- calcium

micronutrients:

- glucose
- magnesium
- phosphate

metabolites:

- creatinine.

Sodium (Na⁺)

| Normal 133–146 mmol/litre |

Sodium is the main extracellular cation – the most common positively charged ion in fluid outside of cell. Abnormal levels increase mortality (Herrod *et al.*, 2010; Kolmodin *et al.*, 2013). Encephalopathy can occur when levels fall to 130 mmol/litre (Overgaard-Steensen, 2010).

Acute hyponatraemia is usually caused by water overload (Reynolds *et al.*, 2006; Spasovski *et al.*, 2014), but can be caused by

- excessive salt loss (e.g. gut, sweating)
- dehydration compensated by fluid shifts.

Little sodium is normally lost in urine, and sodium is reabsorbed in response to the adrenal hormone aldosterone.

With salt deficiency, the logical treatment is to give salt. In sicker patients, this probably needs to be intravenously, in 0.9% saline (Ackrill and France, 2002) or hypertonic saline (Overgaard-Steensen, 2010; Spasovski *et al.*, 2014) infusion, provided cardiac and renal function are capable of handling the fluid load. If caused by fluid imbalance, then fluid status should be normalised. With fluid overload, fluid restriction may be needed, but if patients are not fluid overloaded, fluid restriction can cause dehydration (Sargent, 2005) and distress.

Acute hypernatraemia is usually caused by dehydration (Fisher and Macnaughton, 2006).

Potassium (K⁺)

> **Normal 3.5–5.3 mmol/litre**

Serum potassium normally originates from diet (especially fruit), but as potassium is the main intracellular cation, cell damage and fluid shifts can cause hyperkalaemia. Most potassium loss is normally through the kidneys (with about one tenth lost in stools (Campbell, 2003)), so oliguria or polyruria can cause abnormalities. Potassium is especially important for cardiac and nerve conduction, so abnormalities can be catastrophic.

Mild hyperkalaemia (<6) may be treated with calcium resonium. Normally given orally (it can also be given rectally), calcium resonium is not absorbed, but itself absorbs potassium, which is then excreted when the resonium is passed in stools. Serum potassium >6 is usually treated with glucose and insulin; when insulin transfers glucose into cells, it takes potassium with it. Calcium gluconate (or chloride) is often given concurrently to stabilise cardiac conduction (Nyirenda *et al.*, 2009).

Other treatments for hyperkalaemia include loop diuretics (Nyirenda *et al.*, 2009), which may cause dehydration, and salbutamol (Kemper *et al.*, 1996), which may cause tachycardia. These are generally 'last resort' therapies. Aggressive furosemide or salbutamol therapy for other reasons may similarly cause significant hypokalaemia.

Potassium supplements can be given orally (some oral supplements are bitter, but can be made more palatable with squashes) or intravenously, although in most areas intravenous potassium in restricted to at most 40 mmol/litre IVI. Intravenous potassium can cause phlebitis.

Calcium (Ca⁺⁺)

> **Normal 2.2–2.6 mmol/litre**
> **[corrected]**

While most (99% (Marieb and Hoehn, 2013)) body calcium is normally in teeth and bones, the small amount of serum calcium is important for

- clotting
- cardiac conduction
- vasoconstriction
- cell repair.

Serum calcium originates in diet (especially dairy products) and is lost mostly in urine. Blood/bone balance is regulated by thyroid and parathyroid hormones.

Serum calcium is in two forms:

- ionised (freely available, active)
- protein-bound (inactive).

Normally, 45% is protein-bound (Lough, 2008), but as identified above most sicker patients have protein deficiencies. Reduced binding means more calcium remains active. Therefore laboratories usually *correct* calcium according to measured protein levels, to reflect activity (see Figure 3.1). Ionised calcium is discussed further in Chapter 8.

High calcium is rare. Hypocalcaemis can be treated with oral or intravenous calcium supplements.

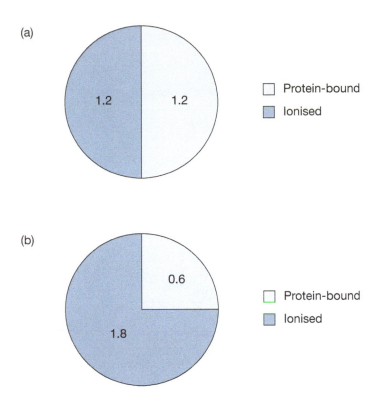

Figure 3.1 Serum calcium. Example of total calcium measured as 2.4 in two people. In (a), half of serum calcium is protein bound. In (b), due to low plasma proteins, only one quarter is protein bound, making ionised levels excessive. Correcting the calcium in (b) would therefore increase the total calcium figure to reflect excessive activity.

Glucose ($C_6H_{12}O_6$)

> **Normal levels – see Table 3.2**

Table 3.2 Normal/target serum glucose

	before meals	2 hours after meal
Non-diabetic	4.0–5.9 mmol/litre	<7.8 mmol/litre
Type 2 diabetes	4.0–7.0 mmol/litre	<8.5 mmol/litre
Type 1 diabetes	4.0–7.0 mmol/litre	<9 mmol/litre
Children with diabetes	4.0–8.0 mmol/litre	<10 mmol/litre

(Diabetes UK www.diabetes.org.uk/Guide-to-diabetes/Monitoring/Testing/accessed 12.04.2015)

Glucose is normally the main energy source for cells. Glycolysis in mitochondria of cells combusts each molecule of glucose with 6 molecules of oxygen to form 36 molecules of adenosine triphosphate (ATP = cell energy):

$$C_6H_{12}O_6 + 6\ O_2 \rightarrow 36 \text{ molecules of ATP}$$

High and low levels can cause confusion (Hare *et al.*, 2008), unconsciousness and death. Low serum glucose should be treated by giving glucose (orally or intravenously). High levels should be treated with hypoglycaemics – severe hyperglycaemia needs intravenous insulin.

Magnesium (Mg^{++})

> **Normal 0.70–1.00 mmol/litre**

Magnesium is widely present in normal diets, especially green leafy vegetables. Magnesium is a calcium antagonist, so vasodilates, reduces heart rate, and bronchodilates. It is excreted in urine, and also lost excessively with vomiting and diarrhoea. Aminoglycoside antibiotics and protein pump inhibitors (PPIs) increase magnesium loss.

Most acute illnesses result in low magnesium levels; about one tenth of hospitalised patients have deficiencies (Parikh and Webb, 2012). Magnesium should therefore be supplemented (if low). This usually necessitates intravenous infusion; during infusions, heart rate and blood pressure should be frequently monitored.

Phosphate (PO$_4^{3-}$)

Normal 0.8–1.5 mmol/litre

Phosphate is needed for production of adenosine triphosphate (cell energy). Low phosphate levels, very common with acute illness, lead to cell failure. Phosphate supplements are usually best given orally. Intravenous phosphate is available, but most preparations take 24 hours to infuse, should be given through a large (preferably central) line, and should not be mixed with any other drug.

Creatinine

Normal 49–90 (female),
64–104 (male) micromol/litre

Creatinine is a waste product of muscle metabolism, and so is produced at a relatively constant rate. It is not reabsorbed by the kidneys, so acutely raised serum creatinine can only be caused by haemoconcentration (dehydration) or renal impairment (failure to clear). Serum creatinine rises once half of nephron function is lost (Kee, 2009). With renal failure, serum creatinine increases by 50–100 micromol/day (ICS, 2007). Creatinine is not per se harmful, so treatment should focus on the problem – dehydration or renal failure.

Implications for practice

- Blood is the main transport mechanism of the body.
- Therefore abnormal function of systems is often reflected in, or caused by, abnormalities in blood.
- Nurses usually have easy access to blood results, and are most likely to be the first recipient if laboratories telephone results, so should be able to interpret core results and know when to escalate concerns.
- For most aspects, think in threes.
- Treat problems, not symptoms.

Summary

Interpreting blood results is often challenging for nurses, but with the acuity of many illnesses, nurses able to make 'first aid' interpretation and recommendations can often hasten interventions to prevent or reduce harm. There are many possible blood tests; this chapter has outlined the core tests usually measured in acute illness. Some further tests are discussed in other chapters. Abnormal levels may be a symptom of disease, may cause problems themselves, or be both a symptom and a problem; and causes may differ between different patients. And as with any measurement, there can always be false positives and false negatives. Results should therefore be interpreted in the context of the individual patient, and treatment should focus on minimising risks.

Useful website

www.harmonypathology.co.uk

Further reading

There are a number of books summarising laboratory results, including Higgins (2013) and Kee (2009), although many predate Pathology Harmony. It is however more useful to practise interpreting results in practice, using a table such as Table 3.1, than to read extensively about them.

Clinical scenario

Mr Henry Stubbings' (see Scenario in Chapter 1) blood results on admission include:

Hb	164 g/L
WCC	24 × 109/L
Plt	185 × 109/L
bilirubin	17 micromols/L
Alk Phos	95 units/L
ALT	32 units/L
T protein	40 g/L
albumin	28 g/L
Na	158 mmol/L
K	3.6 mmol/L
Ca	2.2 mmol/L
Mg	0.68 mmol/L
Phos	0.72 mmol/L
Creat	156 micromol/L

1   Identify which results are abnormal, and list likely causes of abnormalities in this instance.
2   Which results cause you most concern, and why?
3   How would you expect these abnormalities to be treated? Do any of the treatments need specific observations/monitoring?

Table 3.3 Normal ranges (summary)

haemoglobin	140–180 grams/litre (male) $\times 10^9$/litre
	115–165 grams/litre (female) $\times 10^9$/litre
white cell count	4–11 $\times 10^9$/litre
neutrophils (polymorphs)	2.5–7.5 $\times 10^9$/litre
basophils	<0.2 $\times 10^9$/litre
eosinophils	0.04–0.44 $\times 10^9$/litre
lymphocytes (T and B cells)	1.5–4.0 $\times 10^9$/litre
monocytes (scavengers)	0.2–0.8 $\times 10^9$/litre
CRP	<10 mg/litre
platelets	150–400 $\times 10^9$/litre
bilirubin	<21 mmol/litre
alkaline phosphatase (Alk Phos)	30–130 units/litre
alanine (amino)transferase (ALT)	<40 units/litre
aspartate aminotransferase (AST)	<40 units/litre
gamma glutamyl transpeptidase (GGT)	10–48 units/litre
albumin	35–50 grams/litre
total protein (TP)	60–80 grams/litre
PT	10–12 seconds
aPTT	28–34 seconds
INR	0.9–1.1
sodium	133–146 mmol/litre
potassium	3.5–5.3 mmol/litre
calcium (total)	2.2–2.6 mmol/litre (corrected)
glucose	4.0–5.9 mmol/litre (non-diabetic, pre-meal)
magnesium	0.70–1.00 mmol/litre
phosphate	0.8–1.5 mmol/litre
creatinine	49–90 micromol/litre (female)
	64–104 micromol/litre (male)

Part 2

Breathing

Chapter 4

Respiratory failure

Contents

Fundamental knowledge

■ Mucociliary ladder (function of mucus and cilea)

Introduction

Respiratory disease is increasing, is a major cause of hospital admission, and causes more than one in five deaths in the UK (BTS, 2006). As with any system disease, respiratory failure may be acute, chronic, or acute-on-chronic. Treatment in acute hospitals focuses on treating acute problems (including the acute element of acute-on-chronic), but chronic diseases will necessitate continuing management while in acute hospitals.

Oxygen is needed for cells to function; without oxygen, cells fail and die, and when sufficient cells die, the organ they are part of fails, threatening the person's life. Cells produce carbon dioxide, which if not cleared is toxic, and will also kill. Gases move into and out of the lungs by *ventilation*. With healthy ventilation, gases within blood are normal. But respiratory failure causes problems with one or both gases.

Brief overviews of key pathologies

- pneumonia and respiratory tract infections
- asthma
- COPD
- pulmonary oedema
- pulmonary emboli
- neuromuscular
- postural (kyphosis, Parkinson's disease, sleep apnoea)

are included.

Respiratory drive

Like other vital functions, breathing is controlled by the brain-stem. Chemoreceptors (specialised nerve endings that measure chemicals in arterial blood) respond to:

- hypercapnia
- acidosis
- hypoxia.

If any of these are present, more signals reach the brain-stem respiratory centres, which respond by increasing rate and depth of breathing, which typically normalises blood chemistry within minutes (Marieb and Hoehn, 2013).

Carbon dioxide

In health, carbon dioxide creates the main drive to breath. Air is approximately 21% oxygen and 79% nitrogen, with only trace amounts of other gases – 0.04% is carbon dioxide (Barrett *et al.*, 2010). Carbon dioxide in blood has been produced by cells: normal energy production in the mitochondria of cells is by glycolysis – each molecule of glucose combusts with six molecules of oxygen to form 36 molecules of adenosine triphostae (ATP = cell energy). But the atoms from this process normally form six molecules of carbon dioxide and six molecules of water:

$$C_6H_{12}O_6 + 6 \text{ molecules of } O_2 \rightarrow 6\ CO_2 + 6\ H_2O$$

Like other gases, carbon dioxide diffuses across a semi-permeable membrane (the cell wall) from a greater concentration (inside the cell) to a lesser (capillary blood).

Carbon dioxide is a soluble gas, so some is carried by blood in solution:

$$CO_2 + H_2O \leftrightarrow H_2CO_3 \text{ (carbonic acid)}$$

Carbon dioxide is therefore a 'potential' acid – in pure chemistry it is not an acid, as acids must contain hydrogen (see Chapter 8), but it readily forms the main acid of the bloodstream. The hypercapnic and acidosis drives to breathe are therefore (sometimes) linked – excessive blood carbon dioxide causes excessive carbonic acidosis (respiratory acidosis – see Chapter 8).

Abnormal cell metabolism – anaerobic (without oxygen) or from alternative energy sources (mainly fat) – produces less energy and more waste, and often additional waste products.

Carbon dioxide is carried by blood in three ways:

- in solution, as carbonic acid (about 10%);
- by haemoglobin (about 20%); a different part of the molecule to that which carries oxygen, so carbon dioxide does not compete with oxygen within haemoglobin;
- in bicarbonate (HCO_3^-).

(Marieb and Hoehn, 2013)

Carbon dioxide is cleared through expiration; therefore hypoventilation causes hypercapnia. It is also a vasodilator, so hypercapnia increases blood flow to skin, potentially causes the person to look 'flushed'. At higher levels it is neurotoxic, causes twitching, shaking, confusion, drowsiness and eventually coma. See Table 4.1.

Table 4.1 **Signs of hypercapnia**

- shallow/slow breathing
- flushed/pink
- twitching/shaking/confusion/drowsy

Mechanics of breathing

Each breath has three parts:

- inspiration
- pause/hold
- expiration.

Inspiration involves active muscle expansion: the diaphragm moves down and intercostal (rib) muscles move outwards, increasing intrathoracic space, and so making intrathoracic pressure negative in relation to the atmosphere outside the body. This negative pressure draws air into lungs. If larger breaths are needed, 'accessory' muscles are used – clavicles (shoulder) and in extreme cases abdominal muscles. New use of accessory muscles by patients is therefore usually a sign of deterioration. Because inspiration is an active process, it is relatively quick.

The pause (or hold) phase being relatively brief, the greatest proportion of time in each breath is expiration – passive recoil of muscles, forcing air out of lungs. Take a breath, focusing on what proportion is inspiration and expiration; most breaths have an inspiration:expiration (I:E) ratio of 1:2, so if a breath lasts 3 seconds, approximately one second is inspiration, and two are expiration.

Gas exchange

Gas exchange (oxygen, carbon dioxide) in the lungs relies on three factors

- ventilation (V): airflow into alveoli; breath size
- perfusion (Q): pulmonary capillary blood flow
- diffusion: movement across tissues between alveoli and pulmonary capillaries).

Respiratory failure

Respiratory failure can be caused by many diseases, but is classified into two types.
   Type 1 failure (oxygenation failure) is hypoxia and normocapnia:

- hypoxia: PaO_2 <8 kPa
- normocapnia: $PaCO_2$ <6 kPa

(BTS, 2002)

Carbon dioxide is 20 times more soluble than oxygen (Waterhouse and Campbell, 2002). Alveolar epithelium and capillary endothelium are normally 0.1–0.2 micrometers apart (Jain and Bellingan, 2007), but diseases increasing the fluid barrier (e.g. pulmonary oedema, pneumonia) create a greater barrier for oxygen than carbon dioxide (diffusion failure).
   Type 2 failure (ventilatory failure) is hypoxia plus hypercapnia:

- hypoxia: PaO_2 <8 kPa
- hypercapnia: $PaCO_2$ >6 kPa.

(BTS, 2002)

Ventilation

Hypoventilation means little moves into and out of lungs, resulting in little oxygen entering and little carbon dioxide being removed. Hypoventilation occurs if

- breath size (tidal volume) is small – shallow breathing
- respiratory rate is slow (rule of thumb: <10 bpm)
- gas is 'trapped' in alveoli (e.g. tachypnoea).

Tachypnoea is a compensatory mechanism to increase gas exchange. Up to a point, this is effective. But between air entering the airways at the nose/mouth and gas exchange occurring in alveoli is *deadspace* – approximately 150 ml of air from the previous breath (Marieb and Hoehn, 2013). This relatively oxygen poor and carbon dioxide rich air is the first air to reach alveoli. Healthy resting breaths may be 450 ml; with 150 ml deadspace, 300 ml of air reaching alveoli would be good quality (21% oxygen). Faster rates reduce the time of each breath, inevitably reducing breath volume. If breath volume is 200 ml, the same 150 ml deadspace results in only 50 ml of good quality air reaching alveoli. A rule of thumb problem tachypnoea is 25 bpm, where ViEWS/NEWS scores 3.

Perfusion

Capillaries cover almost all the alveolar surface. The average adult has 480 million alveoli (Lumb, 2010), creating a surface area of 70 m^2 (Adam and Osborne, 2005) – more than 40 times skin surface area. This gives alveoli a large functional reserve; extensive perfusion failure occurs before gas exchange is impaired.

Diffusion

In health, gases equalise in 0.25 seconds (Marieb and Hoehn, 2013). A normal resting heart rate of 70–80 bpm means blood remains in capillaries for about 0.75 seconds – two to three times normal equalisation time. Extensive diffusion failure occurs before gas exchange is impaired, and the person desaturates.

Ventilation perfusion mismatch

Normal healthy adult resting minute volume (amount of air inhaled per minute) is about 4 litres. Over the same minute, a healthy adult heart at rest ejects about 5 litres of blood, making normal ventilation:perfusion (V/Q) ratio 4:5. In health, volumes increase and decrease in proportion, maintaining normal ratios. In mild ill-health, V/Q ratio may be maintained by

- reflex vasoconstriction reducing perfusion if alveoli are unventilated (e.g. mucous plug);
- atelectasis (collapse of alveoli) if they are unperfused.

But severe illness provokes inflammatory responses, which prevent reflex vasoconstriction. If airflow is reduced, and inflammation present (e.g. acute exacerbation of chronic obstructive pulmonary disease – AECOPD), V/Q mismatch can occur, resulting in blood returning to the left side of the heart with little gas exchange having occurred. V/Q scans show both airways and bloodflow in the lungs, to assess any mismatch.

Atelectasis

Water placed between two smooth sheets of plastic creates sufficient 'surface tension' to make them difficult to separate. Similarly, when alveoli collapse at the end of expiration, the moist walls tend to stick together. Scattered in the alveolar walls are specialised (type II) cells which release *surfactant*, a chemical which reduces surface tension and so helps alveoli reinflate with the next breath. Premature babies have little or no surfactant production, necessitating exogenous surfactant until they reach term. In adults, surfactant production may be inhibited by:

- hypoxia
- acidosis
- poor perfusion
- smoking
- dry gas (unhumidified oxygen).

Many, or all, of these factors may be present in acutely ill patients.

Work of breathing

The mechanics of breathing involves muscular work. Muscular work consumes energy, which as discussed previously is produced in cells using (normally) oxygen and glucose. Increasing muscular work therefore consumes more oxygen. At rest, healthy adults use 1–3% of total body oxygen for breathing (Hinds and Watson, 2008). But increasing muscular work increases demand: with respiratory disease, work of breathing can consume 25–30% of available oxygen (Hinds and Watson, 2008). To increase oxygen supply, the respiratory centres increase respiratory rate, which as discussed above is effective up to a point (the limit being around 25 bpm).

Treating respiratory failure

Specific underlying causes of failure, such as infection, should be treated, but with two types of respiratory failure there are two broad treatments:

- type 1 (oxygenation failure) needs oxygen
- type 2 (ventilatory failure) needs ventilation.

Giving oxygen is relatively easy (and is discussed further in Chapter 5). Improving ventilation is more challenging, but can be improved by

- sitting upright (Morley, 2002)
- deep breathing/breathing exercises
- bronchodilatation
- (if necessary) mechanical (non-invasive) ventilation (see Chapter 9).

Pulmonary circulation is a low pressure system: Sturgess (2014) cites normal systolic pulmonary artery pressure as 15–25 mmHg, about one sixth of normal systemic arterial systolic pressure. Blood therefore tends to pool at bases of the lungs. Lungs being triangular, the largest area for air is at the base, so air and blood volume are similar as long as the chest is upright. Conversely, lying supine forces maximum airflow to the front of the lungs (air rises), while capillary bloodflow falls with gravity to the back, creating a V/Q mismatch. In health, we cope with this mismatch, but with respiratory dysfunction this V/Q mismatch can precipitate failure. Upright positioning helps restore normal V/Q ratio.

Deep breathing and breathing exercises are often viewed as the domain of physiotherapists, who have much to offer patients with respiratory disease. However, nurses can also usefully remind patients to take deep breaths between physiotherapy treatments. Deep breathing uses distal alveoli which during shallower breathing remain largely unused. Unused alveoli tend to collapse. Frequent deep breathing therefore helps prevent atelectasis. Early mobilisation places patients in an upright position and stimulates deeper breathing, so reduces mortality (Martinson *et al.*, 2001).

Delivering drugs to the site of problems generally optimises their benefits. Nebulised drugs are usually of three types

- bronchodilators (beta-agonists, such as salbutamol)
- steroids (such as ipratropium)
- humidifying agents (such as saline – see Chapter 5).

Unlike upper airways, where patency is maintained by cartilage, lower airways are prone to bronchoconstriction. Drug droplets therefore need to be small enough to reach lower airways, which needs a droplet size of 0.8–3 microns (Papiris *et al.*, 2002). To achieve this, gas flow should be 6–8 litres per minute.

Moisture left in nebuliser pots is a potential medium for bacterial growth, especially pseudomonas. Nebulisers should therefore be cleaned and dried (according to hospital policy) after each use, to prevent nebulising bacteria into the lungs with future use. Nebuliser pots should be disposed of according to hospital policy (many trusts have policies of daily changes); when pots are changed, this should be documented.

Common respiratory problems

Respiratory tract *infections* may originate from inhaled pathogens or organisms migrating/translocating from elsewhere in the body (endogenous infection). Traditionally, the lower respiratory tract was believed to be sterile, although recent studies suggest microbes do normally inhabit the lower airways, and that pneumonia results from disruption of the normal ecosystem (Dickson *et al.*, 2014). The respiratory tract has various non-specific immune defences, such as the mucociliary ladder, and secretion of antibacterial substances, such as lysozyme, in saliva. With ill-health, non-specific immunity may be impaired; smoking damages mucociliary function. Pneumonia ('chest infection') may be acquired in the community, or within healthcare (HCAI, healthcare-associated infection). Usual incubation time for infection is about 48 hours, so infections occurring after 48 hours in hospital are classified as HCAIs. Although any organism can cause pneumonia, bacteria are usually responsible, so initially broad-spectrum antibiotics are usually prescribed, until sputum can be cultured.

Chronic obstructive pulmonary disease (COPD) causes persistent airflow limitation that is usually progressive and is associated with inflammatory responses in airways (GOLD, 2013). It is usually caused by

- bronchitis *or*
- emphysema.

COPD usually results from smoking (Brusselle *et al.*, 2011; GOLD, 2013), is progressive, and eventually fatal. Incidence of COPD is increasing (Martinez *et al.*, 2011); worldwide, it is the fourth leading cause of death (GOLD, 2013). Most people with COPD are managed in the community, but acute exacerbations (usually from chest infections) often necessitate acute hospital admission. Care therefore focuses on curing acute exacerbations, and managing the chronic element. Bronchitis is inflammation of bronchioles, restricting airflow into the lungs. Emphysema (from the Greek for 'puffed up') occurs when chronic distension of alveoli causes loss of elasticity, and therefore failure to adequately ventilate. Less frequently, genetic deficiency of alpha antitrypsin 1 (a protective enzyme) causes early-onset COPD, especially in smokers. Many patients with AECOPD need non-invasive bilevel ventilation on admission to acute hospitals.

Asthma is a chronic inflammatory disorder of the airways (Global Initiative for Asthma, 2012), but hospital admission is usually only necessary with severe acute exacerbations. More often a childhood disease, a significant incidence also occurs in adults, usually before the age of 40 (To *et al.*, 2012). UK incidence of asthma is among the highest in the world (To *et al.*, 2012). Core treatment for asthma is

- oxygen
- bronchodilators
- steroids.

Pulmonary oedema, excess fluid in tissue spaces of lungs, forms a barrier to oxygen transfer. Fluid overload is usually caused either by aggressive fluid therapy or renal failure. Immediate treatment for pulmonary oedema is intravenous diuretics (usually furosemide), and often continuous positive airway pressure (CPAP, to force fluid back into the cardiovascular system (see Chapter 9)).

Pulmonary emboli are a major cause of death, but are often found only at post-mortem. Major pulmonary emboli cause either death or severe breathlessness, necessitating empirical treatment with oxygen and systemic anticoagulants. Smaller emboli usually allow time for confirmatory tests – contrast tomographic pulmonary angiography (CTPA) being the recommended test (Stein *et al.*, 2006). If confirmed, treatment is anticoagulation, with system support.

Various neuromuscular diseases can cause failure of either nerve signals to respiratory muscles, or failure of muscles to respond. In acute hospitals, the ones most often seen are

- Gullain–Barré syndrome
- (exacerbations of) myasthenia gravis.

Progressive neuromuscular diseases are also seen, such as:

- motor neurone disease
- multiple sclerosis.

With progressive diseases, respiratory failure will usually be the eventual cause of death. If there is a treatable cause for exacerbations, such as a chest infection, it is reasonable to treat this; if respiratory failure results just from progression of the disease, palliative care is usually the kinder option.

Abnormal posture, such as kyphosis ('bent spine'), a stoop from Parkinson's disease, or sleep apnoea (airway obstruction caused when lying flat, typically with very obese large-necked people) can cause respiratory limitations. While rarely a cause of hospital admission, such problems can complicate care. In acute hospitals, people with these problems usually benefit from overnight non-invasive bilevel ventilation.

Psychological care

Good psychological care is desirable for humanitarian reasons. But as discussed in Chapter 2, stress has detrimental physiological effects, such as tachycardia and tachypnoea, both of which increase oxygen demand. Reducing distress therefore has physiological benefits. Patients should therefore be kept informed about their condition, and whenever possible involved in decision-making. 'Meet and greet' helps reduce anxieties. Pain relief should be a core value of nursing (see Chapter 20), and anything within reason that helps patients relax should be encouraged. Because sick patients are often hypoxic, memory and understanding may be impaired, so explanations should be given in a way patients can understand, and may need to be repeated. Patients may also have long-standing cognitive impairment, especially if they have chronic respiratory disease (Barclay, 2013).

Implications for practice

- The respiratory system has a large functional reserve; by the time patients become symptomatic, much deterioration has already occurred.
- Respiratory failure causes hypoxia and may cause hypercapnia.
- Positioning upright optimises ventilation.
- With nebulisers, use 6–8 litres/minute gasflow.
- Clean and dry nebulisers after each use; change daily (and record changes).
- Respiratory distress is exacerbated by psychological distress; good psychological care helps reduce stress responses.

Summary

Respiratory disease is a major cause of acute hospitalisation. In health, lungs have a large reserve function, so by the time of admission, much deterioration has already occurred, and crises are often imminent. Many diseases can cause respiratory failure, but respiratory failure is classified into two types: type 1 respiratory failure is an oxygenation failure and so needs oxygen, whereas type 2 is ventilator failure, and needs ventilation – positioning upright usually being the initial strategy, followed by bronchodilatation, and possibly mechanical non-invasive ventilation. Underlying causes of failure, such as infection, should also be treated.

Useful websites

British Thoracic Society
Global initiative for chronic Obstructive Lung Disease (GOLD)
Global Initiative for Asthma (GINA)

Further reading

There are a number of major national and international reports on respiratory diseases, such as NICE (2010a), DOH (2011a), SIGN/BTS (2012), GOLD (2013) and Global Initiative for Asthma (2012), which provide authoritative discussions of treatments, and often pathologies.

Clinical scenario

Mrs Jenny Franks, aged 45, is admitted to your ward with bronchopneumonia. She is known to be asthmatic and a smoker, with no history of chronic obstructive pulmonary disease. She is very anxious about her son, who left home one month ago to study at university. She is found, outside the ward, having suffered a severe asthma attack while smoking a cigarette. Her respiratory rate is now 45 bpm, blood pressure 175/95 mmHg, heart rate 128 bpm. Her oxygen saturation is 83%.

1   Using an A-B-C-D-E assessment, list your initial priorities during Mrs Franks' attack.
    Mrs Franks is prescribed 4 hourly nebulisers of ipratropium and salbutamol, reducing daily doses of initially 40 mg prednisolone. Using a pharmacology text, such as the *British National Formulary*, list the expected effects and potential side effects of these medicines. What observations and other aspects of nursing care might be needed because of these drugs?
2   Drawing on your own experience, material in this chapter and any other material that you have access to, develop an evidence-based plan of care for Mrs Franks for the first 48 hours following this attack.
3   The day following her attack, Mrs Franks' son arrives unexpectedly on the ward, and appears very frightened and anxious. He has already seen his mother, who has given him vague information about what happened. He asks you for information. What information and other care would you give to Mrs Franks' son? Justify your decisions.

Chapter 5

Oxygen therapy

Contents

Introduction

Oxygen is vital for life. Without oxygen, cells die. Supplementary oxygen is therefore a life-saving therapy for many acutely ill patients. But like all drugs, too much oxygen can cause harm and even be fatal (NPSA, 2009). Recent years have seen increasing controversy over oxygen toxicity. Options for delivering supplementary oxygen are discussed (face masks – Venturi, variable performance; nasal; high flow nasal).

Oxygen can harm

The 2009 NPSA report identified 281 serious incident reports related to oxygen therapy in the UK (267 from acute hospitals) over five years. Oxygen was found to have caused nine deaths and contributed to a further 35 deaths. Over the same period, there were 279 litigation claims related to oxygen. There were two causes of harm:

- underuse
- overuse.

Overuse of oxygen caused serious harm in two main groups of patients:

- premature infants
- people with chronic obstructive pulmonary disease (COPD).

As this text is adult-care focused, only the second group are considered here.

Initial target saturations

Oxygen should be prescribed to achieve a target saturation, rather than a specific amount of oxygen being prescribed (BTS, 2008). For most people without COPD, initial target saturation should be 94–98%. For people with COPD, initial target saturation should be 88–92% (BTS, 2008) (see Table 5.1)

Table 5.1 Initial target saturations (BTS, 2008)

Non-COPD	COPD
94–98%	88–92%

Oxygen delivery systems

Unless patients have artificial airways, oxygen can be delivered via

- face mask (or systems than enclose the head)
- nasal cannulae.

Oxygen face masks may be

- fixed performance (high flow, 'Venturi')
- variable performance.

Face mask – fixed performance

Venturi valves jet oxygen through a narrow valve, after which air is entrained. To dilute the pure oxygen sufficiently, a large volume of air is added, creating flows of 30–80

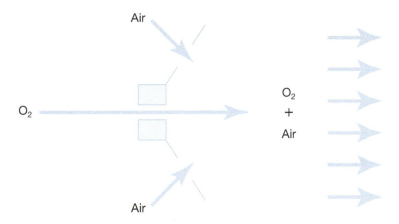

Figure 5.1 Venturi valve

litres/minute into the mask (volume depends largely on the percentage of the valve, but also differs slightly between manufacturers; see Figure 5.1). Normal healthy adult resting minute volume (the amount of air breathed each minute) is about 4 litres, so even on exertion, no-one breathes 30 litres per minute. So more than enough volume is delivered into the mask, creating a flow out of the mask that prevents any significant entrainment of room air into the mask. The patient therefore breathes an accurate ('fixed') percentage of oxygen, provided oxygen flow is set to at least that specified by the manufacturer higher oxygen flow rates deliver the same percentage, but lower may not). Oxygen flow should be measured from the middle of float. Minimum volumes of oxygen that should be used differ between manufacturers, so you should check details on valves available within your Trust.

Valves are colour coded:

- blue 24%
- white 28%
- orange 31%
- yellow 35%
- red 40%
- green 60%.

Most clinical areas only stock a selection of these; the orange (31%) is seldom used, or stocked.

Due to the large volumes delivered into the mask, Venturi systems have often been called 'high flow'. However, the term 'high flow' is also now used for a different system, discussed below, so to prevent confusion, it is safest to call these systems 'Venturi' rather than 'high flow'.

Time out 5.1

From your ward/department's store-room, identify which percentage Venturi valves are stocked, and what the minimum litre flow for each is.

Reservoir (non-rebreathe) face masks

(See Figure 5.2)

Pure oxygen flows into the reservoir, above which is a one-way valve. Negative pressure inspiration causes this valve to open, and so nearly all the volume breathed in is pure oxygen from the reservoir. There will however be slight dilution from the dead-space air created by the face mask – air which, being from the last expiration, will be relatively oxygen poor and carbon dioxide rich. Gas inhaled will therefore be less than 100% oxygen – Jevon (2007) suggests it is approximately 85%. The one-way valve prevents exhaled

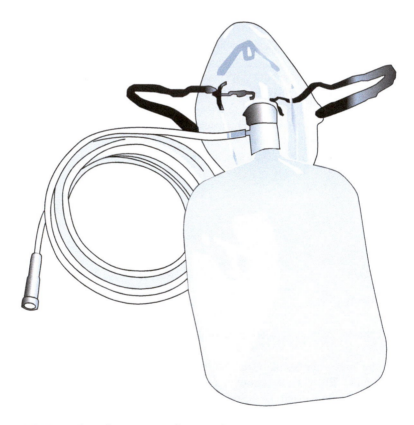

Figure 5.2 Non-rebreathe reservoir face mask

air entering the reservoir, hence 'non-rebreathe'. Litres set on the flow meter should be sufficient for the whole volume of the patient's breath. Although 10 litres may be sufficient for some patients, their minute volume is unlikely to be known, so if a reservoir mask is needed, 15 litres should be used.

Variable performance face masks

(See Figure 5.3)

These deliver oxygen from the flow meter directly into the face mask. Depending on how much volume the person breathes, pure oxygen is therefore diluted with a variable volume of air, making the performance (percentage) variable. Manufacturers' instructions often indicate that each litre of oxygen adds approximately 4% to the 21% already in air (Morton and Remphe, 2013). However, as with all masks, there is 'dead-space' within the mask (dead-space was discussed in Chapter 4); anecdotal reports suggest variable performance masks need a minimum flow of 5 litres to clear the deadspace, which would make oxygen delivered around 40%. These masks are therefore probably unsuitable for use with COPD.

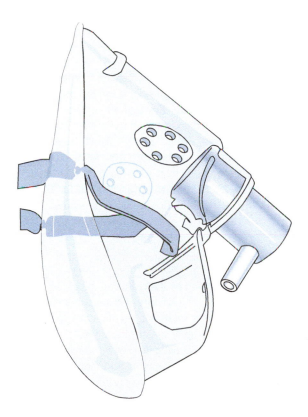

Figure 5.3 Variable performance masks.

Nasal cannulae

Nasal cannulae (also called speculae or 'specs') are variable performance, delivering a few litres of pure oxygen which is then diluted with air to make up the volume breathed. Ewens (2001) suggests inhaled oxygen is 24–44%, partly depending on set litres. Each litre of oxygen adds approximately 4%. However, nasal oxygen is ineffective if patients are mouth-breathing; with deterioration, mouth breathing becomes more likely. Most people will tolerate 1–3 litres of nasal oxygen, but higher flows are generally uncomfortable. Increased needs suggest the person may be deteriorating, and so nasal oxygen may be inappropriate.

Most patients find nasal cannulae more comfortable than face masks. Nasal oxygen also allows the person to eat, drink and talk without face masks getting in the way. So if nasal oxygen will suffice, it is generally preferable to face mask oxygen.

Nasal cannulae easily become displaced, resulting in one (or sometimes both) prongs being outside the nostril. Not only does this reduce the oxygen delivered into airways, but it often jets dry oxygen onto the corneal surface, which can cause damage (corneal ulcers). If cannulae cannot be supported unaided, paper-based tape can usually secure them to the cheeks. Cannulae can also cause skin damage above ears; if skin looks sore, loose swabs can prevent friction.

High flow nasal oxygen

(See Figure 5.4)

These systems deliver a high flow of fixed performance heated humidified oxygen via large nasal cannulae. Air is entrained through a filter, and oxygen percentage can be titrated to an inbuilt oxygen analyser. Typically, flows of 40–60 litres per minute are used. As this flow far exceeds volumes inhaled, most flow into the nostril will flow back out through the mouth, creating a CPAP effect of between 2–8 cmH$_2$O in the oropharynx (Corley et al., 2011), varying both with flow and between individual patients. This helps prevent and reverse atelectasis. Because the system is heated and humidified, it is well-tolerated (Price et al., 2008; Turnbull, 2008), and may prevent need for non-invasive ventilation (Maggiore et al., 2014). In practice, high flow equipment is often called by brand names, such as Vapotherm™, AirVO™ (or its precursor Optiflow™).

Commencing oxygen

In an emergency, patients are likely to be hypoxic, and hypoxia kills, so oxygen therapy should be commenced at high levels (e.g. 15 litres via a non-rebreathe face mask). Oxygen should then be titrated down to target saturation. In non-emergency situations, it is safest to start low (24 or 28%) and titrate up to target saturations.

Traditionally, concern about COPD patients relying on their hypoxic drive to breathe has limited oxygen therapy for these patients to no more than 28%. The BTS (2008) suggest that up to 50% rely on their hypoxic drive, although Bateman and Leech (1998) had suggested an incidence of only 10–15%. However, with acute exacerbation of COPD, preventing tissue hypoxia overrides concerns about carbon dioxide retention, so oxygen should be given to achieve target saturations of 88–92% (GOLD, 2013). As oxygen should

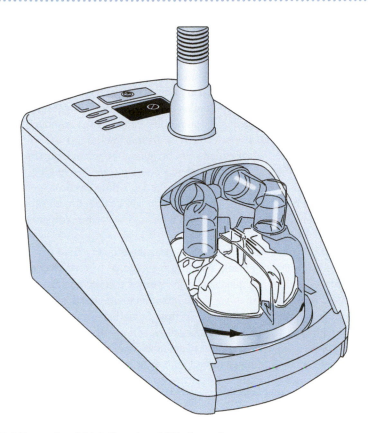

Figure 5.4 Example of high-flow humidified nasal oxygen

be given to target saturation (88–92% for COPD), more should only be given if patients are hypoxic, and if hypoxic, they should retain their hypoxic drive. Outside of crises, it is therefore safest to usually restrict oxygen with COPD patients to 24 or 28%; if needing more than this, the patient is deteriorating, and so urgent senior help should be sought.

Traditionally, high-concentration oxygen has been commenced with cardiac arrest. Cabello *et al.* (2010) suggested this could increase mortality, and that oxygen should only be given if patients were hypoxic. There is some evidence that oxygen can *cause* coronary vasoconstriction (Conti, 2011). However, randomised controlled trials on this issue are non-existent (they would be unethical). After Cabello *et al.*'s recommendation, the UK Resuscitation Council 2010 guidelines stated that in all cases of peri-arrest oxygen should be given.

Humidification

Inhaled room air in the UK is usually 50% humidified (Ballard *et al.*, 1992); it can hold double the moisture it already contains. Warmer air can contain more. The human airway normally warms air to body temperature, and fully humidifies it. Most of this warming and humidifying occurs in the upper airway, especially the nasal cavity. With nasal breathing, air is about 36°C and 80–90% humidified by the carina, but only 60–70% humidified with mouth breathing (Dutta *et al.*, 2006).

Oxygen is a dry gas (0% humidified), and so will absorb moisture from the airways. In addition to causing discomfort, this will dry mucus and damage cilia, making the person more prone to developing infection. Bateman and Leech (1998) suggest that flows of up to 4 litres/minute are probably adequately humidified by the airway, although this assumes the person is not dehydrated. Prolonged (more than a few hours) use of higher flows should therefore be humidified. If patients are breathing though a tracheostomy, oxygen should always be humidified (see Chapter 5 in *Intensive Care Nursing*).

Of delivery systems discussed above, only the high flow nasal oxygen has in-built humidification. With other systems, humidification can be added with saline nebulisers (BTS, 2008). Face masks can be humidified with cold water humidifiers (called 'large volume nebulisers' by the BTS, 2008).

Patients should be encouraged to drink (unless there is any fluid restriction or they are nil by mouth). If unable to drink, mouthcare should be offered frequently (e.g. 2–4 hourly). Patients with nasal cannulae should be warned that oxygen can cause drying of their nostrils, and they may wish to use some lubricant to prevent this. Face mask oxygen can cause drying, and possibly cracking, of lips. Some balm may be useful. The only lubricant stocked by most acute hospitals is yellow soft paraffin or white petroleum jelly ('Vaseline®'); concerns have been expressed about the flammability of these, but Winslow and Jacobson (1998) failed to make these ignite even with a flame-thrower.

Oxygen and transfers

If patients need oxygen during transfer, sufficient oxygen should be taken to allow for increased needs, or unexpected problems (lifts can break down). Following untoward incidents, the Medicines and Health Regulation Authority (MHRA, now disbanded, but was part of the DOH) issued an alert in 2009; it advises

- at 4 litres a minute, a size D cylinder would last 85 minutes, while a size PD would last 75 minutes;
- at 10 litres per minute, a D cylinder would last 34 minutes, a PD cylinder 30 minutes;
- at 15 litres, a size D cylinder would last 23 minutes, a PD cylinder 20 minutes.

Oxygen toxicity

Oxygen toxicity was first described by Joseph Priestley in 1775; nineteenth-century animal experiments confirmed that oxygen could cause tissue damage. Once oxygen therapy became practical in the twentieth century, evidence of oxygen toxicity from practice accumulated.

Oxygen in air consists of paired atoms (O_2). Normally, cells use whole molecules; but sometimes a single oxygen atom is released. This oxygen 'radical' is highly reactive, and can cause tissue damage. Normally about 1% of oxygen molecules are converted to reactive oxygen species (ROS) (Galley, 2011). A healthy body contains many antioxidants (among the hundreds of antioxidants are vitamins C and E, and even haemoglobin)

(Mak and Newton, 2001). In ill-health, more oxygen radicals are released, and there are likely to be fewer antioxidants. Oxidative stress has been implicated in more than one hundred diseases (Pierce *et al.*, 2004). Hyperoxia, from excessive oxygen therapy, increases ROS release (Knight *et al.*, 2011). The amount and time for oxygen toxicity are debated, but are traditionally considered to be more than 60% for more than 24 hours (Hinds and Watson, 2008). However, in the context of probable tissue damage from insufficient oxygen, the risk of possible damage from excessive oxygen is probably a lower priority. Oxygen should therefore be given to achieve a target saturation.

Implications for practice

- Oxygen is needed by cells; without oxygen, cells die.
- Oxygen is a drug, so must be prescribed (in emergencies, prescription can be retrospective).
- Prescription should be to a target saturation, not an absolute amount of oxygen.
- In emergencies, commence with high concentrations, and reduce down to target saturation; in non-emergency situations, commence low and increase to achieve targets.
- Long-term use of high concentration oxygen should be humidified.
- Ensure sufficient oxygen is available for transfers.

Summary

Oxygen is vital for life. Oxygen therapy is frequently needed for sicker patients, and can be life-saving, but it also exposes patients to potential harm. Nurses are accountable for their actions, and so should be aware of safety issues surrounding oxygen and its administration.

Useful website

www.brit-thoracic.org.uk

Further reading

National (BTS, 2008) and local guidelines for oxygen therapy guidelines should be followed. Readers should also be aware of guides from manufacturers of equipment used in their hospitals.

Clinical scenario

Mrs Roberta Jones is admitted with an acute exacerbation of COPD. She used to smoke heavily, but stopped two years ago. On arrival in A&E her vital signs are

RR 35 bpm (shallow)
pulse 90 bpm (irregular)
BP 150/90 mmHg (MAP 109)
T 36.4°C
SpO_2 86% on 2 litres nasal oxygen.

She is agitated, and mumbles random words.
   She lives alone, and is largely housebound. The next of kin, her daughter, lives 200 miles away.

1   Using A-B-C-D-E assessment, identify main concerns for Mrs Roberts, Calculate her NEWS/ViEWS.
2   Which vital signs cause you particular concern, and why?
3   What treatments will be likely to benefit Mrs Roberts during the early stage of her time in hospital?

Chapter 6

Airway management

 Contents

Fundamental knowledge

- Upper airway and tracheal anatomy
- Respiratory failure

Introduction

Airway obstruction is likely to cause respiratory arrest, so airway is the first stage in ABCDE assessment. Airway obstruction may be audible, either with the ear alone or with a stethoscope. This chapter describes commonly-heard lung sounds, principles of establishing and maintaining a clear airway, and use of artificial airways, especially temporary tracheostomies. Suction technique is discussed.

Lung sounds

Although abnormal breathing sounds may be clearly audible, auscultation with a stethoscope is a valuable respiratory assessment. Most stethoscopes have a

- 'bell' (smaller) *and a*
- 'diaphragm' (larger).

The bell is useful for focused sounds, such as heart sounds, but for diffuse sounds, such as from the lungs, the diaphragm should be used. Become familiar with normal (healthy) sounds first, then listen to the patient's lung sounds as part of assessment. Most readers, and their family/friends/colleagues, are likely to have healthy lungs. There are also various audio aids for lung sounds (see Useful websites below).

Although lung sounds can be heard clearly on the back, many patients will need assistance to sit upright, so it is often more practical to place stethoscopes on the front of patients' chests. Compare sounds of one lung with the other. Begin with the bronchi (usually about the fourth intercostal space just to the side of the sternum). In health, breathing should sound like air passing through a large tube. Then compare the mid zones of each lung (mid thorax, angled down from bronchi). This sounds similar to the bronchi, but quieter (same quality, less quantity). Then listen to bases (anywhere between the nipple line and mid axilla); air entry is quietest at the bases (same quality, least quantity).

Common abnormalities that may be heard include:

- wheezing
- crackles.

Wheezing suggests bronchoconstriction, indicating need for bronchodilators. With crackles, listen carefully to assess whether they occur just on inspiration or both inspiration and expiration. Crackles that occur on inspiration, but not expiration, usually indicate resistance to alveolar expansion, such as from lung consolidation. Crackles occurring on both inspiration and expiration are usually from fluid (usually sputum) inside the airways, so may benefit from

- deep breathing and coughing
- respiratory physiotherapy (to mobilise secretions)
- saline nebulisers (to mobilise secretions)
- deep suction (if crackles can be heard in the bronchi).

Stridor, almost complete airway obstruction, is audible without a stethoscope. Urgent help should be summoned, as it is a peri-arrest situation.

Maintaining a clear airway

Reduced level of consciousness may cause the tongue to fall back, obstructing the airway. Airway patency may be re-established through positioning, such as the jaw thrust used in basic life support. Reduced consciousness may also impair cough and gag reflexes, enabling any fluids such as saliva or vomit to be aspirated into the lungs. Unconscious patients lacking cough reflexes should be nursed in the 'recovery' position (see Figure 6.1) to facilitate gravity drainage of secretions, and any orophayngeal secretions that do not drain should be removed with deep suction (see below).

With reduced consciousness, a Guedel airway may be useful to prevent the tongue falling back and occluding the airway. One the patient is sufficiently conscious to spit out the airway, they are usually sufficiently conscious to safely maintain their own airway.

Tracheostomies

A tracheostomy (= stoma in the trachea, created by a *tracheotomy*) may be:

- temporary
- permanent
- minitracheostomy.

Patients with acute severe respiratory disease or who are being weaned from invasive ventilation may benefit from a temporary tracheostomy to reduce *deadspace*. In practice, most ward patients with temporary tracheostomies are transferred from Intensive Care Units. Permanent tracheostomies are usually formed when cancer necessitates removal of part of the airway.

Originally, tracheostomies were *surgical*, a stoma being created through surgical incision. Permanent tracheostomies are still created surgically, and with difficult airways or other problems surgical approaches may be used. But most temporary tracheostomies

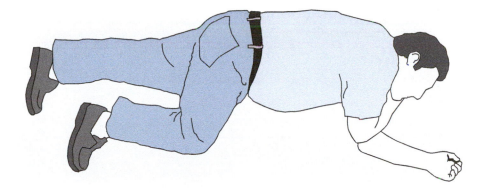

Figure 6.1 Recovery position

are now created using *percutaneous* dilatation (Nolan and Kelley, 2011), a needle hole being stretched until a tube can be inserted. In acute hospitals, tracheostomies are usually created percutaneously in the Intensive Care Unit, to facilitate weaning from artificial ventilation. Once self-ventilating, patients may then be transferred to wards with the temporary tracheostomy still in place.

Deadspace

As identified in Chapter 4, deadspace air (normally about 150 ml) dilutes oxygen of inhaled air and causes rebreathing of exhaled carbon dioxide. While not usually problematic with healthy breathing, shallow breathing (small breath volumes) means deadspace (poor quality) air forms a disproportionately large part of air reaching alveoli. Tracheostomies halve deadspace, making weak breaths more effective.

Tube sizes

Normal adult tracheostomy sizes are: 7.0, 7.5, 8.0 and sometimes 8.5 and 9.0 mm internal diameter. Sizes are printed on the external bladder and neckplate. Tube size should be recorded clearly in patients' notes, but nurses caring for patients with tracheostomies should also check the tube size each shift.

Inner cannulae

Temporary tracheostomies usually have (two) inner tubes. These should be changed at least 4 hourly with productive coughs, and at least 8 hourly in all patients (ICS, 2014). Inner tubes are single patient use, so should be cleaned (with water) and dried after removal. If secretions are minimal, and tube patency maintained, specialist staff (e.g. Critical Care Outreach) may advise less frequent changing of inner tubes.

Problems

Tracheostomies may create various problems for both patients and staff (see Table 6.1).

Table 6.1 Tracheostomies – problems

- communication
- nutrition
- cough reflex impaired
- ulceration
- infection
- loss of normal airway functions (humidification, warming, filtering of air)

Communication

Speech is created by air passing through vocal cords. Tracheostomy tubes are inserted below vocal cords, so if cuffs are inflated they usually prevent sound being formed. Loss of speech isolates patients, so nurses should explain that the tube causes loss of speech, and that the voice will return following its removal.

Alternative ways to communicate may include

- mouthing words and lip reading
- writing boards and pens
- sign/alphabet boards
- speaking valves/tubes.

Speaking valves (see Figure 6.2) or tubes necessitate cuff deflation, so patients must be able to protect their own airway (cough, swallow). Speech therapists should be included in the multidisciplinary care team.

Some patients with deflated cuffs or with sufficient cuff-leak find placing fingers over their tube restores their voice. However, human skin is covered with commensals which, in the respiratory tract, could become pathogens, so finger occlusion should be discouraged.

Tubes with fenestrations (holes in the side) allow air to pass through vocal cords. Fenestrated tubes should have both fenestrated and unfenestrated inner tubes. Fenestrated inner tubes normally remain in place to enable speech. For suction, unfenestrated inner tubes should be inserted to prevent catheters passing through fenestrations and damaging delicate tracheal tissue (NHS Quality Improvement Scotland, 2007).

Nutrition

The oesophagus and trachea being virtually adjacent, tracheal tubes can make swallowing difficult (Romero *et al.*, 2010; NCEPOD, 2014; ICS, 2014), especially if the cuff remains inflated (Amathieu *et al.*, 2012). Swallowing should be assessed before commencing oral fluids/diet, ideally by a speech and language therapist. Nurses should observe patients when eating or drinking in case aspiration occurs. Nutrition should be monitored, supplementing with liquid or nasogastric feeding if necessary, and involving dieticians.

Impaired cough reflex

Effective coughs rely on closure of the glottis creating sufficient pressure in lungs to force the glottis open and rapidly expel mucus. Tracheostomy tubes prevent complete glottis

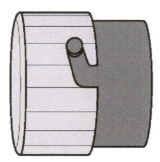

Figure 6.2 **Speaking valve**

closure, often making cough reflexes weak. Deep suction may be needed to clear secretions.

Most adult wards will only stock up to three sizes of suction catheters:

- FG 10 (black)
- FG 12 (white)
- FG 14 (green)

Suctioning can cause mechanical damage to the delicate airway tissue, so the smallest size that will be effective should be chosen. FG 10 should clear watery secretions, such as saliva or loose sputum, but for thicker secretions FG 12 may be needed. FG 14 catheters are not recommended for use with tracheostomies.

Suction causes trauma, so pressure should be limited; common practice is no more than 20 kPa. Tenacious secretions may benefit from mobilisation with saline nebulisers, mucolytics (ICS, 2014) or chest physiotherapy. If frequent suctioning is likely to be needed, a nasal airway can spare the patient repeated trauma from catheters. NCEPOD (2014) cite National Tracheostomy Safety Project minimum of 8 hourly suction for patients with tracheostomy, but ICS (2014) recommend individually assessing suction needs and encouraging patients to expectorate, without recommending a suction frequency. Blocked tubes should be removed, after which suction can be applied through the stoma (ICS, 2014).

Minitracheostomy

This is not an airway; it is a very narrow tube allowing access for suction (FG 10 catheter or smaller). Rarely used, they are useful if patients are able to breathe adequately through their normal airway but are likely to have problems with secretion clearance (Beach *et al.*, 2013).

Ulceration

Pressure sores, usually associated with visible skin near bony prominences, can develop wherever sustained pressure exceeds perfusion pressure of capillaries supplying oxygen and nutrients to that tissue. Most tracheostomies on wards have deflated cuffs, but if cuffs are inflated they place continuous pressure on very delicate tracheal epithelium. When pressure sores heal, scar tissue remains which, being inelastic, could cause chronic respiratory limitation.

Excessive cuff pressures can cause tracheal necrosis. Cuff pressure, measured with a manometer (like tyre pressure gauges) which attaches to the external bladder, should not exceed 25 cmH$_2$O (ICS, 2014). Pressure should be checked each shift and whenever air is removed from or added to the cuff. Pressure should be checked at least 8 hourly (ICS, 2014) and documented at least once each shift (NCEPOD, 2014).

Infection

Like most surgical wounds, tracheal stomas should be kept clean and redressed. Dressings should usually be changed daily, or more frequently if soiled, but nurses should check surgical/medical notes before performing the first dressing.

Changing tracheostomy dressings *always* requires two people, to prevent loss of the tracheostomy and possible respiratory arrest. The second person, standing on the other side of the patient, assists by holding the tube, so acts under supervision and need not be a qualified nurse.

Redressing tracheostomies requires:

- standard dressing pack (including sterile swabs)
- sterile saline (0.9%)
- sterile tracheostomy dressing
- clean tracheostomy tapes.

Dressing is easiest if patients lie supine, which makes them less likely to cough.

Tracheostomies can damage skin and other body tissue. Sores may develop around the site of the stoma. These are most likely to be caused by

- pressure
- irritant fluids

and may form a source for infection from micro-organisms colonising the respiratory tract.

The warm moist area underneath neckplates can easily be colonised by micro-organisms. A swab may need to be sent for culture (MC+S). Excessive secretions may necessitate a soft suction catheter to remove them. The stoma should be cleaned thoroughly with saline (ICS, 2014). Current medical practice varies about whether or not neckplates are stitched to the skin. If stitches are used, sterile cotton buds or forceps and swabs may be needed. Buds with loose cotton may leave fibres which could be inhaled, so should be avoided.

Once clean and dry, stomas are covered with a commercially produced keyhole dressing. If stitched, forceps may be needed to draw the dressing fully under the neckplate. Check manufacturer's instructions for which side of the dressing should be placed against the skin.

Most Trusts use commercially produced tube holders. These should be placed tightly enough to allow two fingers to slide beneath them (Docherty and Bench, 2002), adequately supporting the tracheostomy tube without being uncomfortably tight for the patient.

Dressing changes should be recorded together with relevant observations:

- How clean is the site?
- Colour and amount of secretions?

Loss of normal airway functions

The human airway

- warms
- humidifies *and*
- filters inhaled air.

Most of these functions take place in the deadspace (discussed above). Reducing deadspace by up to half significantly impairs all three functions, so artificial alternatives are needed to replace them.

Heat/moisture exchanger humidifiers (e.g. 'Swedish nose' – see Figure 6.3) reflect warmth and moisture back into the airways, and filter inspired air, but if oxygen is inserted into the sideport users should check flow does not bypass the humidifying membrane. Heated water humidification is more effective, and is available on some high-flow systems.

Inadequate humidification can cause airway obstruction/arrest from dry, sticky mucus plugs. Tracheostomies should therefore always be humidified (ICS, 2014).

Occlusion

As with any arrest situation, help should be summoned urgently. If suction fails to clear the airway, the tracheostomy cuff should be deflated with a syringe to allow some air to bypass the tube. As much oxygen as possible should be given, preferably 100%.

The tracheostomy tube should now be removed, so cut/remove tapes and any stitches, using scissors – there is not usually time to fetch a stitch cutter. The tracheostomy tube should be easy to remove. Stomas are usually well formed by seven days (Bodenham and Barry, 2001), so should provide the patient with a reasonable airway, although a replacement tube should be inserted as quickly as possible. New stomas may collapse quickly, necessitating more rapid insertion of a replacement tube.

Two spare tubes (one the same size as the patient's, and one a size smaller) should be kept near the patient's bedside, together with a pair of tracheal dilators. With a well-formed stoma, a new tube of the same size should be easy to insert. If the stoma is newly formed, appears to be collapsing, or if there is any difficulty with trying to insert a tube of the same size, there are two options:

- inserting the smaller tube (which can be replaced later in a planned, controlled procedure);
- using tracheal dilators to enlarge the stoma.

In an emergency, it is usually quicker, and so safer, to opt for the smaller tube.

Once the patient has a patent airway, a doctor (preferably an anaesthetist) should urgently review the patient.

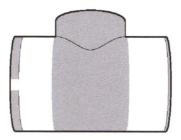

Figure 6.3 Heat moisture exchange (HME) humidifier ('Swedish nose')

Should tracheostomies occlude, removal of the inner tube usually restores patency. If removing the inner tube fails to establish a patent airway, suction should usually be attempted. If this fails, the old tube should be removed and replaced, ideally with a tube of the same size. If a similar size tube cannot be inserted, either the stoma may be dilated with tracheal dilators, or a tube a half-size smaller should be inserted.

Emergency equipment

The tracheostomy is the patient's only airway, so emergency equipment needs to be quickly and easily accessible. NCEPOD (2014) recommend that wards caring for patients with tracheostomies should have a difficult airway trolley, identical to ones in the hospital's theatres, and that endoscopy equipment should be immediately available.

Emergency equipment near the beside (and during transfers) should include:

- suction (working and ready to use)
- suction catheters (including Yankeur)
- gloves, aprons and eye-protectors
- spare tubes: one the same size and one a size smaller
- tracheal dilators
- rebreathing bag and tubing
- catheter mount or connection
- syringe
- disconnection wedge
- tube holder and dressing
- resuscitation equipment.

(ICS, 2014)

Much of the kit may be included with a 'tracheostomy box' supplied by Critical Care Outreach.

Remembering individual professional accountability (NMC, 2015), staff caring for patients with a tracheostomy should ensure emergency equipment is easily accessible at the start of their shift, including that suction equipment is working.

Signs and outline careplans should be displayed at bedheads of patients with tracheostomies (NCEPOD, 2014).

Planned removal

Removing tracheostomies significantly increases work of breathing, by up to one third (Chadda et al., 2002), causing potential dyspnoea. Removal is normally a medical decision, and should be performed by someone competent both in removal and airway management. Respiratory function should be monitored closely following removal.

Implications for practice

- Temporary tracheostomies reduce airway deadspace, so can significantly reduce work of breathing.

- The upper airway warms, moistens and filters air; bypassing most of the upper airway creates potential risks and problems.
- Although the cough reflex normally remains, tracheostomies weaken the strength of coughs, so patients often need suction to clear airway secretions.
- Thick, dry secretions can occlude the tracheostomy, causing respiratory arrest.
- Staff caring for patients with temporary tracheostomies should know how to re-establish an airway as quickly as possible.
- Emergency equipment should be checked each shift.
- Unless the patient is adequately clearing their own airway secretions, suction should also be performed at least once each shift, as near the start to enable individualised planning of care for that shift.

Summary

Temporary tracheostomies can provide a useful medical treatment for severe acute respiratory limitations, but they create many actual and potential problems for patients. Nurses should therefore know the potential risks created and how to minimise the problems created by tracheostomies. Critical Care Outreach services should usually be involved in the team caring for patients with tracheostomies (Lewis and Oliver, 2005).

Useful websites

Various websites offer the opportunity to listen to lung sounds, including
www.easyauscultation.com/lung-sounds.aspx
http://solutions.3m.com/wps/portal/3M/en_EU/3M-Littmann-EMEA/stethoscope/littmann-learning-institute/heart-lung-sounds/lung-sounds/

Further reading

St George's Healthcare Trust (originally 2006, now regularly updated for internet access) and ICS (2014) provide authoritative guidelines for tracheostomies, while NCEPOD (2014) provides a useful review of national practice.

Clinical scenario

Mr Thomas Fraser was admitted to hospital three weeks ago with a severe acute exacerbation of COPD, initially requiring artificial ventilation in ICU, where a percutaneous temporary tracheostomy was inserted. He is now self-ventilating, but still has the tracheostomy (cuff deflated), and has now been transferred to your ward.

1   From reading this chapter, and your own experiences, list actual and potential problems the tracheostomy might cause Mr Fraser. Identify any equipment that will be needed. Where it is not stocked in your own workplace, identify where you could obtain this equipment.

2   Identify nursing observations that should be performed in relation to Mr Fraser's tracheostomy. Include frequency of observations. From this book, and any other available sources, identify the evidence-base for this aspect of care.

3   Over the following week Mr Fraser's condition slowly deteriorates; aspiration is suspected. Mr Fraser is breathless, hypoxic and appears frightened. List options for treatment. Unfortunately Mr Fraser's condition has caused acute disorientation, so his ability to make informed decisions are limited. You may therefore have to be his advocate. As Mr Fraser's nurse, decide how far, if at all, you would advocate escalation of treatment.

Chapter 7

Intrapleural chest drainage

Contents

Fundamental knowledge

- Pleural anatomy

Introduction

Chest drains can remove any abnormal collection of fluid or air from the thorax. As there are two main organs in the chest (the heart and lungs), chest drains are almost always used to treat problems with either of these organs. Cardiac drains are widely used following cardiac surgery, but this chapter describes chest drains used to treat pulmonary problems.

Small collections of air or fluid may resolve spontaneously or be removed by needle aspiration. Larger collections necessitate intrapleural chest drains, more often just called 'chest drains'. Although chest drains have been used for over a century, there is surprisingly little research-based evidence (MacDuff *et al.*, 2010). There are however UK national guidelines, published by the BTS; sections authored by Havelock *et al.* (2010) and MacDuff *et al.* (2010) are especially useful. Chest drains are the catheters inserted into the patient's pleura. Insertion is usually a medical role. Indwelling drains are connections to collection chambers, which are usually managed by nurses (and often incorrectly called 'chest drains'). This chapter focuses on nursing management of collection chambers and related care of patients.

Patients needing chest drainage are usually breathless and hypoxic, so their respiratory function (rate, depth, saturations) should be closely monitored, and they often need supplementary oxygen both before and following insertion of drains. Respiratory observations should therefore be performed frequently, at least every 4 hours. Chest-drain specific observations are discussed below.

Physiology

Lungs are covered by two pleura: the outer (*parietal*) pleura is attached to respiratory muscles, while the inner (*visceral* or *pulmonary*) is attached to the lungs. On inspiration, respiratory muscles move outwards, increasing intrathoracic space which makes intrathoracic pressure negative compared with atmospheric (air) pressure. This draws the parietal pleura outwards. Between the two pleura is a film of 2–5 ml of fluid (Roskelly *et al.*, 2011); this creates sufficient *surface tension* ('stickiness') to draw the visceral pleura outward, expanding lung volume, and so drawing air from the atmosphere into alveoli.

In health, intrapleural pressure remains slightly negative, ranging between minus 2 and minus 6 cmH$_2$O (Hough, 2001). This constant negative pressure helps keep alveoli patent and prevents atelectasis. If intrapleural pressure equalises with intrapulmonary or atmospheric pressure, lungs collapse, causing respiratory distress.

Pneumothorax

A pneumothorax is air or gas in the pleural space (*pneuma* = air). The term is often incorrectly used in clinical practice to include fluid collections (haemothorax = blood, pyothorax = pus). Collections may be *mixed* (e.g. air and blood). Precise cause may affect where the drain is inserted, but principles of nursing management and care are identical for all types, so this chapter follows common nursing usage of 'pneumothorax' to describe all collections. Air (or fluid) enters through a hole, which may be

- primary (spontaneous) *or*
- secondary (to lung disease or trauma).

As long as the hole allows air to both enter and escape, the pneumothorax is

■ open.

A small, open pneumothorax may self-resolve without intervention, but collections are often large enough to necessitate needle aspiration or chest drainage. But if the hole creates a one-way valve, allowing air to enter on inspiration, but preventing it escaping on expiration, the pneumothorax is described as

■ tension,

enlarging with each breath, and potentially compressing the heart, causing pulseless electrical activity (PEA) cardiac arrest. Tension pneumothorax is a medical emergency, necessitating urgent drainage.

Pleural effusion

Pleural effusions are fluid collections in the pleural space that have accumulated through capillary leak, not a ruptured pleura. Effusion may be from

■ exudate *or*
■ transudate.

Exudate is oedema-like leak caused by either increased hydrostatic pressure or low osmotic pull in the intravascular compartment (see Chapter 10), so is protein poor. Transudate is caused by inflammation, so is protein-rich, and often looks cloudy.

Effusions tend to be smaller than pneumothoraces, so more often self-resolve, or can be resolved by needle aspiration. Large effusions may need chest drain insertion.

Chest drains

In the past, wide-bore drains were often used (typically 24–32 FG). Narrower tubes are generally as effective, and cause less pain and fewer complications, so FG 10–14 are recommended (Davies *et al.*, 2010; Fysh *et al.*, 2010; Galbois *et al.*, 2012). Wider tubes remain available, and may occasionally be preferred for draining a haemothorax (Light, 2011).

An open tube between the pleura and atmosphere creates potential for air (and micro-organisms) to re-enter the pleura. Traditionally, this has been prevented by placing the exit of the tubing under water ('under water seal drain' – UWSD). UWSDs are still used, but are increasingly being replaced by dry systems, which use a one-way mechanical valve.

Suction

Traditionally, external suction was used in the belief it increased drainage. However, there is no evidence it did (Havelock *et al.*, 2010), and external suction may cause pulmonary oedema (MacDuff *et al.*, 2010). If external suction is used, the amount suggested in literature ranges from usually –10 to –40 kPa, with most authors recommending –20 kPa. However, few of these recommendations are evidence-based, and in contrast to previous editions, current UK national guidelines (MacDuff *et al.*, 2010) suggest external suction should not routinely be used.

Changing chambers

Changing collection chambers may introduce infection, so they should only be changed when full, or there is some other specific indication (Allibone, 2003; Durai *et al.*, 2010). Changing chambers should use aseptic non-touch technique. The drain will need to be clamped, to prevent air entry into the pleura. Drains should be clamping for the minimum time necessary to change chambers.

Dressing

Dressings should be bio-occlusive, comfortable and prevent disconnection. Roskelly and Smith (2011) recommend dry dressings around the insertion site, and avoiding heavy strapping which would prevent chest wall movement. Jones (2011) recommends transparent adhesive dressings. Keyhole dressings, such as manufactured for vascular devices, are useful; if two are placed opposite each other, the drain can exit through a central hole, with a further (non-keyhole) transparent dressing on top to secure the drain. Dressing used should be recorded clearly in care plans.

Pain management

Pain is a common problem, unnecessary pain causing 15 of 58 NHSLA chest-drain-related claims between 1995 and 2006 (NPSA, 2008). Although smaller bore drains are less painful than wider ones (MacDuff *et al.*, 2010), pain may be caused by:

- the drain itself
- wound site
- inflammation
- pulling from tubing.

To reduce pain, patients will often limit breathing and avoid coughing (Gray, 2001), which predisposes them to developing chest infections. Nurses should therefore

- ensure analgesia is prescribed
- ask patients if they have any pain
- observe for nonverbal signs of pain
- assess effectiveness of analgesia given
- if analgesia is ineffective, inform medical staff.

Observations

In addition to 'basic' respiratory observations, such as rate and depth of breathing and oxygen saturation, nurses should observe

- Swinging or suction
- **Bubbling**
- **Draining**.

Swinging

Provided external suction is not used, fluid should swing with respiration. Cessation of swinging suggests either that the problem has resolved, or the drain is blocked (Sullivan, 2008). Suction creates a constant negative pressure, and so drains on suction should not swing. Suction pressures should however be monitored.

Bubbling

Bubbling only occurs if air is being drained. Sudden cessation of bubbling suggests drain blockage. Coughing, which creates positive intrathoracic pressure, may dislodge clots. Otherwise, a blocked tube is a medical emergency, potentially causing tension pneumothorax and PEA arrest. If suction is used, excessive turbulence indicates excessive negative pressure (Bar-El *et al.*, 2001).

Draining

If fluid is drained, the level in the chamber should be marked, along with the time and the date at least each shift. Type of drainage should be recorded (e.g. blood, pus), and volume included in the daily fluid balance. Rapid drainage is both painful and may cause pulmonary oedema (Roskelly *et al.*, 2011). Initial drainage should be limited to no more than 1500 ml within the first hour; after this volume, the drain should be clamped for an hour (Havelock *et al.*, 2010).

Oxygen

Loss of lung volume often causes hypoxia, necessitating supplementary oxygen. There is limited, dated evidence that high concentration oxygen hastens resolution of high pneumothoraces (Northfield, 1971), possibly due to reduced nitrogen concentration (nitrogen is more easily absorbed) (Light and Lee, 2010). Giving high concentration oxygen for this reason is supported by national guidelines (BTS, 2008; MacDuff *et al.*, 2010).

Positioning

Patients should be encouraged

- to sit upright, to improve drainage
- to breathe deeply, to prevent chest infection
- to mobilise.

Patients should be actively involved in managing their drains, and be aware not to raise the chamber to chest height.

Flushing

Collection chamber tubing is wide, so unlikely to block. However, narrow-bore drains are prone to blockage (Medford and Maskell, 2005). Davies *et al.* (2010) discourage routine flushing of tubing, but recommend flushing blocked catheters with 20–30 ml sterile saline. Flushes into/towards pleural space should not be performed by nurses (unless it is part of their specialist role).

Clamping

Clamping can convert an open pneumothorax into a life-threatening tension pneumothorax. Drains should only be clamped

- if disconnected
- when changing collection chamber
- if there is excessive drainage (see above)
- moving the chamber above the patient is unavoidable
- briefly, following any drug instillation (e.g. 1 hour for sclerosants (Roberts *et al.*, 2010)).

There is no evidence that clamping before removal is beneficial; any request to clamp prior to removal should be documented, together with duration for clamping (Havelock *et al.*, 2010).

Clamped drains should be closely supervised by nursing staff familiar with management of chest drains, and unclamped if the patient develops respiratory distress (Havelock *et al.*, 2010).

Complications

Thirty per cent of patients with chest drains experience complications (Ball *et al.*, 2007). There are three main groups of complications:

- insertional (e.g. pain, tissue damage)
- positional (inadequate drainage, subcutaneous emphysema)
- infectious.

(Jones, 2011)

Any concerns should therefore be reported to medical staff.

Subcutaneous emphysema

Also called surgical emphysema or tissue emphysema, this is where air or gas collects in tissues. Although any air leak may cause tissue emphysema, the most likely chest drain cause is an eye of the drain being outside the pleural cavity (Lefor, 2002). As air rises, this usually collects in the chest or in the neck, and while it usually benign (Papiris *et al.*, 2004), resolving spontaneously, it can cause discomfort, cause necrotising fasciitis, inhibit breathing, and obstruct the airway (Kesieme *et al.*, 2012). When touched, 'crackling' can be felt.

Infection

Five of 17 chest-drain-related UK deaths between 1995 and 2006 were from infection (NPSA, 2008). All procedures involving disconnection or the wound should therefore be aseptic.

Removing chest drains

Removal is painful (Puntillo *et al.*, 2014), so appropriate analgesia should be given. Most chest drains are not sutured in, making removal simple. If sutured, 'mattress' sutures should have been used. A mattress suture comprises two sutures to the skin (not connected to the drain) and one around the drain (not connected to the skin). The three sutures are then tied together. So, when the three sutures are cut, they will need to be tied again following removal of drain. This necessitates two people (Havelock *et al.*, 2010).

Drains should be removed with a firm, brisk movement (Havelock *et al.*, 2010), either when intrathoracic pressure is either positive (valsalva manoeuvre, like straining at stool) or neutral (on expiration) (Havelock *et al.*, 2010), to prevent air being drawn in through the open wound by negative pressure inspiration. After removal, an occlusive dressing, such as hydrocolloid, should be placed on the wound site. Respiratory function should be closely monitored following removal, as pneumoraces may recur.

Implications for practice

- External suction is not recommended; if used, pressures should be between minus 10–20 cmH$_2$O.
- Patients with chest drains usually need strong analgesics, and usually also benefit from anti-inflammatory medicines; offer analgesia for removal.
- Check dressings each shift.
- Observe for swinging, bubbling, draining.
- Mark fluid level at least each shift (on the chamber); include volume in daily fluid balance.
- Patients should be encouraged to mobilise, having been taught how to safely manage their drain bottle.
- A clamped drain can cause a tension pneumothorax and PEA cardiac arrest; tubing should therefore only be clamped if unavoidable, and then for the minimum time necessary, with a registered professional in the immediate vicinity of the patient.

Summary

Intrapleural chest drains are a useful medical solution to a large (>20%) pneumothorax. They expose patients to potential risks, which nursing care should anticipate and minimise. Patients with chest drains should therefore be cared for in wards where staff are familiar with management of chest drains (Havelock *et al.*, 2010). Respiratory function and the drainage system should be closely observed.

Further reading

Core further reading is the national guidelines from the British Thoracic Society (BTS, 2010), published as six documents, of which Davies *et al.* (2010), Havelock *et al.* (2010) and Roberts *et al.* (2010) are the most useful. The Marsden Manual (Roskelly and Smith, 2011) offers useful nursing advice. There is also an article by Sullivan (2008), although this predates current national guidelines. Many manufacturers support their products with informative websites.

Clinical scenario

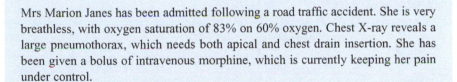

Mrs Marion Janes has been admitted following a road traffic accident. She is very breathless, with oxygen saturation of 83% on 60% oxygen. Chest X-ray reveals a large pneumothorax, which needs both apical and chest drain insertion. She has been given a bolus of intravenous morphine, which is currently keeping her pain under control.

1 With the help of colleagues from work, list the items that will be needed for insertion of a chest drain.
2 You are asked to assist the doctor inserting the drain. Identify what is expected of you, both by the doctor and to care safely for your patient.
3 Devise a plan of care to manage Mrs Janes' chest drain for the first twelve hours following insertion.

Chapter 8

Blood gas interpretation

Contents

Introduction

Arterial and venous blood gases are often taken from deteriorating patients. This chapter focuses on arterial results, with indications of whether results can be inferred from venous gases. If measuring venous gases, it is however wise to follow trends from venous samples only.

Many results may be included on a blood gases printout, but there are four groups of results (not always placed together):

- pH
- respiratory function
- metabolic function
- electrolytes and metabolites.

This chapter follows this sequence, using a 5-step analysis:

1 pH
2 respiratory ($PaCO_2$, PaO_2, saturation)
3 metabolic (bicarbonate, base excess)
4 compensation
5 electrolytes and metabolites (most covered in chapter 3)

Generally accepted normal ranges are identified, together often with ideal figures. Core aspects of analysis are identified; further aspects of blood gas, including some results not discussed in this chapter, can be found in the parallel chapter of *Intensive Care Nursing*. Abbreviations are listed in Table 8.2, at the end of this chapter.

STEP 1: pH

Normal (arterial): 7.35–7.45
Ideal: 7.4

---

pH ('puissance d'hydrogène' – power of hydrogen) is a scale to identify acidity or alkalinity of chemicals. The scale ranges from 0 (strongest possible acid) to 14 (strongest possible alkali), with a chemically neutral point of 7.0 (pure water). Blood is chemically slightly alkaline, so arterial blood below 7.35 is described as *acidosis*, while pH >7.45 is *alkalosis*. Significantly lower pH can be found is some parts of the body (e.g. stomach, urine), but blood pH below 6.8 or above 7.8 is usually rapidly fatal (Hennessey and Japp, 2007). Blood pH is the sum of respiratory and metabolic acid/base balance. To maintain homeostasis, the body attempts to *compensate* for an imbalance of one with an equal and opposite reaction with the other (see step 4 below). pH imbalance may therefore be *respiratory*, *metabolic*, or *mixed*.

Like other gases, hydrogen moves from areas of greater concentration to lesser. Cell metabolism produces acids, making normal intracellular pH about 7.0 (Atherton, 2003; Chesler, 2005). As hydrogen ions diffuse into capillary blood, venous blood has a lower pH than arterial – normally about 7.35 (Marieb and Hoehn, 2013).

STEP 2: RESPIRATORY

Blood gases contain various measures of respiratory function; three are discussed here:

- $PaCO_2$
- PaO_2
- saturation (SaO_2).

$PaCO_2$ (**P**artial pressure **a**rterial **C**arbon dioxide)

> **Normal: 4.6–6.1 kPa (British Thoracic Society, 2008)**
> **Ideal: 5.3 kPa**

Carbon dioxide is another waste product of cell metabolism, and is potentially toxic. Clearance depends on rate and depth of breathing (ventilation), so $PaCO_2$ indicates

- ventilation.

Carbon dioxide is a highly soluble gas, so one way blood transports carbon dioxide is in solution, as carbonic acid (see Chapter 4). Carbon dioxide therefore also indicates

- respiratory acid/base balance.

Excessive carbon dioxide (>6.1 kPa) results in excessive carbonic acid, and therefore a respiratory acidosis.

low CO_2 (<4.6 kPa)	high CO_2 (>6.1 kPa)
hyperventilation respiratory alkalosis	hypoventilation respiratory acidosis

The UK measures gases in the systeme international unit of kilopascals (kPa). Some countries, such as the USA, measure in millimetres of mercury (mmHg). 1 kPa = 7.4 mmHg.

Measuring PCO_2 of venous blood probably has little value, although Treger *et al.* (2010) suggests it correlates with arterial levels.

PaO$_2$ (**P**artial pressure **a**rterial **O**xygen)

> **Normal: 12.0–14.6 kPa (British Thoracic Society, 2008)**

Partial pressure of oxygen is the pressure which oxygen exerts in the volume of blood; it therefore effectively indicates the amount of oxygen available to diffuse into tissue cells, whereas saturation (below) indicates haemoglobin carriage of oxygen.

The normal range (above) is for healthy individuals. However, people who have chronic obstructive pulmonary disease (COPD) will be used to lower levels, and are less likely so survive if PaO$_2$ exceeds 10 kPa (Howard, 2009).

If levels are below those desired, supplementary oxygen should be given. With high levels, supplementary oxygen should be reduced; oxygen toxicity is discussed in Chapter 5.

If assessing for home oxygen therapy, gases should be taken when any supplementary oxygen has been removed for at least 20 minutes. Home oxygen therapy is only indicated if

- PaO$_2$ ≤7.3 kPa or SaO$_2$ ≤88% twice over three-week period or
- PaO$_2$ 7.3–8.0 kPa or SaO$_2$ 88% if evidence of
  - pulmonary hypertension
  - peripheral oedema suggesting congestive cardiac failure or
  - polycythemia (haematocrit >55%).

(Gold, 2013)

In acute care, oxygen should not be removed for taking blood gases (Burt and Arrowsmith, 2009), as this both puts patients at potential risk of hypoxia, and negates information from PaO$_2$ about whether oxygen therapy is optimal.

Measuring PO$_2$ of venous blood has no value.

Saturation (SaO$_2$)

> **Normal arterial: 97–98%**
> **Target saturation: 94–98 % for most patients, 88–92%**
> **with COPD (British Thoracic Society, 2008)**

Arterial blood gas saturation measurements are essentially identical to those from pulse oximeters, except that blood gas analysers use far more colours, and so unlike pulse oximeters remain accurate in the presence of carbon monoxide.

Haemoglobin (Hb) molecules consist of four 'chains', each of which can carry one molecule of oxygen (O$_2$). Most haemoglobin in arterial blood is normally fully saturated (HbO$_8$), with a few molecules being only 75% saturated (HbO$_6$). Haemoglobin has a high affinity for oxygen, but usually allows one molecule to dissociate in capillaries, and so normal venous saturation is 70% (Garry *et al.*, 2010). Unless patients are moribund, arterial blood should not be near 70% saturated, and so saturation is useful for confirming whether samples are venous or arterial. In the presence of normal arterial/peripheral saturation, venous saturation can indicate tissue oxygen delivery and/or uptake of oxygen. This is discussed further in *Intensive Care Nursing*.

As with peripheral saturation, blood gas saturation is limited by the amount of haemoglobin available – 100% of half the amount is a significant reduction. Haemoglobin is measured by blood gases.

Oxygen will only reach cells if it can dissociate from haemoglobin. Factors such as alkalosis and hypothermia reduce oxygen dissociation, making saturation high but PaO_2 low; conversely, acidosis and pyrexia increase dissociation, lowering saturation but increasing PaO_2. This is discussed further in *Intensive Care Nursing*.

STEP 3: METABOLIC

Smaller analysers, such as some used in the community, may only provide one metabolic measurement; most hospital machines provide two:

- bicarbonate
- base excess.

Bicarbonate (HCO_3^-)

> **Normal: 22–29 mmol/litre (Pathology Harmony)**
> **(mmol/litre = milliequivalents/litre, abbreviated as mEq/L)**

Bicarbonate is the main 'buffer' in blood, inactivating the hydrogen ions needed to form acids. It is produced in many parts of the body, especially the gut, and mainly the liver. Low bicarbonate levels (<22 mmol/litre) result in insufficient buffering, and therefore metabolic acidosis. High levels (>29 mmol/litre according to Pathology Harmony, but many texts cite 26 mmol/litre as the upper normal limit) are metabolic alkalosis.

Severe acidosis is often fatal, so in the past was treated with aggressive infusion of intravenous sodium bicarbonate. However bicarbonate, like sodium, does not significantly enter cells (where metabolic acids are produced). Paradoxically, bicarbonate can dissociate into carbon dioxide and a hydrogen and oxygen radical; carbon dioxide can diffuse freely into cells, worsening intracellular acidosis. The Resuscitation Council (2010) therefore advise not to 'routinely' give sodium bicarbonate.

Venous and arterial bicarbonate are, for practical purposes, comparable (Treger *et al.*, 2010).

Base excess (BE)

> **Normal: +2 to minus 2**
> **Ideal: 0**

'Base' is another word for 'alkali', so an excess of base is a metabolic alkalosis. Base excess can be negative, which means metabolic acidosis.

Bicarbonate is the main alkali in blood, so base excess is largely derived from bicarbonate. The two metabolic measurements should therefore reflect each other.

Standardised measurements

Most analysers will print a single bicarbonate result and a single base excess result, usually both results being standardised. But some analysers may print both actual and standardised measurements. Actual are levels which have been actually measured in the sample, whereas standardised are the actual measurements adjusted to what they would have been in ideal conditions. Ideal conditions are:

- temperature 37.0°C
- carbon dioxide 5.3 kPa.

Bicarbonate, and the base excess largely derived from it, are viewed as metabolic measurements. However, bicarbonate is not purely metabolic in origin; a small quantity of bicarbonate derives from carbon dioxide ($CO_2 + H_2O \leftrightarrow H_2CO_3 \leftrightarrow HCO_3^- + H^+$). Carbon dioxide levels are affected by temperature (most places no longer temperature correct gases). Therefore standardising measurements (suffix of 'std' or prefix of 'S') removes any respiratory element, significant if carbon dioxide levels are grossly abnormal. If both measurements are printed, the standardised ones should normally be used.

Summary of metabolic acid/base balance

Acidosis	Alkalosis
↓ HCO_3^-	↑ HCO_3^-
↓ BE	↑ BE

STEP 4: COMPENSATION

Because of the narrow limits for compatibility with life, homeostasis attempts to maintain arterial pH at 7.4. Any imbalance is countered, if possible, with an equal and opposite reaction to restore pH. So, for example, a metabolic acidosis will be countered if possible by a respiratory alkalosis.

Usually, acidosis is the problem; any alkalosis is therefore usually compensatory. Respiratory compensation is rapid – acidosis stimulating increases in rate and depth of respiration, lowering carbon dioxide levels to create a respiratory alkalosis. Metabolic compensation is slower, often talking several days. Metabolic compensation can also persist for days after the respiratory problem has been resolved, leading to possible 'metabolic overshoot' alkalosis.

So, if pH is normal, either

- both sides (CO_2 and SBC/SBE) are normal *or*
- the problem is fully compensated.

If pH is abnormal, compensation is either

- incomplete *or*
- failed.

STEP 5: ELECTROLYTES AND METABOLITES

Almost all analysers will measure sodium, potassium and glucose. These were discussed in Chapter 3. Various other electrolytes and metabolites may be measured, depending on assays included in the analyser. For practical purposes, arterial and venous levels are similar.

Calcium (Ca^{++})

Normal (ionized): 1.2 mmol/litre (Parikh and Webb, 2012)

As identified in Chapter 3, blood calcium is in two forms: ionized (or 'free', active) and protein-bound (inactive). Laboratory U+Es measure total calcium. But blood gas analysers measure ionized calcium, and therefore levels will be approximately half of laboratory levels.

Chloride (Cl^-)

Normal: 95–108 mmol/litre (Pathology Harmony)

Chloride levels are often neglected in healthcare, and few analysers include this measurement. The hyperchloraemia of 0.9% saline can cause metabolic acidosis, but identifying chloride as the cause of the problem is only possible if chloride is measured; chloride is often the 'forgotten' electrolyte – often not measured, with few people being aware of its normal range, or potential effects. Chloride is discussed further in Chapter 25.

Lactate

> **Normal: <1.0 mmol/litre (Dellinger RP *et al.*, 2013) *or***
> **0.6–2.5 mmol/litre (Pathology Harmony)**

Many analysers do not measure lactate, as its inclusion is both problematic and expensive. However, lactate is a valuable marker of anaerobic metabolism, typically caused by perfusion failure. Lactate is discussed further in Chapter 13.

Diagnosing the problem

Like any observation, blood gas results should be interpreted in the context of the patient. The history of the present condition will usually indicate whether acid base imbalance is respiratory or metabolic in origin. But as the only commonly seen cause of significant primary alkalosis is panic-induced hyperventilation, acidosis can usually be assumed to be the problem, with any alkalosis being compensatory.

Respiratory acidosis is caused by hypercapnia from hypoventilation. This may be due to chronic disease – acute exacerbations are a common cause of hospital admission. But hypoventilation may also be acute, such as respiratory depression from opioids. Three examples of hypercapnic respiratory failure are illustrated in Table 8.1.

Table 8.1 Three examples of hypercapnic respiratory failure

	$PaCO_2$	pH	HCO_3^-
Chronic	↑	normal	↑
Acute	↑	↓	normal
Acute-on-chronic	↑	↓	↑

The chronic hypercapnic respiratory failure, being normal for the patient, is fully compensated by metabolic alkalosis.

The acute respiratory failure (e.g. opioid overdose) has not had sufficient time to develop metabolic compensation, and therefore respiratory acidosis causes overall acidosis.

The acute-on-chronic mixes both the acute and chronic pictures, with an overall acidosis resulting from the acute element.

Both the acute and the acute-on-chronic patients need to improve ventilation (position, bronchodilators, non-invasive ventilation). Commencing non-invasive ventilation for the chronic picture would be futile, and might induce overall alkalosis.

Metabolic acidosis can have varied causes, including

- *kidney disease* (hydrogen ions not excreted)
- *liver failure* (little bicarbonate produced)
- *tissue acids* (e.g. lactic, ketoacids)
- *hyperchloraemic*.

Table 8.2 (Some) abbreviations used in blood gas printouts

A = alveolar
C = content
F = fractional concentration in dry gas
I = ideal
P = pressure, or partial pressure
Q = volume of blood
S = standardised
T = total
a = arterial
c = capillary *or* calculated
e = estimated
v = venous

Implications for practice

- Interpret results using the 5-step systematic approach (pH, respiratory, metabolic, compensation, electrolytes and metabolites).
- Significantly deranged blood pH is incompatible with life, therefore if possible the body compensates to restore arterial pH to 7.4.
- Acidosis is usually the problem; any alkalosis is usually compensatory.
- Most results from venous gases are comparable with arterial results, although it is safest to follow trends from one type.
- Except for the gases themselves (oxygen, carbon dioxide) many venous results have similar ranges to arterial.
- Interpret results in the context of the patient.

Summary

Blood gases can provide useful information about patients' conditions, although are usually only taken when patients deteriorate. Venous blood gases are being increasingly used in various contexts, including diabetic ketoacidosis (see Chapter 26). Interpreting results is a skill, which like all skills improves with practice; once patient needs have been met, return to the results, and using the 5-step approach analyse them in the context of the patient.

Further reading

Practice, rather than extensive reading, is the best way to develop skills. Hennessey and Japp (2007) and Foxall (2008) provide handbooks with many scenario-based examples.

Exercises

Using the 5-step approach, analyse the following results:

1

pH	7.341
PCO_2	5.42 kPa
PO_2	21.7 kPa
HCO_3–sdt	21.5 mmol/l
SBE	–3.5 mmol/l
ctHb	134 g/l
SO_2	100%
K^+	3.2 mmol/l
Na	148 mmol/l
Ca^{++}	1.14 mmol/l
Cl^-	126 mmol/l
Glucose	12.7 mmol/l
Lactate	2.4 mmol/l

The patient: a 34-year-old type 1 diabetic originally admitted with diabetic ketoacidosis, now stabilised, with insulin being infused as per protocol; polyuria persists; supplementary oxygen 40%.

2

pH	7.247
PCO_2	6.71 kPa
PO_2	9.93 kPa
HCO_3 –std	21.4 mmol/l
SBE	–5.9 mmol/l
tHb	112 g/l
SO_2	96.4%
Na^+	136.6 mmol/l
K^+	5.6 mmol/l
Ca^{++}	1.11 mmol/l
Cl^-	109 mmol/l
Glucose	3.0 mmol/l
Lactate	0.66 mmol/l

The patient: a 90-year-old female 2 days following major gut surgery, receiving 28% oxygen; BP 100/60 mmHg, peripherally cold.

3

pH	7.354
PCO_2	2.18 kPa
PO_2	29.30 kPa
SO_2	99.5%
HCO_3–std	15.7 mmol/l
BE	−7.8 mmol/l
Na^+	154.5 mmol/l
K^+	5.93 mmol/l
Ca^{++}	1.02 mmol/l
Cl^-	114 mmol/l
Glucose	2.4 mmol/l
Lactate	1.74 mmol/l

The patient: 48-year-old male, respiratory arrest leading to PEA in ambulance; sample taken following return of spontaneous circulation; receiving oxygen 15 litres/minute via non-rebreathe reservoir mask.

Chapter 9

Non-invasive ventilation

Contents

Fundamental knowledge

- Respiratory anatomy and physiology
- Respiratory failure (see Chapter 4)

Introduction

Ventilation is the movement of air in and out of the lungs. Failure of ventilation is therefore life-threatening, often necessitating mechanical support. Pedantically, the term 'non-invasive ventilation' should only be applied to equipment which cycles between inspiratory and expiratory support; in practice, the term is also used to include systems providing single pressure support. This chapter follows common practice by including

- continuous positive airway pressure (CPAP)
- bilevel non-invasive ventilation (bilevel NIV).

High flow nasal oxygen, which effectively supplies low-level CPAP, was discussed in Chapter 5. In many Trusts, equipment may be called by brand names, such as BiPAP™ for bilevel NIV.

Technically, CPAP is not ventilation, as it hinders, rather than helps, expiration. It is however included in this chapter because

- it is a useful respiratory support
- understanding CPAP helps explain bilevel NIV
- increasingly, the same machines are used for both modes.

This chapter frequently refers to the authoritative RCP/BTS/ICS (2008) guidelines for NIV.

CPAP

Continuous positive airway pressure, sometimes called by its mechanical ventilation equivalent name positive end expiratory pressure (PEEP), closes the airway circuit before the end of expiration, when pressure falls to a preset minimum positive pressure. This traps residual volume within the circuit, which includes the patient's lungs. Air trapped in alveoli

- prevents collapse (*atelectasis*)
- enables oxygen exchange to continue

while the positive pressure in airways before collapsed alveoli helps reinflation (reverses atelectasis). CPAP therefore improves oxygenation, so is useful for type 1 respiratory failure. CPAP is also useful for treating pulmonary oedema (see below).

While improved oxygenation makes CPAP useful for type 1 failure, the same pressure that supports inspiration inhibits expiration. Carbon dioxide clearance from lungs depends on expired volume. The 'gas trapping' caused by CPAP may inhibit carbon dioxide removal, worsening hypercapnia. This limits the usefulness of CPAP for treating hypercapnic respiratory failure, such as from acute exacerbations of COPD.

Some hospitals use positive pressure ventilators intermittently for physiotherapy, usually to reverse atelectasis, especially post-operative. Modes include Intermittent Positive Pressure Breathing (IPPB; the 'Bird®'), CPAP and Bilevel NIV. Negative pressure cuirasses, which cover the front of the thorax, are sometimes used to mobilise sputum. Pryor and Prasad (2008) devote a chapter to NIV, but elsewhere include only passing mentions of intermittent interventions.

Bilevel NIV

Bilevel non-invasive ventilators essentially provide two alternating levels of CPAP – a higher one on inspiration, and a lower one on expiration:

- IPAP = inspired positive airway pressure
- EPAP = expired positive airway pressure.

The higher pressure of IPAP assists inspiration, delivering larger volumes for less effort by the respiratory muscles. In addition to inhaling larger volumes, and so more oxygen, reducing the *work of breathing* (respiratory muscles use less oxygen and energy) leaves more oxygen for other parts of the body. The lower pressure of EPAP enables more of the inhaled volume to escape, compared with CPAP. This assists more carbon dioxide clearance. Increasing the difference between IPAP and EPAP (sometimes termed *pressure support*) increases carbon dioxide clearance. Bilevel NIV is therefore useful for treating type 2 respiratory failure – in practice, in acute hospitals, this usually means acute exacerbations of COPD. Bilevel NIV is sometimes called by the brand name of whatever system is used within the hospital (e.g. BiPAP®). Most bilevel machines can also deliver CPAP.

Cautions

CPAP and bilevel NIV provide useful supports for people with respiratory failure, but being noninvasive provide no protection for the airway; patients must therefore be able to maintain their own airway. Positive pressure should not be used

- if patients are vomiting, as it may force gastric acid into lungs, causing pneumonitis;
- if there is airway obstruction from an inhaled object, which it would similarly force down the airway;
- with an undrained pneumothorax, which it will enlarge causing tension pneumothorax and cardiac arrest;
- where it may damage susceptible tissue, such as facial burns/trauma or recent upper gastrointestinal surgery;
- when copious respiratory secretions are present, as it will inhibit clearance.

(RCP/BTS/ICS, 2008)

Settings

Settings vary between machines, but common options are listed below; many are available on both CPAP and bilevel modes.

Pressures are usually commenced low, partly to increase acceptance (RCP/BTS/ICS, 2008), and partly to minimise risks. Typical (custom and practice) initial pressures are 5 cmH$_2$O for CPAP and IPAP 10 cmH$_2$O and EPAP 4 cmH$_2$O for bilevel NIV.

Trigger senses respiratory effort, causing the cycle to change from EPAP to IPAP. This enables machines to follow patients' own breathing, which is physiologically more comfortable than machine-imposed cycles.

Ramp which commences at low pressures and automatically ramps pressure up over a set time. This allows patients to adjust to target pressures, and improves acceptance.

Rise time is the time each breath takes to reach maximum inspiratory pressure. Middle settings are usually best, but with tachypnoea (>30 breaths/minute), shorter rise time helps ensures full IPAP, and so lung volume, is reached in the relatively short inspiratory phase. With obstructed airways, slower rise time is likely to cause less distress.

Rate setting is only for back-up apnoea breaths. It should therefore be set low enough so as not to interfere with the patient's own breaths – if the rate setting is higher than the patient's, the machine will control breathing. A rule of thumb setting is half the patient's own rate, provided this will offer sufficient breaths in the event of apnoea. Rate setting may need to be decreased when the patient's rate reduces.

Oxygen may be available directly through the machine, or need to be added into the circuit from a standard oxygen flow metre.

Although apnoea back-up enables most machines to function as mechanical ventilators, this is an emergency safety measure, and should not be used to routinely ventilate apnoeic patients – not least because NIV provides no airway protection.

Masks

(See Figure 9.1)
For both CPAP and bilevel NIV masks should be fitted accurately; there is usually a range of sizes, so users should know how to fit locally used disposables. In acute hospitals face masks are usually used (Nava and Hill, 2009), although other options typically include

- full head mask
- helmet
- nasal mask
- mouth-piece.

Patients unable to tolerate face masks may comply with other options. Nasal masks should only be used if patients breathe through their nose, while mouth-pieces necessitate mouth-breathing. There also 'full face masks', larger than the standard face mask; many patients

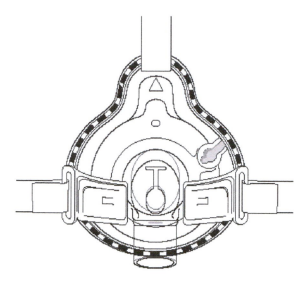

Figure 9.1 **Face mask with head harness**

find these less claustrophobic, and although eyes are inside the mask, eye complications do not seem to be significant.

Most machines compensate for leaks, but leaks should be small, and at the base of masks not up into eyes, as this may cause conjunctivitis (Zandiah and Katz, 2010). Most machines measure leak volumes, but feel around the mask for leaks. Condition of facial skin should be observed and recorded both before starting NIV and during use; sores often occur on the bridge of the nose (Nava and Hill, 2009; Carron *et al.*, 2013). If skin looks friable, or shows signs of pressure sore development, hydrocolloids or other protective dressings are useful. Some discomfort may be unavoidable, but whenever possible nurses should relieve or reduce discomfort, for example by repositioning the mask.

Deterioration

Many patients benefit from NIV, but about a quarter deteriorate further, necessitating escalation (intubation and ICU admission) or palliation. Which patients will deteriorate is unpredictable (Poponcik *et al.*, 1999), so NIV should be attempted (Jolliet *et al.*, 2001), monitored closely, and if necessary be replaced by invasive ventilation within four hours of commencing NIV (RCP/BTS/ICS, 2008). NIV can reduce need for intubation (Nava *et al.*, 2011), but if intubation is necessary, delay can prove fatal (Esteban *et al.*, 2004).

Failure rate for NIV exceeds 16% (Carron *et al.*, 2013), either from patients refusing the treatment or it not being effective, so plans to commence NIV should also include clear plans for action if NIV fails (Telfer *et al.*, 2007; RCP/BTS/ICS, 2008) – including whether NIV is 'ceiling treatment', and whether resuscitation or palliative care is appropriate. The ICU/Critical Care Outreach team should be involved in planning.

Which patients may benefit?

Non-invasive ventilation is used in community settings mainly to treat

▨ sleep apnoea (McMillan *et al.*, 2014).

In acute hospitals, non-invasive ventilation is usually used to treat

▨ acute exacerbations of chronic obstructive pulmonary disease (COPD)

although other uses include treating

▨ pulmonary oedema
▨ severe pneumonia

and in critical care for

▨ weaning from invasive ventilation (Burns *et al.*, 2009)
▨ post-operative support (Glossop *et al.*, 2012)
▨ neuromuscular disease, such as Guillain–Barré syndrome.

NIV for neuromuscular disease and chest wall deformity may need to be continued in the community. Discussion below is restricted to use of NIV; more general discussion of many of these pathologies was included in Chapter 5.

COPD

Bilevel NIV significantly improves survival from acute exacerbations of COPD (RCP/BTS/ICS, 2008; Nava and Hill, 2009; Parola *et al.*, 2012), making this the most common indication for NIV in acute hospitals. Bilevel NIV should be the first-line intervention with respiratory failure in COPD, initiated as soon as respiratory acidosis occurs (arterial pH <7.35, $PaCO_2$ >6 kPa) (RCP/BTS/ICS, 2008; Nava and Hill, 2009). Underlying causes should also be treated concurrently – for example, suspected infection should be investigated (sputum specimen) and treated with antibiotics.

Pulmonary oedema

Positive pressure within alveoli hastens return of interstitial oedema into pulmonary circulation (Nava and Hill, 2009; Weng *et al.*, 2010), although does not improve survival (Gray *et al.*, 2008). Combined with diuretic therapy to remove the fluid from the body, treatment times often need to be limited to a few hours.

Pneumonia

Jolliet *et al.* (2001) and Baudoin (2002) recommend using NIV for severe pneumonia. While few other studies address this issue, bilevel NIV is widely used for type 2 respiratory failure, and is an effective treatment for severe hypoxaemia (Ferer *et al.*, 2003), which could be caused by severe pneumonia.

Sleep apnoea

Sleep apnoea causes poor sleep for both sufferers and carers, and tissue hypoxia to sufferers. Overnight positive pressure ventilation (CPAP or bilevel) significantly improves sleep (McMillan *et al.*, 2014), so enabling more daytime activity (Patel *et al.*, 2003). It may also restore hypercapnia as the main respiratory drive. While normally managed in the community, these people may be admitted to acute hospital for respiratory crises or non-respiratory problems, so need overnight NIV.

Complications

Hypotension

Positive intrathoracic pressure reduces ventricular filling and so, unless compensatory mechanisms occur, reduces blood pressure. Problems from reduced perfusion pressure may be offset by improved oxygenation, including to the myocardium. For some patients, NIV improves cardiac function (Nelson *et al.*, 2001; Sin *et al.*, 2000; Yin *et al.*, 2001).

At low pressures, this effect is usually insignificant, but CPAP above 10 cmH$_2$O can cause significant hypotension (Carron *et al.*, 2013). Bilevel NIV does not appear to cause significant hypotension (Somauroo *et al.*, 2000). However, when commencing positive pressure NIV, blood pressure should be closely monitored, such as setting automated non-invasive blood pressure monitors on 5 or 10 minute cycles for 30 minutes, and using appropriate alarm settings to warn staff about hypotension.

Renal

Hypotension may compromise all systems but kidneys are at high risk from

- (volume-responsive) acute kidney injury
- ischaemia (acute tubular necrosis).

Hydration and perfusion should therefore be optimised.

Endocrine

Stress increases hormone release:

- renin-angiotensin-aldosterone cascade (hypertension; see Chapter 10)
- antidiuretic hormone (oliguria)

while positive intrathoracic pressure reduces plasma atrial natriuretic peptide (see Chapter 10), predisposing to oliguria. Together, these hormones can cause various problems, including oedema – systemic and pulmonary. Pulmonary oedema worsens hypoxia.

Gut

With swallowing, some air enters the stomach. Both the trachea and oesophagus lead off the oropharynx, so positive pressure in upper airways causes more air to be swallowed, while impeding its escape (Carron *et al.*, 2013). Air in the stomach can cause gastric distension which

- splints the diaphragm, reducing breath size and making breathing more difficult
- provokes discomfort, nausea and/or vomiting

and if not removed

- creates flatus (Parsons *et al.*, 2000).

If gastric distension is problematic a nasogastric tube should be passed and left on free drainage. The bag may need frequent emptying. Anti-emetics and peppermint should be prescribed to relieve discomfort.

Psychological

Many people find NIV, especially CPAP, uncomfortable and distressing. While some patients may overtly refuse it, others may covertly resist its use by removing, or attempting to remove, it frequently. Like many other respiratory interventions, little or no benefit is gained until about 20 minutes. Frequent removal is not therapeutic, but also indicates patients are not willing to consent to treatment, and are becoming distressed. The stress response causes detrimental physiological effects, including tachypnoea, tachycardia, hypertension, hyperglycaemia and fluid retention (see Chapter 2). So to prevent harmful distress, and potential claims of assault, frequent removal should be recognised as an indication for discontinuation.

Approaching patients with face masks and NIV headgear may provoke fear. Having explained what NIV can offer, whenever possible patients should be offered the mask to hold in their hands and place it against their own face. Slowly building up the gas flow (*ramp*) may also help tolerance. If patients are comfortable with the treatment, they are more likely to accept it (Jarvis, 2006); if patients reject the treatment, they are unlikely to consent to further attempts. As nurses usually commence NIV, and adjust equipment, success or failure of NIV largely depends on nursing management (Jarvis, 2006).

Like many respiratory interventions, commencing NIV relies largely on inspired guesses, using close monitoring and subsequent adjustments to achieve optimal effect.

Observation

Non-invasive ventilation is usually commenced because patients cannot adequately breathe by themselves. Therefore patients receiving NIV should be closely observed. Observation should include

- respiratory rate, heart rate
- level of consciousness, patient comfort
- chest wall movement, ventilator synchrony, accessory muscle use.

(RCP/BTS/ICS, 2008)

Pulse oximetry indicates oxygenation, so should be continuously monitored for at least the first 12 hours of NIV (RCP/BTS/ICS, 2008). Hypoxia may cause

- confusion, drowsiness or agitation
- compensatory tachycardia.

But oximetry does not measure carbon dioxide or haemoglobin levels (see Chapter 2). Visual observations indicating poor ventilation (hypercapnia) include

- very slow or fast respiratory rate (<10 or >30 breaths per minute)
- shallow chest wall (or accessory muscle) movement.

The mainstay of carbon dioxide measurement in clinical practice remains blood gas analysis (see Chapter 8):

- arterial
- capillary
- transcutaneous.

Transcutaneous gases, usually measured on the ear, differ slightly from arterial, but generally have close correlation (Cox et al., 2006), so provide continuous or frequent monitoring of trends. Attempts to develop pulse co-oximeters (pulse oximeters that also measure carbon dioxide) have so far not yielded reliable technology (Bolliger et al., 2007). RCP/BTS/ICS (2008) recommend earlobe capillary sampling, citing recent studies supporting its reliability with carbon dioxide levels. An arterial blood gas should be taken with the initial capillary gas if identifying comparability; thereafter, capillary gases provide a useful trend of improvement or deterioration.

RCP/BTS/ICS (2008) recommend arterial gas sampling within 1 hour of commencing NIV, within 1 hour of subsequent changes, and within 4 hours if the patient is not clinically improving. NIV has failed so should be replaced by invasive ventilation (RCP/BTS/ICS, 2008) or terminal care.

Weaning

Chronic respiratory disease usually necessitates weaning rather than suddenly stopping NIV. Once pH is within normal range (above 7.35), underlying cause of the disease are resolving, and respiratory rate has normalised, weaning should commence (RCP/BTS/ICS, 2008). This should be pre-planned, using increasing periods off the ventilator.

Implications for practice

- CPAP is useful for type 1 respiratory failure.
- Bilevel NIV is useful for type 2 respiratory failure.
- NIV should be a first line treatment for type 2 respiratory failure.
- Respiratory acidosis causing blood pH of 7.25–7.35 in an indication for NIV.
- Patients receiving NIV should be closely monitored and observed, which necessitates sufficient numbers of staff with sufficient knowledge and skills of using NIV to safely care for the patient.
- When commencing NIV, plans should be made for treatment options if NIV fails. There are usually only two options:
  - invasive ventilation (usually in ICU)
  - palliative care.
- ICU or critical care outreach should be involved with plans for escalation.
- If 6 hours of treatment has not resulted in significant improvement, treatment should be changed to one of the above options.

Summary

Non-invasive ventilation has significantly improved outcome from respiratory failure, so is used in various wards specialising in respiratory care, and sometimes elsewhere. Patients with chronic respiratory disease may have previously experienced successful treatment with NIV, expecting nursing staff to be as familiar with the treatments as they are. CPAP, although technically not ventilation, can be a useful respiratory support for type 1 respiratory failure, especially when caused by pulmonary oedema. Bilevel NIV is useful for ventilatory (type 2) respiratory failure. However, NIV will not be successful for all patients, so patients should be closely observed, monitored and reviewed.

Further reading

RCP/BTS/ICS (2008) guidelines are the single most important resource for all UK staff using NIV. Readers should be familiar with NIV and other relevant protocols of their own hospital.

Clinical scenario

Jack Adams, aged 74, is admitted with an acute exacerbation of COPD. On arrival in A&E he was breathless and cyanosed. Arterial blood gas analysis showed pH 7.27, PaO_2 7.2, $PaCO_2$ 8.3 kPa. Bilevel NIV is commenced and he is transferred to the medical assessment ward for further observation.

1   List the nursing observations that should be made. Identify which observations should be continuous, and suggest an initial frequency for observation which will be intermittent.

2   Using A-B-C-D-E assessment, identify problems that Mr Adams is likely to, or may experience as a result of NIV. Suggest ways these problems could be resolved or minimised.

3   After two days of NIV support and other medical treatments, Mr Adams' condition improves sufficiently to consider removing ventilatory support. Make a list of criteria that you would use before removing or weaning NIV. Identify the rationales for these criteria. Analyse the evidence on which these are based, and how reliable you consider that evidence to be.

Part 3

Cardiovascular

Chapter 10

Perfusion

Contents

Introduction

The cardiovascular system is the body's main transport mechanism. It carries gases, nutrients and waste, as well as many things that are important for homeostasis – heat, infection control mechanisms, control factors and hormones. So if perfusion fails, multiple problems threaten various aspects of function. But most importantly, if perfusion fails, cells do not get what they need – oxygen, glucose, and removal of potentially toxic waste. Cells can survive short periods of perfusion failure by resorting to anaerobic metabolism and metabolism of alternative energy sources, but both produce less energy and more waste. Therefore prolonged ischaemia leads to cell death. When insufficient cells remain for function, systems fail, and risk of morbidity and mortality escalate.

Some hormones which affect perfusion are discussed. By definition, hormones are chemicals released by a gland into the bloodstream; hormones target other organs/systems, and despite their small quantities, have powerful effects.

Normally, cells die through *apoptosis* (autophagy – '*cell cleaning*'), sometimes called 'programmed cell death' or 'cell shrinkage' – an implosion-like process ensures intracellular contents are safely enclosed in cell membranes for safe disposal, rather like disposing of soiled dressings safely in yellow waste bags. Pathological cell death, *necrosis*, resembles an explosion, with potentially toxic intracellular contents spreading into surrounding tissue. Failure of autophagic clearance can cause remodelling, such as in

- cancer
- neurodegeneration
- cardiomyopathy
- auto-immune diseases.

(Sridhar *et al.*, 2012)

Blood pressure

Arterial blood pressure results from three factors:

- heart rate
- stroke volume
- arterial/arteriole resistance (systemic, or peripheral, vascular resistance).

$$BP = HR \times SV \times SVR$$

Hyper- or hypo-tension therefore results if one or more of these factors is abnormal. While blood pressure and heart rate are easily measured, stroke volume and arterial resistance are not.

Stroke volume

Stroke volume is the amount of blood ejected when the ventricles contract. In health, right ventricular stroke volume matches the left. An average healthy left ventricle holds about 130 ml of blood, but not all of this blood is ejected. Normal stroke volume is about 70–90 ml (Barrett *et al.*, 2010). Cardiac output, the amount of blood ejected by the left ventricle over a minute, is

heart rate × stroke volume

So if resting pulse is 70 bpm and resting stroke volume is 70 ml, 70 × 70 = 4900 ml; as these are approximations, average resting healthy cardiac output is about five litres/minute.

Chapter 2 identified the value of feeling pulses for strength; stroke volume is significantly reduced if pulses are weak/thready, and significantly increased if they are bounding (Campbell and Jackson, 2011).

Ventricles fill during diastole; during systole, valves between atria and ventricles should close, while active contraction prevents filling. Systole is the active phase of the cardiac cycle; diastole is whatever time is left between systoles. While the time of each systole will reduce with tachycardia, reduction in each systolic time is disproportionately less that increase in rate. Barrett *et al.* (2010) suggest that with heart rates of 60 bpm diastolic time is 0.62 seconds, while at rates of 200 bpm diastolic time is 0.14 seconds. So tripling heart rate reduces diastolic time (ventricular filling time) by three quarters. At heart rates of 200 bpm there will be much less blood in the ventricles each time they contract, therefore stroke volume will be far smaller.

An average healthy left ventricle holds about 130 ml of blood, but at rest normal stroke volume is about 70 ml, rising to about 90 ml on exercise. Normal ejection fraction is therefore >55% (Jowett and Thompson, 2007). Ejection fraction is measured with echocardiography, and can usefully indicate viability of heart function.

From arteries, blood flows into arterioles – short but highly muscular vessels; arterioles normally regulate flow into capillaries, where perfusion occurs.

Tunica intima

The inner layer of all blood vessels, and for capillaries the only layer, is tunica intima. This is squamous epithelium (squamous = scale-like), smooth thin cells that overlap, like fish scales.

Being smooth, tunica intima facilitates bloodflow and helps prevent thrombus formation. Being thin, and with potential gaps where cells overlap, tunica intima is semi-permeable, so gases, nutrients and waste can cross between blood and cells. But tunica intima is also chemically active, releasing many chemicals that maintain haemostasis. Some of these chemicals were mentioned in Chapter 3, for example

- prostacyclin (keeps platelets inactive)
- thromboplastin and platelet activating factor (trigger clotting).

It also releases chemicals that regulate vascular muscle:

- nitric oxide (vasodilates, also anti-inflammatory (Sahin *et al.*, 2012))
- endothelin (vasoconstricts)

and chemicals that assist inflammatory responses:

- leukotrienes (increase capillary permeability).

Tunica intima can therefore affect vascular resistance.

Systemic vascular resistance

Capillary refill time (CRT – see Chapter 2) is affected by bloodflow and resistance. Prolonged CRT therefore indicates either poor flow or high resistance (or both). Bloodflow is indicated by pulse strength, so CRT is useful to assess SVR. Other indicators of abnormal SVR are peripheral colour and warmth, and diastolic blood pressure (low DBP = vasodilatation = low SVR).

Capillary perfusion

From arteries, blood flows into arterioles – short vessels, but the blood vessels that have proportionately the greatest amount of muscle, and so are most able to regulate bloodflow.

Capillaries are crucial to perfusion, as it is at capillary level that delivery occurs. Cells need oxygen, and oxygen (not being very soluble) is carried by haemoglobin. But average erythrocyte diameter is 8 micrometres, while the average capillary diameter is 5–6 (Patel and Burnard, 2009). Erythrocytes therefore have to change their shape to pass through capillaries; their 'donut shape' enables them to do this, until with age their membranes become less pliant, and they are trapped in capillaries – see Chapter 3. As erythrocytes squeeze through capillaries, the haemoglobin which carries oxygen is essentially adjacent to capillary walls; as oxygen is not very soluble, this means oxygen molecules have very little fluid to pass through before entering cells. However, as identified in Chapter 3, nearly all (99%) blood cells are red cells, and red cells are essentially haemoglobin, so simplistically, blood is mainly haemoglobin and water (plasma). Therefore higher haemoglobin creates the paradox that although it carries more oxygen, bloodflow through capillaries, where oxygen is delivered, is impaired. This may explain Hebert *et al.*'s (1999) finding (subsequently confirmed by McLellan *et al.*, 2003) that optimal survival in sicker patients occurs with haemoglobin 70–90 grams/litre (an alternative explanation might be that bacteria need iron to survive, and low haemoglobin deprives them of this, so inhibits sepsis).

Capillaries being semi-permeable, water and small solutes (essentially, plasma minus plasma proteins) leak into the space between capillaries and cells, the interstitial fluid (see Chapter 23). In the average healthy person, about 24 litres (nearly five times the 5 litre total blood volume) leaks out of capillaries in 24 hours. This transports nutrients, such as glucose, into vicinity of cells.

Capillary occlusion

Intracapillary pressure is often cited as 32/28, making capillary occlusion pressure (mean capillary pressure) 30 mmHg. These figures, the basis for design of much pressure-relieving equipment, originate from Landis (1930). This study remains valid, but figures cited were mean (average) pressures of healthy volunteers. So, some patients may have lower capillary pressures, making them more susceptible to capillary occlusion, and perfusion failure.

Normotension – central nervous system regulation

The average healthy 70 kg person has about 5 litres of blood. As long as a 5 litre volume is contained with a 5 litre space, normal pressure is maintained. More volume than space causes hypertension, while more space than volume causes hypotension.

In healthy, the body maintains haemostasis and perfusion by matching space to volume. The main mechanisms for this are regulated by the brain-stem, which primarily maintains cerebral perfusion (see Chapter 17). The central nervous system therefore needs feedback about blood pressure (afferent nerves) and a mechanism to resolve the problems (endocrine).

The cardiac centres of the brain-stem receive some information through chemoreceptors (discussed in the context of respiratory regulation in Chapter 4), but more through baroreceptors, specialised nerve endings that sense pressure in arterial walls, especially the arch of the aorta and the carotid arteries – blood that will be flowing to the brain-stem itself. Baroreceptors respond to sustained changes in

- mean arterial pressure *and*
- pulse pressure.

So, when we get up in the morning, rising from the horizontal to vertical position, and gravity is suddenly placed against bloodflow to the brain-stem, the pressure drop stimulates responses to maintain cerebral perfusion. Delayed baroreceptor response causes postural hypotension, a problem found in up to 30% of older people (Low, 2008), usually resulting from chronic hypertension causing baroreceptor damage. Comparing lying and standing blood pressure, part of falls risk assessment, therefore indicates baroreceptor health.

Baroreceptors respond to mean arterial pressure (see Chapter 2) and pulse pressure. Pulse pressure is the pressure created by pulse: systolic minus diastolic.

Time out 10.1

Ideal BP is often cited as 120/80 mmHg. What would this make the pulse pressure?

If a patient's BP is 165/90, what is their pulse pressure? What difference do you notice between the two pulse pressures? What do you think is the main reason for this difference?

While the two diastolic blood pressures in the above time out exercise are similar, the second systolic pressure is far higher. As pulse volumes are unlikely to be dramatically different, wide (high) pulse pressure resistance indicates high resistance, almost invariably caused by poor vascular tone from atherosclerosis (Task Force, 2013). Narrow pulse pressures (e.g. 20) are caused by either

- hypovolaemia *or*
- poor cardiac output.

Patient context usually makes the cause obvious – e.g. post-operatively it is likely to be hypovolaemia, whereas with heart failure it is likely to be poor cardiac out. Pulse pressure is visibly obvious on charts by proximity between systolic and diastolic marks.

Hypotension sensed by baroreceptors triggers the neurohormonal response of adrenocorticotrophic hormone (ACTH) release, the stress response described in Chapter 2. ACTH stimulates release of adrenaline (and other hormones), and adrenaline stimulates both alpha receptors (vasoconstriction) and beta receptors (increased heart rate and blood pressure). While cardiac beta-stimulation with adrenaline is largely limited to cardiac arrest and critical/coronary care units, beta-blockers are widely used to treat hypertension. However, beta stimulation is used in another context: smooth bronchial muscle dilates with beta stimulation, hence the tachycardic effect of salbutamol.

Normotension – other mechanisms

Two other mechanisms regulate systemic blood pressure:

- the renin-angiotensin-aldosterone cascade
- antidiuretic hormone
- natriuretic hormones (including peptides).

The kidney is especially sensitive to perfusion failure. If it is not perfused, oliguria quickly occurs. To protect itself from hypoperfusion, the kidney releases the hormone renin in response to low bloodflow. Renin targets the liver, where it converts the prohormone (inactive hormone) angiotensinogen into angiotensin 1. Angiotensin 1 is a mild vaso-constrictor, but primarily targets lungs, where it is converted by angiotensin converting enzyme into angiotensin 2, a very powerful vasoconstrictor. This increases systemic blood pressure, so provided renal hypoperfusion was caused by hypotension, resolves the trigger. Chronic kidney disease is often accompanied by extensive vascular disease (Moody *et al.*, 2013), including renal artery stenosis, so the trigger for renin release, and chronic hypertension, remains.

Angiotensin and aldosterone are produced and act synergistically (Vinson and Coghlan, 2012). Among other functions, aldosterone regulates sodium reabsorption by the kidney. The significance of aldosterone follows from the next mechanism.

Another neuroendocrine mechanism is antidiuretic hormone, released by the pituitary gland. This increases water reabsorption by the kidney, which together with the sodium (salt) reabsorbed by aldosterone, forms saline, so increasing intravascular volume.

Natriuretic factors (or peptides; type A, type B) are chemicals released by the right atrium of the heart in response to increased stretch. They increase sodium loss through the kidneys (natrium – Na^+ = sodium), so resolving the hypervolaemia that has caused stretching.

Circadian rhythm

The body's daily rhythm (circa dies = about the day), regulated by the suprachiasmatic nuclei in the hypothalamus and controlled through hormones, normally ebbs about 03.00–04.00 and peaks about 18.00 (Redón *et al.*, 2001). Bloodflow and blood pressure mirror this rhythm. Bloodflow is therefore most sluggish at the ebb (Tanaka *et al.*, 2004), hence 'night cramps' and the high incidence of myocardial infarction between 06.00–11.00 following peak release of adrenaline and cortisol (Soo *et al.*, 2000; Scheer and Shea, 2014). Unnecessary stimulation, such as early morning washes, at this high risk time, and especially in high-risk patients, could precipitate crises.

Coronary perfusion

Perfusion is vital to all cells and systems, but failure to perfuse myocardium causes cardiac arrest. The first two arteries to leave the aorta are coronary arteries (right, left). The left coronary artery soon divides into the left anterior descending and the circumflex (left posterior) arteries. These three coronary arteries supply myocytes with oxygen and glucose.

Myocytes have more mitochondria than any other cells (Neubauer, 2007), so have exceptionally high oxygen demand, extracting nearly all available oxygen (Barrett *et al.*, 2010). Oxygen supply can only be increased by

- vasodilatation
- tachycardia.

Vasodilatation relies on release of nitric oxide from endothelium. But diseased vessels produce little nitric oxide, so compensatory tachycardia is likely. Compensatory tachycardia is generally effective provided heart rate does not exceed 130 bpm (Hinds and Watson, 2008). But tachycardia increases myocardial work (oxygen demand), so when stroke volume is significantly reduced, oxygen demand exceeds supply, provoking ischaemic pain (angina). Unfortunately angina is a late symptom of coronary artery disease, rarely occurring until coronary arteries are three-quarters occluded (Task Force, 2010).

Implications for practice

- Perfusion provides cells and organs with what they need – oxygen, nutrients, waste removal.
- If perfusion fails, compensatory mechanisms are exhausted.
- Unresolved ischaemia leads to pathological cell death (necrosis).
- So cardiovascular disease/problems compromise all body systems and quality of life.
- Minimum mean arterial pressure for perfusion is 65 mmHg, but people who are normally hypertensive will need higher MAP.
- Wide pulse pressure indicates cardiovascular disease.
- Oliguria is an early sign of perfusion failure.

Summary

Various vital signs, and clinical assessment, indicate perfusion, but the most significant is mean arterial pressure. Perfusion is vital for all tissues; poor perfusion causes tissue damage, and eventually death. Perfusion failure should therefore be urgently reversed, so concerns should be escalated quickly.

Further reading

Jowett and Thompson (2007) remains the key text on cardiac nursing. The European Society of Cardiology provides authoritative guidelines on many cardiovascular diseases.

Clinical scenario

Mrs Margaret Bowles, aged 68, is admitted for investigations, having suffered frequent chest pains for the last three days. She is a type 2 diabetic, has angina, smokes, and suffers from frequent night cramps. She appears mildly jaundiced.
   Vital signs are

T	36.4°C
BP	106/89 mmHg (MAP 95)
pulse	122 bpm (irregular)
resps	23 bpm
SpO$_2$	89% (on air)
responds to voice	
blood sugar	11.8 mmol/litre

1   What is Mrs Bowles' NEWS/ViEWS score? What actions does this suggest? Use A-B-C-D-E assessment, list your main concerns.
2   What risk factors does Mrs Bowles have for perfusion failure? Are they any signs of perfusion failure?
3   What further investigations are needed? How would you care for Mrs Bowles during her first 24 hours in hospital?

Chapter 11

Heart failure

Contents

Fundamental knowledge

- Cardiovascular anatomy and physiology; structure of blood vessels
- Renin-angiotensin-aldosterone cascade (see Chapter 10)

Introduction

Heart disease is the most common cause of hospital admission in older people (NICE, 2014a). Heart failure may be caused by problems with the structure or function of the heart (von Klemperer and Bunce, 2007), has reached epidemic proportions in developed countries, with incidence increasing (Adler *et al.*, 2009; Kim and Han, 2013). Despite recent reductions in mortality, coronary heart disease remains the single largest cause of death in the UK (Townsend *et al.*, 2012).

Heart failure may be acute, chronic, or acute-on-chronic. Acute heart failure typically occurs from acute cardiac events, such as myocardial infarction or severe sepsis. It is sometimes called 'decompensated' heart failure, because the failing heart ejects small pulses, while compensatory mechanisms fail to sustain blood pressure. Hypotension usually causes hypoperfusion, progressing to cardiogenic shock (see Chapter 13), usually necessitating transfer to coronary or intensive care units. This chapter focuses primarily on chronic and acute-on-chronic failure, both of which are a major burden on public health, causing and complicating many acute hospital admissions. Acute heart failure is discussed further in the next chapter, although pathophysiology of acute and chronic failure share much in common.

Chronic heart failure is typically progressive and compensated, chronic vascular disease progressively increasing vascular resistance. Compensatory tachycardia maintains perfusion at the cost of hypertension. Once decompensation occurs, heart failure becomes an end-stage (terminal) disease.

This chapter outlines what heart failure is, how it can affect individuals, and nursing care both for acute crises and for health promotion during recovery/rehabilitation. Hypertension, an almost inevitable cause of heart failure, is discussed. A brief overview of some commonly used drugs is included, with their main effects and side-effects. However, this is not a pharmacology text; many more drugs are available, and each drug can have many other side effects.

Hypertension

Hypertension is sustained systolic blood pressure ≥140, and/or diastolic blood pressure ≥90 mmHg (Task Force, 2013). Prolonged pumping against high resistance causes compensatory hypertrophy, but progressive hypertrophy eventually usually results in failure. Left-sided failure, the more common type, usually results from vascular disease (Lakasing and Francis, 2006), such as atherosclerosis, arteriosclerosis, peripheral vascular disease. Progressive strain causes left ventricular hypertrophy. Stroke volume may increase, but even if this and heart rate remain unchanged, increased systemic vascular resistance increases blood pressure.

Chronic hypertension increases resistance against which the left ventricle pumps, so chronic hypertension almost inevitably causes chronic left ventricular strain, left ventricular hypertrophy, and eventually left ventricular failure.

Primary hypertension is rare; hypertension is usually secondary to vascular disease – hardening of arteries and arterioles, often diagnosed as peripheral vascular disease. In the UK over half of over 60s are hypertensive (Bunker, 2014). The single most significant factor in development of vascular disease is smoking (Townsend et al., 2012), but other significant modifiable factors include excessive alcohol intake and diet, especially saturated fats (Townsend et al., 2012). Lack of exercise (Townsend et al., 2012), stress (Todaro et al., 2003) and environmental pollutants also often contribute to disease.

In health, normotension is maintained by balancing release of endogenous vasodilators and vasoconstrictors, most of which are released by vascular endothelium (see Chapter 10). But diseased vessels release less nitric oxide (Kalanuria et al., 2012), the main endogenous vasodilator. Nitric oxide is also anti-inflammatory, antithrombotic, and antiproliferative (Sahin et al., 2012). Failure of adequate nitric oxide production therefore significantly contributes to complications of heart failure.

Vascular disease increases resistance, and so systolic blood pressure. Therefore pulse pressure (systolic minus diastolic) rises significantly, and is a quick indicator of the extent of vascular disease. Reducing systolic blood pressure by as little as 10 mmHg significantly reduces morbidity and mortality from coronary heart disease and vascular events such as stroke (Law *et al.*, 2009). Mortality risk may be assessed by comparing systolic blood pressure of both arms – differences exceeding 10 mmHg indicate increased 10-year mortality risk (Clark *et al.*, 2012).

Cardiomyopathy

Damaged heart muscle will not pump effectively. Developing the World Health Organization and International Society and Federation of Cardiology 1995 classification system, Elliott *et al.* [2008] classify types of cardiomyopathy as

- hypertrophic
- dilated
- restrictive
- arrhythmogenic right ventricular

but also include 'unclassified cardiomyopathies'

- left ventricular non-compaction
- Takotsubu

the most common type being *dilated*. Cardiomyopathies are summarised in Table 11.1.

Table 11.1 The main cardiomyopathies

	Effects	Main causes	Incidence
Hypertrophic	Ventricular (left and/or right) hypertrophy, usually asymptomatic	Genetic [Spirito and Autore, 2006]	Rare; usually young people
Dilated	Dilates (enlarges) both ventricles, so impaired systolic function; progressive	Usually alcohol [Adam *et al*, 2008]; also street drugs such as cocaine [Hall and Henry, 2006], metabolic disorders, autoimmune disease, pregnancy	Most common type; usually older people
Restrictive	Heart normal size or slightly enlarged, but filling restricted	Endomyocardial fibrosis; primary disorder	Rarest type of cardiomyopathy
Arrhythmogenic right ventricular	Progressive replacement of (especially right) ventricular muscle with fat/fibre	Genetic	Rare

A recently (in 1990) identified cardiomyopathy is acute stress cardiomyopathy; its many other names include 'apical ballooning syndrome' or 'Takotsubu' (after Japanese octopus pots, which it visually resembles) (Rotondi and Manganelli, 2013). This usually occurs in women over 50 years of age (Kyriacou, 2012), and can mimic acute myocardial infarction, but without significant biomarker release (Gianni *et al.*, 2006). Usually triggered by major stress, such as bereavement, most people recover spontaneously (Gianni *et al.*, 2006), so it is often considered benign (Rotondi and Manganelli, 2013), needing only supportive intervention. But it can cause prolonged QT syndrome, and sudden cardiac death, so may need an implantable cardiac defibrillator (Rotondi and Manganelli, 2013). One fifth suffer complications, such as cardiogenic shock, which may necessitate intervention such as intra-aortic balloon pump (Akashi *et al.*, 2008). Incidence is uncertain, but of those initially diagnosed with acute myocardial infarction incidence is generally about 2% (Gianni *et al.*, 2006) and 6% in women (Rotondi and Manganelli, 2013).

Symptoms

The heart uses more energy than any other organ (Neubauer, 2007), extracting nearly all oxygen delivered by the coronary arteries. This leaves little reserve if demand increases. Sustained increased demand causes compensatory responses – tachycardia (Mehta and Cowie, 2006) and muscle enlargement, but both of these further increase oxygen and energy demand, so structural changes accelerate. Tachycardias up to 130 beats per minute are usually compensatory, and usually effective (Hinds and Watson, 2008). But structural changes in the heart, together with vascular resistance to output, progressively reduce cardiac output, and so tissue perfusion.

Left-sided heart failure causes pulmonary vascular congestion, causing

- pulmonary oedema
- breathlessness
- limited exercise tolerance.

(Mehta and Cowie, 2006)

Pulmonary vascular disease and/or pulmonary oedema impairs gas diffusion, so blood returning to the left side of the heart is often poorly oxygenated. Breathlessness hinders normal activities of living, including eating and drinking, so patients may be malnourished and dehydrated. Malnourishment may cause emaciation, but a significant factor contributing to many patients developing heart failure, and breathlessness, is obesity. Breathlessness is often especially bad at night, so patients often complain of poor sleep.

Right-sided heart failure may follow from left-sided failure (von Klemperer and Bunce, 2007), but may also result from pulmonary disease. Blood pressure in the pulmonary circulation is considerably lower than systemic blood pressure, pulmonary artery systolic pressure typically being 15–25 mmHg (Sturgess, 2014); together with proximity and relatively small volume of pulmonary vasculature, this means right ventricular workload is normally considerably less than left ventricular workload. However, pulmonary hypertension significantly increases right ventricular workload, causing right-sided hypertrophy. Right atrial hypertrophy often causes atrial fibrillation (Mehta and Cowie, 2006), further compromising myocardial oxygenation and systemic perfusion, although provided medical management is optimised atrial fibrillation does not reduce survival in patients with heart failure (Tveit *et al.*, 2011).

Heart failure is a syndrome, so diagnosis is made by the overall clinical picture, and not through any single test, although NICE (2014a) recommend initial testing for acute heart failure with either B-type natriuretic peptide (normal <100 ng/litre) or N-terminal pro-B-type natriuretic peptide (NT-proBNP; normal <300 ng/litre). Other tests often used to contribute towards diagnoses include

- echocardiography – checks heart size and function, including ejection fraction (EF);
- chest X-ray – views heart size and shape;
- cardiac catheterisation – measures pressures in right heart chambers;
- biopsy – views tissue cells.

Nurses should ensure their patients have given informed consent for procedures, and where significant risks are attached to procedures, that these have been explained to patients. Procedures may require specific preparation, so nurses should check local requirements for planned procedures. Nurses should also check if there are any special post-procedure instructions.

Other information contributing to diagnosis includes

- vital signs (heart rate, blood pressure, respiratory rate)
- 12-lead ECG
- blood results (U+Es, FBC, LFTs)
- weight.

Treatment aims are to improve both

- life expectancy, and
- quality of life.

(NICE, 2010b)

Acute admission

Patients admitted with acute-on-chronic heart failure are almost invariably fluid overloaded, so diuretic therapy is usually necessary (Krum and Abraham, 2009). Heart failure however creates the paradox that while the venous system and other fluid compartments are usually overloaded, arteries are often underloaded, making arterial blood pressure low. The kidney is very susceptible to hypotension, so once heart failure causes acute admission there is high risk of volume responsive acute kidney injury (see Chapter 24). Cardiac function (throughput) is usually optimised by giving vasodilators, such as glyceryl trinitate (GTN), to reduce cardiac workload (Krum and Abraham, 2009).

Key drug groups used to control heart failure are usually

- diuretics
- antihypertensives
- lipid-lowering ('statins').

But because of likely complications of heart failure, various other cardiac and non-cardiac drugs are also often needed for

- rate control
- thrombosis prevention.

Diuretics

Heart failure typically causes venous congestion and so oedema. Diuretic therapy reduces both oedema and preload, enabling the failing heart to function more effectively. Three main groups of diuretics are used

- loop (e.g. furosemide, bumetanide)
- thiazide (e.g. bendroflumethiazide, metolazone)
- potassium-sparing (e.g. amiloride).

Loop diuretics inhibit reabsorption in the Loop of Henle, so not only reduce renal reabsorption of water, but also significantly reduce renal reabsorption of potassium. Loop diuretics can therefore cause hypokalaemia. Hypokalaemia can impair cardiac conduction, causing escape ectopics and dysrhythmias. Urine is formed from arterial blood, but excess water is mainly either in veins or tissues (oedema); diuretics can therefore cause hypovolaemia, stimulating thirst. Fluid restriction may therefore be necessary; this often increases patients' distress.

Anti-hypertensives

Anti-hypertensives significantly reduce incidence of heart failure (Beckett *et al.*, 2008), so are useful for long-term management, although the arterial hypotension that often accompanies acute admission may contraindicate their use. The main groups of anti-hypertensive drugs are

- ACE inhibitors
- beta-blockers
- aldosterone antagonists
- angiotensin receptor blockers
- calcium antagonists.

Blood pressure is the sum of cardiac output multiplied by systemic vascular resistance; drugs that reduce either therefore reduce blood pressure.

Angiotensin converting enzyme (ACE) activates angiotensin I into the powerful vasoconstrictor angiotensin II (see Chapter 10). ACE inhibitors ('prils') therefore reduce vasoconstriction.

Beta stimulation to the heart increases rate and contractility, so beta blockers ('-olol's; carvedilol) reduce cardiac output, and should be prescribed for all patients with heart failure (Hernandez *et al.*, 2009).

Aldosterone increases renal reabsorption of sodium, and so contributes to the fluid overload of heart failure. Aldosterone antagonists, such as spironolactone, increase renal sodium loss, and so diuresis.

Angiotensin receptor blockers (ARBs), such as losarten, are alternatives for ACE inhibitors (NICE, 2010b).

Calcium both increases cardiac conduction and vasoconstricts. Calcium channel blockers (e.g. nifedipine, amlopidine, diltiazem) therefore reduce both aspects that create blood pressure.

Statins

Atherosclerosis is a cyclical problem with a complex pathology. It usually begins in child-hood (Kalanuria *et al.*, 2012), and is mainly caused by plaque formation from lipids such as cholesterol and low-density lipoproteins (LDLs). Lipid-lowering drugs ('statins') both inhibit plaque formation, and significantly reduce existing plaque (Jensen *et al.*, 2004), therefore reducing cardiovascular events (Taylor *et al.*, 2011; Heart Protection Study Collaborative Group, 2012).

Current UK recommended lipid levels are

- total cholesterol (TC) <5 mmol/litre in healthy people, <4 in high risk patients;
- low density lipoprotein (LDL) <3 mmol/litre in healthy people, <2 in high risk patients.

(NHS Choices, accessed 2014)

Statins cannot be used with liver failure, so liver function should be monitored. Other significant side effects of statins include

- gastrointestinal (pain, nausea/vomiting, flatulence, diarrhoea, constipation)
- headache
- muscle damage.

(Ford, 2013)

Depending on symptoms experienced by patients, various other cardiac (and non-cardiac) drugs may be needed. Atrial fibrillation and angina frequently co-exist and need treating. Statins are potentiated by amiodarone and some other drugs (Hilmer and Gnjidic, 2013), so pharmacy advice should be sought with concurrent medication.

Atrial fibrillation

New atrial fibrillation should be reversed (rhythm control), but atrial fibrillation from heart failure is often chronic; what cannot be cured should be controlled:

- rate control <110 bpm
- anticoagulation (INR 2.5, to reduce stroke risk).

Atrial fibrillation, together with therapeutic drugs, is discussed in Chapter 14.

Non-pharmacological treatment

In addition to drugs, helping people with chronic heart failure largely focuses on symptom relief. Although care will vary between patients, likely aspects of nursing care include

- close monitoring of vital signs, fluid balance and daily weight
- oxygen therapy
- rest
- fluid management
- salt restriction (limiting hypervolaemia)
- health promotion.

British Thoracic Society (BTS, 2008) guidelines recommend oxygen therapy to achieve target saturations of 94–98% provided hypercapnic respiratory failure is not also present; if the person also has COPD target saturation should be 88–92% until an arterial blood gas has been obtained.

Changes in volume of body water are indicated by changes in daily weight. Daily weight increase are almost always an indication for medical review of drug therapy. Fluid management often necessitates restriction, so fluid balance should be closely monitored.

Health promotion should focus on avoiding risk factors. Advice may vary with the causes of heart failure (see Table 11.1), but lifestyle changes should include:

- weight control
- exercise
- sodium restriction
- potassium enhancement
- moderate alcohol
- diet – increase fruit and vegetables, low-fat dairy, restrict saturated fats.

(Chobanian, 2009)

With alcohol-related dilated cardiomyopathy, stopping drinking, nutritious diet and vitamin B supplements can reverse the myopathy (Adam *et al.*, 2008). Most acute hospitals offer management programmes for people with heart failure. While heart failure limits lifestyle, rest should be carefully planned to include gently increasing activity and exercise, based on advice from physiotherapists and/or specialist cardiac nurses.

Prognosis

Chronic heart failure is a progressive disease, with high mortality (NICE, 2010b). Five per cent of people with heart failure have end-stage disease (Adler *et al.*, 2009). With end-stage disease, palliative care/referral should be initiated (Adler *et al.*, 2009).

Even before its end-stage, heart failure typically causes progressive limitations to activities of living which are physically, socially and mentally disabling. More than one fifth of people with heart failure suffer from depression (Rutledge *et al.*, 2006). Although precise prognosis for each patient may not be fully predictable, nurses can offer useful advice to help people with heart failure limit their problems, and limit the progression of the disease. People admitted to acute hospitals with established chronic heart failure usually have an eventually terminal disease, so although acute problems can often be treated, the team (including the patient) should discuss appropriateness of interventions in the light of likely prognosis. Possible considerations include

- what the patient's wishes are
- whether the patient has made a living will
- what should be ceiling treatment
- whether a *do not attempt cardiopulmonary resuscitation* order should be instigated, and if so how long it should remain in effect.

People with heart failure often have a poor understanding of their condition, and need both specialist information and psychosocial support (Aldred *et al.*, 2005), such as counselling. If active treatment is appropriate, patients should be aware of their long-term prognosis so they can plan for their future – some patients may wish to make a 'living will' to limit potentially futile treatment in the future.

Implications for practice

- Chronic heart failure is a progressive syndrome.
- Acute admission may be caused by acute or decompensated heart failure.
- Vital signs and daily weight are important for monitoring acute episodes.
- Heart failure needs pharmacological management; key groups of drugs are beta-blockers, ACE inhibitors, thiazide diuretics, angiotensin receptor blockers, and calcium antagonists (Task Force, 2011).
- Long-term follow-up and management in the community will be necessary after discharge.
- Lifestyle changes (exercise, diet) can significantly slow progression, so health promotion should be emphasised.

Summary

Chronic heart failure is a common, complex and progressive syndrome. It exerts a high human cost on its victims, and is the leading cause of hospital admission in older people (NICE, 2014a). Not surprisingly, heart failure is therefore a major health target for politicians. However, the insidious nature of the disease means that most initiatives will take many years to show any benefits, and the effects of political changes on many unhealthy aspects of UK lifestyle are often questionable. Heart failure is therefore likely to remain a burden to individuals, healthcare and society for some years.

Further reading

Task Force (2013) and NICE (2010b; 2014a) provide authoritative guidance, while Townsend *et al.* (2012) provide much raw data, with useful comments. Taylor *et al.* (2011) review statins. Elliott *et al.* (2008) provide useful descriptions of cardiomyopathies.

Clinical scenario

Alan Burnside, aged 78, is admitted via his GP for investigations for suspected heart failure. Increasing breathlessness has limited his mobility, and he now seldom leaves his house. His wife is his main carer.

Vital signs on arrival are:

blood pressure 168/98 mmHg
pulse 115 bpm
respiratory rate 36 bpm
temperature 37.6°C

He has experienced difficulty in passing urine, and is currently unable to supply a sample for testing. His ECG reveals atrial fibrillation.

1 Using NEWS/ViEWS, calculate Mr Burnside's score. Identify actions required by the score. Is there any additional information you need before proceeding?
2 List further investigations which you, as Mr Burnside's nurse, are likely to initiate within the first 24 hours of his admission to an acute hospital.
3 Completing his admission paperwork, you also begin preparing his discharge planning. From what you know so far, what aspects are likely to need attention for discharge? Identify relevant aspects of care.

Chapter 12

Acute coronary syndromes and recovery from acute heart failure

Contents

Fundamental knowledge

- Cardiac anatomy and myocyte physiology

Introduction

Myocardial infarction (MI, or AMI – acute myocardial infarction) is heart muscle necrosis caused by ischaemia, identified through clinical features, such as

- ECG
- elevated biomarkers, such as troponin
- imaging
- pathology.

(Thygesen *et al.*, 2012)

Worldwide, it is a major cause of mortality and morbidity. Over half of deaths occur within 1 hour of symptoms (Power, 2014), such as angina, so rapid identification and treatment are vital.

If there are any cardiac concerns, an ECG should be recorded. This may show clear evidence of myocardial infarction, such as ST segment elevation or a new left bundle branch block (see Chapter 14). This is classified as a

- STEMI (ST elevation myocardial infarction).

In the absence of clear diagnosis from an ECG, biomarkers such as troponin should be measured. If positive, this indicates infarction:

- NSTEMI (Non ST elevation myocardial infarction).

If negative, the patient should be treated as having

- unstable angina (see below)

until this can be excluded. These are the three acute coronary syndromes (ACS) – see Table 12.1.

Table 12.1 The Acute Coronary Syndromes (ACS)

- STEMI
- NSTEMI
- Unstable angina

Myocardial infarction is classified into five types (see Table 12.2).

Table 12.2 Types of myocardial infarction (Thygesen et al., 2012)

1: Spontaneous
2: Secondary to ischaemic imbalance
3: Cardiac death due to myocardial infarction
4+5: Caused by revascularisation procedures

Angina

Type 2 myocardial infarction is usually preceded by angina. During the relatively early stages of atherosclerosis, plaque has a thin fibrous cap which can easily rupture, causing cholesterol to escape and a thrombus to form. In coronary arteries, this is called *unstable angina* (Ford, 2013) as it is likely to cause occlusion and myocardial infarction. With time, the cap becomes more fibrous and less likely to rupture (*stable angina*).

Chest pain may be cardiac or non-cardiac in origin. Even if it is cardiac, there are many cardiac causes other than angina/myocardial infarction (Jowett and Thompson, 2007). However because of the high risk of imminent death if chest pain is caused by angina, any chest pain should be presumed to be cardiac until proven otherwise.

The pain of angina is caused by myocardial ischaemia. If ischaemia is reversed, the myocardium recovers; if not reversed, ischaemia is likely to progress to infarction. In an attempt to reverse ischaemia, myocardium triggers a compensatory tachycardia which, as identified in Chapter 10, is usually effective up to about 130 bpm. But progressive ischaemia triggers faster rates, which both increase oxygen demand and reduce supply.

Infarction

Most infarctions are caused by plaque (Kalanuria *et al.*, 2012) – coronary artery disease (CAD), atherosclerosis of the coronary arteries. Infarction can also be caused by coronary artery spasm.

Like most cells, myocytes normally store adenosine triphosphate (ATP – cell energy – see Chapter 1), so can survive a period of ischaemia. Myocytes can usually survive up to 20–40 minutes before extensive irreversible damage occurs (Burke and Virmani, 2007). However, absence of bloodflow to the brain necessitates immediate cardiopulmonary resuscitation.

When infarction occurs, there is a central zone of damage with little or no flow; any dead tissue in this area is permanently lost. But around this central zone is a marginal zone where there is some viable tissue (Burke and Virmani, 2007). This zone may either be successfully reperfused, or infarct. Reperfusion of any tissue causes potentially toxic chemicals, such as cytokines and oxygen radicals, which have accumulated in the ischaemic area to be flushed into the circulation. Although potentially occurring after reperfusion of any tissue, they are especially problematic following myocardial infarction, as they can cause 'myocardial stunning', resulting in ventricular tachycardia and other dysrhythmias (Gretch *et al.*, 1995). Reperfusion injury can cause up to half of the final infarct size (Yellon and Hausenloy, 2007).

Early perfusion reduces reperfusion injury. Giving nitrates, typically glyceryl trinitrate (GTN) reduces reperfusion injury (Dezfulian *et al.*, 2009) by stimulating production of nitric oxide, the endogenous vasodilator released from vascular endothelium (Sahin *et al.*, 2012). In the context of infarction, GTN is usually infused intravenously, but with angina sublingual GTN may relieve pain by restoring perfusion.

Cardiac biomarkers

Cell damage causes release of intracellular enzymes, and sometimes other chemicals, into the blood. Therefore detecting abnormally high levels of enzymes from a specific type of cell suggests extensive damage to tissue, although as with any result there can always be false positives and false negatives. Many cardiac biomarkers have been marketed, but troponin (I or T) remains the recommended test (Task Force, 2011), and the one almost invariably used. There is no standard range for troponin, as methods of measurements differ (Pathology Harmony, 2011), although anecdotally many laboratories seem to accept 50 ng/litre. Troponin levels generally correlate with extent of damage (higher level = more damage).

There can be a delay between infarction and significant serum levels occurring, so if negative levels should be retested; NICE (2010c) recommend 10–12 hours after symptoms, but assays being now more sensitive, Thygesen *et al.* (2012) recommend 3–6 hours later. More than one third of troponin positive results are false (Blich *et al.*, 2008), caused by problems such as

- renal dysfunction
- cardiac strain from lung disease
- cardiomyopathy and other cardiac disease.

(Task Force, 2011)

Troponin binds to protein, so may remain elevated for up to two weeks following infarction (Task Force, 2011).

Creatine kinase (CK) is less cardiac-specific than troponin, being also released by brain and skeletal muscle tissue. Normal levels are 40–320 (male) and 25–200 (female) units/litre (Pathology Harmony, 2011). Unlike troponin, CK returns to baseline in 2–3 days (Lough, 2008). CK is often used to assess muscle injury, especially if there are concerns about rhabdomyolysis, but may be useful to distinguish between recent (last 2 days) and less recent (last 2 weeks) infarcts.

Inpatient treatments

STEMI is usually caused by complete coronary artery occlusion (Task Force, 2011), so after initial resuscitation is ideally treated with primary percutaneous coronary intervention (pPCI), to restore flow through occluded coronary arteries (DOH, 2008a; Task Force, 2010a; McLenachen *et al.*, 2010). If pPCI facilities are not available or practical, thrombolysis or open heart surgery may be used. pPCI revascularisation is achieved with dilation using cardiac catheterisation, almost invariably inserting a drug-eluding stent (DES) to maintain patency.

NSTEMI and unstable angina are usually treated conservatively – supporting failing systems with possible later percutaneous or other coronary interventions. Both may warrant transfer to a Coronary Care Unit.

Many therapeutic drugs are likely to be used, including many discussed in Chapter 11, and

- clopidogrel (anti-platelet) (Chua and Ignaszewski, 2009)
- aspirin 75–150 mg daily (NICE, 2010c).

This chapter has focused on pathophysiology, but nursing patients who have suffered myocardial infarction should provide holistic care, including

- meeting activities of living that patients are unable to perform themselves;
- ensuring effective pain relief (opioids are often needed);
- monitoring for complications and effectiveness of medical treatments;
- psychological support for patients and their families.

Therapeutic hypothermia

Early therapeutic hypothermia has recently been promoted to limit initial injury (NICE, 2011b), especially for out-of-hospital arrests (Nunnally *et al.*, 2011), but recent evidence (Nielsen *et al.*, 2013) found no benefit from this practice.

Prognosis

Most patients will experience some complications following myocardial infarction, such as

- cardiogenic shock, in 7% (Cook and Windecker, 2008);
- early death, within 30 days (50%) (Ratcliffe and Pepper, 2008));
- depression (Ellis *et al.*, 2005; Lichtman *et al.*, 2014).

Survivors often have residual

- left ventricular failure
- other morbidities, including psychological.

As any complications can occur at any time, patients should be observed and monitored closely until discharge. During rehabilitation, nurses have an important role in promoting health education (see Chapter 11). As with many other conditions, morbidity and mortality are increased if patients with acute coronary syndromes suffer depression (Davidson *et al.*, 2010; Lichtman *et al.*, 2014), so psychological care improves physiological outcome.

Implications for practice

- Cardiac chest pain needs rapid treatment, so presume chest pain is cardiac until proven otherwise (take ECG and, unless a clear STEMI, send Troponin).
- Nitrates dilate coronary arteries, so glyceryl trinitrate (often given sublingually) may relieve angina.
- Most patients experience some complications following infarction; these can occur at any time during hospitalisation, so patients should be observed and monitored closely.
- Recovery on ward should include health promotion, such as advice on lifestyle and diet.

Summary

Coronary heart disease is the single main cause of death in the UK (Townsend *et al.*, 2012). If symptoms, such as angina, occur, myocardial infarction is likely to follow quickly. Angina should therefore be relieved if possible with nitrates. Any chest pain should be suspected as being cardiac in origin until proven otherwise, so an ECG should be recorded, and unless this clearly identifies a STEMI, serum troponin should be tested.

If the patient has had a STEMI, they should be transferred for pPCI, or other appropriate treatments. A NSTEMI or unstable angina will be treated initially with medicines, although may warrant percutaneous interventions later.

On rehabilitation to general wards, nursing care has an important role in supporting the patient's recovery (activities of living, pain relief, health promotion, psychological care) and monitoring for complications.

Useful website

European Society of Cardiology

Further reading

Readers should be familiar with local guidelines for the acute coronary syndromes. European Society of Cardiology guidelines, especially Thygesen *et al.* (2012), provide authoritative resources. UK resuscitations guidelines are scheduled for 2015, shortly after publication of this book. Readers should be familiar with current guidelines.

Clinical scenario

James Ellis, a 54-year-old company representative, was admitted to A&E with central chest pain five days ago. An ECG showed clear ST elevation, so he was treated successfully with a primary percutaneous coronary intervention. He is now in recovery, and transferred to the ward where you are working. His next-of-kin is his wife; he has two adult children who live about 200 miles away.

1   Find the acute coronary syndrome guidelines for your hospital, and list recommended treatments for Mr Ellis.
2   List the main complications Mr Ellis might experience during hospitalisation, and what you would do to prevent/identify these.
3   Identify aspects of health promotion advice you would offer Mr Ellis and his family.

Chapter 13

Shock

Contents

Fundamental knowledge

■ Cardiac anatomy, including pericardium
■ Ejection fraction (see Chapter 10)

Introduction

Shock is a life-threatening medical emergency. The Intensive Care Society (ICS, 2002) define shock as systolic blood pressure below 80 mmHg sustained for more than one hour. If pressure is insufficient to perfuse tissues, cell hypoxia leads to cell failure, necrosis (see Chapter 12) and organ failure. Early recognition and treatment of shock therefore reduces mortality and morbidity. Nurses may be the first staff to recognise shock, through observation of patients and vital signs, so should know how to manage crises as first responders.

Chapter 10 defined normotension as matching blood vessel volume with blood vessel capacity. Shock is therefore a mismatch between the two. So treating shock needs to

- increase (arterial) blood volume
- reduce blood vessel capacity (vasoconstrict)
- or both.

In most clinical areas, vasoconstriction is impractical. Increasing arterial volume necessitates either volume replacement or improving cardiac throughput, depending on the type of shock.

Shock causes cell hypoxia (Hinds and Watson, 2008), so 'first aid' treatment for shock is giving oxygen. Intravenous fluid resuscitation may also be needed to ensure oxygen is delivered to cells. Apart from blood pressure and (often) compensatory tachycardia, most early symptoms of shock are non-specific. Patients are often breathless, peripherally pale and cold, oliguric, and hypoxic. However, compensatory mechanisms may mask or delay some of these signs. After initial hypotension, compensatory vasoconstriction and tachycardia may restore blood pressure. But vasoconstriction is mediated by the neuroendocrine 'stress' response (see Chapter 2), which cannot be sustained for prolonged periods. As hypotension returns, tachycardia induced by myocardial hypoxia (see Chapter 10) accelerates, typically to counter-productive rates. Blood pressure progressively falls, peripheral shutdown increases; once perfusion fails to main organs, the refractory, or irreversible, stage of shock leads inevitably to death.

Sturgess (2014) identifies four types of shock:

- hypovolaemic: inadequate preload
- cardiogenic: pump failure
- obstructive: obstructed bloodflow
- distributive/vasodilatory ('low resistance'): peripheral (capillary) dilatation.

Before discussing each type, some common features of and approaches to all types are outlined. Pathophysiology of shock begins at cell level, and can be challenging to understand, so a clinical scenario 'snapshot' is included for each type. Where these snapshots remind you of patients whom you have nursed, reflect on their care, and recall how their shock was treated.

Initial management is likely to be supervised by medical staff, but on-going management is often devolved to nurses: monitoring and observations are important to identify whether prescribed treatments are effective, or whether further medical assistance needs to be sought. Nursing observations of vital signs are likely to be needed frequently, often at least hourly. Key medical treatments specific to each type of shock are identified, but individual patients may also need support for individual problems, with psychological support and nursing care for activities of living they are unable to perform for themselves.

1: HYPOVOLAEMIC

Hypovolaemic shock is caused by loss of circulating volume. Causes may be obvious, such as through massive bleeding. Bleeding is the leading cause of death with trauma

(Alam and Rhee, 2007). Excessive loss can also occur through urine, such as with diabetic ketoacidosis (see Chapter 27). Some patients are admitted with severe dehydration, for which causes often need to be investigated.

Snapshot

Frank Stanfield, aged 82, has elective total hip replacement surgery. He has heart failure, chronic hypertension, and permanent atrial fibrillation, for which he is warfarinised. Perioperative blood loss is large, 3 litres being returned via a cell-saver. Additional loss is not replaced due to concerns about overload with heart failure. Post-operatively he is hypotensive, tachycardic and oliguric.

Immediate treatment will be

- fluid resuscitation
- stopping the source of volume loss, if possible
- supporting failing systems.

With effective compensatory mechanisms for hypotension (see Chapter 10), people may survive rapid loss of up to two fifths of their blood volume; if compensatory mechanisms are poor, which is likely in many hospitalised patients, losing a fifth or less of blood volume may be fatal (Hall, 2011). Strickler (2010) suggests that irreversible shock often occurs once one quarter of blood volume is lost. Major haemorrhage can be stabilised with tranexamic acid (TXA) (Roberts *et al.*, 2011).

2: CARDIOGENIC SHOCK

Cardiogenic shock is caused by failure of the heart to pump an adequate volume of blood into the aorta. Five to 10% of survivors of myocardial infarction suffer cardiogenic shock (Unverzagt *et al.*, 2014). Although myocardial infarction is the most common cause, it can also be caused by mitral regurgitation and congenital cardiac defects (Smith and Bigham, 2013). Cardiogenic shock has mortality rates of 50–70% (Cook and Windecker, 2008), and is the commonest cause of post-myocardial infarction death (White, 2002).

Snapshot

Charles Ellis, aged 68, is admitted to A&E with inferior myocardial infarction. He has been successfully resuscitated by paramedics, but on arrival in the department is hypotensive (BP 73/58 mmHg), tachycardic (138 bpm) and breathless (32 bpm). Cardiogenic shock is diagnosed. He is transferred to CCU for dobutamine infusion and possible intra-aortic balloon pump.

Cardiogenic shock occurs when more than two fifths of the left ventricle is damaged (Von Rueden *et al.*, 2013). Damage may be from dead, ischaemic or oedematous muscle. Left ventricular failure (low stroke volume and ejection fraction) cause congestive cardiac failure, pulmonary oedema, and therefore impaired oxygenation. Venous overload causes raised jugular venous pressure. Typically, attempted compensatory tachycardia increases myocardial oxygen demand at the same time as oxygen supply is reduced, making a second infarction likely. At least 40% of left ventricular myocardium already being non-functional, further damage usually results in insufficient functional left ventricular myocardium, and rapid death (Hinds and Watson, 2008).

With its progressively worsening pathology and high mortality, cardiogenic shock is challenging to treat. Treating heart failure (overload – see Chapter 12) may reduce myocardial oxygen demand, but inotropes (beta agonists, such as dobutamine) are usually needed to improve cardiac output and myocardial oxygenation. These however also increase myocardial workload. An intra-aortic balloon pump may be needed to augment myocardial oxygenation, although mortality benefits are unproven (Thiele *et al.*, 2012). Neither of these therapies is usually available outside coronary care units or other specialised areas, so patients usually need urgent transfer to appropriate departments; both therapies are discussed further in *Intensive Care Nursing.*

Ejection fraction and other aspects indicating prognosis can be measured with echocardiography. Residual myocardial damage usually leaves survivors with poor quality of life, so given the high mortality, palliative care may often be the kindest option available.

3: OBSTRUCTIVE

Obstructive shock occurs when there is an obstruction to bloodflow between the vena cava and the aorta. This can occur with positive pressure ventilation, including non-invasive (see Chapter 9). It is more likely to be caused by cardiac tamponade.

Like lungs, the heart is surrounded by two tough, fibrous layers, called pericardia. Between them is a small film of fluid, usually 10–20 ml. Bleeding, typically from the highly vascular myocardium, into this space compresses ventricular filling, so reducing cardiac output.

Tamponade can be traumatic or spontaneous. Traumatic tamponade is caused by injury to the pericardium, typically from stabbing, rib fractures or thoracic surgery. It usually occurs quickly, and so is rapidly life-threatening, but as the cause is often obvious, treatment is likely to be quickly available. Spontaneous tamponade usually occurs if the pericardium if friable, typically from pericarditis. It may be less immediately obvious, but is also likely to develop less quickly.

Snapshot

Frances Evans, aged 56, is admitted to A&E following a road traffic accident. Chest X-ray confirms multiple rib fractures. She is hypotensive and breathless, has a raised JVP, and her CXR shows a large heart shadow. Ultrasound confirms a pericardial effusion.

Other than the mostly non-specific signs of shock, together with risk factors, the earliest signs are often identified through medical examination: raised jugular venous pressure, rising significantly on inspiration, together with muffled heart sounds. Pericardial distension causes a large heart shadow on chest X-rays, often triangular in shape. Diagnosis is typically confirmed with echocardiography.

Treatment is through needle aspiration, under ultrasound or radiographic guidance. The needle should remain in place to remove any further accumulation until drainage is less than 50 ml/day (Spodick, 2003).

4: DISTRIBUTIVE

This most diverse and potentially complex group of pathologies is caused by maldistribution of blood into peripheral circulation (capillaries). Normally, one quarter of capillaries are open at any time (Deroy, 2000), with only 5% of total blood volume in capillaries (Barrett *et al.*, 2010). Excessive arteriole vasodilatation significantly increases capillary blood volume, causing arterial hypotension. This significantly reduces diastolic blood pressure, often to pressures such as 40 mmHg.

Many pathologies can cause distributive shock. The most common causes, and those discussed here, are

- anaphylaxis (chemical)
- spinal
- sepsis/systemic inflammatory response syndrome.

Anaphylaxis

This is caused by excessive defensive responses. Antibodies (lymphocytes: T cells, B cells – see Chapter 3) recognise an antigen, such as a therapeutic drug, and initiate an antigen-antibody inflammatory response. Many pro-inflammatory vasoactive mediators are released; most significantly, mast cells and basophils release histamine (Owen *et al.*, 2013), which triples capillary flow (Deroy, 2000), and also causes bronchoconstriction (Finney and Rushton, 2007). Incidence of anaphylaxis is increasing (Resuscitation Council, 2008; Gibbison *et al.*, 2012)

Initial management is to call for help, stop any suspected antigen and give oxygen (Simons *et al.*, 2011). The first-line drug for anaphylaxis is adrenaline (Simmons *et al.*, 2011; Zilberstein *et al.*, 2014). Traditionally, antihistamines (chlorphenamine – Piriton™) and steroids (hydrocortisone) have also been given, although these should be considered second line drugs (Zilberstein *et al.*, 2014) as their efficacy is unproven (Simons *et al.*, 2011). Fluid resuscitation may also be needed, as a third of blood volume may extravase within ten minutes (Zilberstein *et al.*, 2014).

Spinal

Spinal cord injury can damage the pathway for sympathetic nervous system signalling (Hoffman and Hausman, 2013). Paradoxically, the parasympathetic nervous system (vagus nerve) often escapes unscathed. The often uncountered bradycardia and vasodilatation causes profound hypotension within hours of injury (Hoffman and Hausman, 2013), which is often unresponsive to inotropes, such as adrenaline. Spinal shock occurs more often with higher spinal cord injury: cervical injury incidence 19%, thoracic injury incidence 7%, lumbar injury incidence 3% (Guly et al., 2008). Spinal shock can occur within hours of injury (Hoffman and Hausman, 2013).

Initial treatment is aggressive fluid therapy, to fill the dilated space. Outcome from spinal injury is optimised if patients are transferred to spinal injury units.

Sepsis and systemic inflammatory response syndrome

Sepsis is a systemic response to infection in the bloodstream (Dellinger et al., 2013). A medical emergency (Czura, 2011), sepsis is often described as a continuum:

- sepsis
- systemic inflammatory response syndrome (SIRS – described below)
- severe sepsis (sepsis with organ failure)
- septic shock (sepsis with shock).

Systemic inflammatory response syndrome is an inflammatory response occurring throughout the cardiovascular system. The body's own inflammatory response causes vasoactive chemicals to be released, resulting in systemic vasodilatation, capillary leak, and disruption of haemostatic mechanism regulated by vascular endothelium, including clotting. While severe sepsis typically causes SIRS, the majority of cases of SIRS are from non-septic causes (Horeczko et al., 2014), such as from severe (sterile) pancreatitis and major burns.

Snapshot

Janet Thompson, aged 49, had chemotherapy one week ago, and is now leucopenic. On arrival in hospital she is pyrexial, tachycardic, hypotensive, agitated, oliguric.

Mortality and morbidity from sepsis is high: sepsis causes one in seven hospital deaths (All-Party Parliamentary Group on Sepsis, 2014). Early recognition and treatment saves lives (Parliamentary and Health Service Ombudsman, 2013), but sepsis is a complex condition that is often difficult to understand, recognise and treat. The source of sepsis may be almost anywhere in the body; the micro-organism responsible may be bacterial, viral, parasitic, or fungal; presentation and progression can differ significantly between different patients, and because symptoms are non-specific (Capuzzo et al., 2012), sepsis may be misdiagnosed as some other condition.

Following the first international guidelines for severe sepsis (Dellinger et al., 2004) the Surviving Sepsis Organisation (2007) introduced a sepsis screening tool triggered by the Signs and Symptoms of Infection (SSI – see Table 13.1) and the 'Sepsis Six' first hour care bundle (see Table 13.2). There was also a six hour 'resuscitation' bundle with ICU-focused care.

Table 13.1 Signs and symptoms of infection

Are any two of the following present and new to the patient?

- temperature >38.3 or <36 °C
- heart rate >90 beats per minute
- respiratory rate >20 breaths per minute
- white cells <4 or >12 × 10^9/litre
- acutely altered mental state
- hypoglycaemia (>6.6 mmol/litre) unless diabetic

(Surviving Sepsis Organisation, 2007)

Table 13.2 'Sepsis Six' first hour care bundle

- oxygen
- blood cultures
- antibiotics
- fluids
- lactate and haemoglobin
- urinary catheter and hourly output monitoring

(Surviving Sepsis Organisation, 2007)

In place of the SSI, the third international guidelines (Dellinger *et al.*, 2013) list seven generable variables, five inflammatory variables, one haemodynamic variable, seven organ dysfunction variables, and two tissue perfusion variables. The one and six hour bundles were replaced by three and six hour care bundles (see Table 13.3). Downloadable from the Surviving Sepsis website (www.survivingsepsis.org; www.survivingsepsis.org/SiteCollectionDocuments/Implement-Bundle-Card.pdf).

Table 13.3 Three and six hour severe sepsis care bundles (Dellinger *et al.*, 2013)

3 hour bundle:
- measure lactate
- obtain blood cultures before giving antibiotics*
- broad spectrum antibiotics*
- 30 ml/kg crystalloid for hypotension or if lactate >4 mmol/litre

6 hour bundle:
- vasopressors (if hypotension does not respond to initial fluid resuscitation) to maintain MAP ≥65 mmHg
- if persistent arterial hypotension despite initial fluid resuscitation or initial lactate >4 mmol/litre, measure CVP (aim ≥ 8 mmHg) and SvO_2 (aim ≥70%)
- remeasure lactate if initial measure was elevated

*elsewhere the 2013 Guidelines set maximum target times of 45 minutes for taking blood cultures and one hour for giving antibiotics.

The signs and symptoms of infections and the actions of 'Sepsis Six' are included in the 2013 guidelines, but with very many other variables. Although promoted nationally (Parliamentary and Health Service Ombudsman, 2013; All-Party Parliamentary Group on Sepsis, 2014), using the Sepsis Six is difficult to reconcile with the 2013 guidelines.

Treating distributive shock

Like other types of shock, distributive shock is likely to cause cell hypoxia, necessitating oxygen; hypovolaemia from vasodilatation often necessitates aggressive fluid resuscitation. Reversible causes should be remedied, so sepsis necessitates blood cultures (within 45 minutes) and antibiotics (within 1 hour; most Trusts have local protocols for recommended antibiotics).

NICE (2012a) has issued guidance for neutropenic sepsis. Management for neutropenic sepsis is similar to that for sepsis from other causes, although deterioration is often more rapid. Protective isolation is usually necessary.

As with all types of shock, nurses have a central role in both giving prescribed treatments and monitoring their effects. Ineffective treatment, or any deterioration, should be urgently reported to medical staff.

Implications for practice

- Shock is sustained hypotension, and so causes perfusion failure to all organs.
- Unreversed shock is likely to lead to organ failure; shock is therefore a medical emergency.
- Treatment should focus on microcirculatory resuscitation – delivering oxygen to cells.
- For hypovolaemic and septic shock this necessitates intravenous fluids, but with cardiogenic and obstructive shock, fluid input will usually be restricted.
- Readers should be familiar with local policies for managing shock.

Summary

Shock is a life-threatening medical emergency, which if unreversed causes cell hypoxia, failure and death. First aid for shock is therefore to give oxygen. Depending on the cause (type) of shock, it may need volume resuscitation or improvement of cardiac throughput. Nurses have a key role in recognising shock, acting as first responders, administering prescribed treatments, and monitoring their effectiveness.

Useful websites

European Society of Cardiology
Surviving sepsis (*www.survivingsepsis.org/Pages/default.aspx*)

Further reading

Readers should be aware of local (Trust, Network) guidelines for managing various types of shock; nationally and internationally, there are sometimes guidelines for specific aspects of medical therapy, but there is a surprising lack of current guidelines for most types of shock. The Resuscitation Council (UK) has published guidelines for anaphylaxis (update scheduled 2016). Calls at congress (2012, 2013) of the European Society for Cardiology for guidelines on cardiogenic shock have so far not led to publication. British Committee Standards for Haematology 2006 guidelines for massive blood loss do not appear on their website, and do not seem to have been replaced. Some further reading relevant to these topics is included in Chapters 12 and 25.

Key documents on sepsis are Nice (2012a), Dellinger *et al.* (2013) and Parliamentary and Health Service Ombudsman (2013).

Clinical scenario

Mrs Geraldine Evans, aged 74, was admitted for investigations into her heart failure. She has a past medical history of hypertension (established) atrial fibrillation and mild renal impairment. On day 3 she becomes more breathless, feels 'terrible', and looks ashen. Her vital signs are now

RR	34 bpm
HR	142 bpm (irregular)
BP	84/52 (MAP 63) mmHg
T	34.4°C

With the aid of diuretics, urine output had previously been satisfactory, but she is now anuric.

1   What type of shock would you suspect from this information? List your initial concerns and actions.
2   Using A-B-C-D-E assessment, identify medical treatments and investigations that are likely to be needed to reverse the shock?
3   You are working with a year 3 student nurse. Write a few paragraphs summarising what you think has happened in the way you might explain events to the student.

Chapter 14

Interpreting cardiac rhythms

Contents

Fundamental knowledge

- Cardiac anatomy (including coronary arteries)
- Basic electrophysiology, including normal conduction pathways (SA node, AV node, bundle of His, branch bundle, Purkinje fibres)

Introduction

This chapter commences by revising normal cardiac conduction, and how this is represented on electrocardiograms (ECGs). A framework for interpreting rhythms is offered. The more common dysrhythmias are discussed

- atrial fibrillation
- atrial flutter
- atrioventricular node blocks
- bundle branch block
- ventricular tachycardia
- ventricular fibrillation
- systole
- pulseless electrical activity

and likely treatments suggested. Ectopics (atrial, junctional and ventricular) are included.

Acutely ill patients may have chronic dysrhythmias, or develop acute dysrhythmias in response to disease or treatments. For example, about 7% of general surgical patients develop new dysrhythmias post-operatively (Walsh *et al.*, 2007). Level 2 patients may need continuous bedside monitoring or 12 lead electrocardiograms (ECGs). If monitoring or recording ECGs, nurses should be able to recognise common dysrhythmias, and know what, if any, treatments are likely to benefit their patients to enable earlier and optimal intervention. Monitoring, without staff able to interpret monitoring, induces a dangerously false sense of security. This chapter therefore provides a framework for ECG interpretation, describes common dysrhythmias, and key interventions/treatments. Drugs listed are those commonly used; other drugs may also be effective. Like any skill, ECG interpretation needs repeated practice. The appendix lists some commonly used drugs to treat dysrhythmias. The chapter begins with 'basics'; if these are unfamiliar, further descriptions can be found in texts such as Hampton (2013a).

The graph

When no electrical activity is recorded, the graph is horizontal (isoelectric). An upward line from the isoelectric line is a *positive deflection*, while a line downward is a *negative deflection*. ECGs represent three-dimensional electrical activity of cardiac conduction on a two dimensional graph.

With standard settings

- height represents voltage: 1 cm = 1 millivolt (2 large squares, or 10 small squares);
- length represents time: 1 small square = 0.04 seconds, 1 large square = 0.2 seconds.

Figure 14.1 shows a normal sinus rhythm complex.

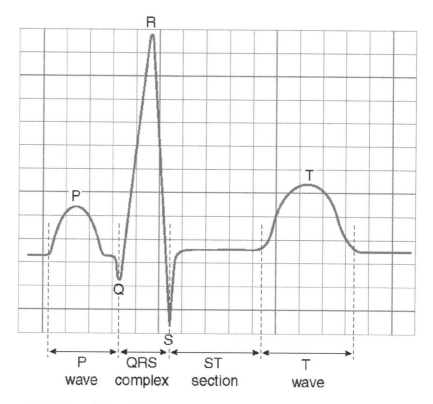

Figure 14.1 **Normal sinus rhythm**

Cardiac muscle contraction follows electrical activity, except with pulseless electrical activity (PEA). With PEA, whatever rhythm is displayed does not produce a pulse.

Electrodes

The six limb leads use three electrodes:

- right arm (red)
- left arm (yellow)
- left leg/hip (green).

Positions can be memorised as 'traffic lights'. These three electrodes produce the six limbs leads ('views'):

- I right arm to left arm
- II right arm to left leg
- III left arm to left leg
- aVR: right arm
- aVL: left arm
- aVF: left leg (**F**oot).

12-lead ECGs and 5-electrode monitors use a fourth limb electrode on the

- right leg (black)

(see Figure 14.2).
5-electrode limb-lead monitors also use

- 4th intercostal space to right of sternum, modified C1 (white).

The six chest (precordial) leads each use a single electrode (see Figure 14.3):

- C (or V) 1: 4th intercostal space (right of sternum) – red
- C2: 4th intercostal space (left of sternum) – yellow
- C4: 5th intercostal space, mid-clavicular line – brown
- C6: 5th intercostal space mid axilla – purple
- C3: between C2 and C4 – green
- C5: 5th intercostal space between C4 and C6 – black.

With normal (healthy) hearts:

- C1 = right atrium
- C2 = right ventricle
- C3 = sternum or left ventricle
- C4 = left ventricle
- C5 = left ventricle
- C6 = left atrium or ventricle

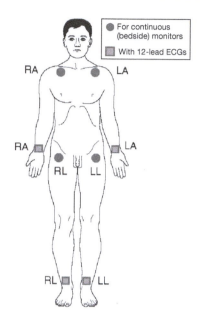

Figure 14.2 Electrode placement – limb leads

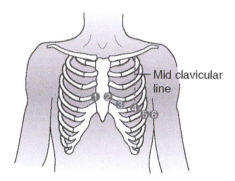

Figure 14.3 Electrode placement – chest leads

So, remembering where leads 'view' the heart, the

- lateral   leads are   I, aVL, C5, C6
- anterior   leads are   C1, C2, C3, C4
- inferior   leads are   II, III, aVF.

Reading ECGs

ECGs contain much information in a small graph, so are best deciphered in logical stages, using a framework such as Table 14.1.

Table 14.1 Framework for reading ECGs

Reading the ECG:

Regularity:
Is the rate regular?
If not, is the rate:
    regularly irregular (is there a pattern?)
    irregularly irregular (no pattern)?

1: P wave:
Does the P wave appear before the QRS?
Is there one P wave before every QRS?
Is the shape normal?
Are P waves missing? (check for pacing spikes)

2: PR interval:
Is the PR interval 3–5 small squares?

3: QRS complex:
Is the QRS width within 3 small squares?
Is the QRS positive or negative?
Is the axis normal?
Does it look normal?

4: ST segment:
Does the isoelectric line return between the S and the T?
If not, is it:
    elevated (>1 mm above isoelectric line)
    depressed (<0.5 mm below isoelectric line)?

5: T wave:
Does the T wave look normal?

6. QT interval
Is the QT interval <1/2 preceding R-R interval?
Is QTc within 0.4 seconds (2 large squares)?

Tachycardia (>100 bpm):
narrow complex (usually with P waves) = atrial (supraventricular)
broad complex (without P wave) = ventricular

When analysing 12-lead ECGs, start with one lead, usually the 'rhythm strip' – a single lead usually running the whole printout length, usually II or C1.

Begin by looking at regularity of rhythms. Using scrap paper, mark two R waves (peaks), then move the paper to see if all R-R intervals are the same. If they are, the rhythm is

■   regular.

Regular rhythms can be pathological (e.g. ventricular tachycardia). If the rhythm is irregular, is it

- regularly irregular (is there a pattern?)
- irregularly irregular (no pattern)?

P wave

This represents atrial depolarisation.

- Is there a P wave?

It should be followed by ventricular depolarisation, so

- Does the P wave appear before the QRS?
- Is there one P wave before every QRS?

Atrial muscle mass is small, so voltage (height) is limited. The shape should however be rounded, above the isoelectric line:

- Is the shape normal?

Abnormal P waves, with normal QRSs, indicate atrial (supraventricular) problems.

PR interval

Atria have no specialised conduction pathway, so impulses are conducted from one muscle fibre to another. This makes conduction across atria relatively slow in proportion to muscle size. Impulses are then normally delayed at the atrioventricular (AV) node. So PR intervals, from the beginning of P wave to the beginning of QRS, should be 3 to 5 small squares (0.12–0.2 seconds):

- Is the PR interval 3–5 small squares?

Prolonged PR intervals, often from atrioventricular node disease, delay conduction (see *First degree block* below).

Q wave

The first negative deflection represents septal depolarisation. Normally, Q waves are either small or absent. Deep (>2 small squares) Q waves indicate myocardial infarction, although not all myocardial infarctions cause deep Q waves. Where deep Q waves do occur, (30-day) mortality is higher (Wong *et al.*, 2006). So although largely useful for retrospective diagnosis, for example in community settings, Wong *et al.* (2006) suggest deep Q waves may be an indication for more aggressive therapy.

QRS complex

From the atrioventricular node, impulses pass down the Bundle of His, which divides into left and right branches, the left bundle further dividing into anterior and posterior hemibranches (or fascicles). From these three branches, impulses spread through Purkinje fibres to ventricular myocytes.

The QRS represents ventricular depolarisation. Although tall (due to the large muscle mass of ventricles), it is narrow (less than three small squares). It should be positive (mainly above the isoelectric line), except in right-sided leads (aVR, C1, C2).

- Is QRS positive or negative?
- Is its width within three small squares?
- Does the QRS look normal?

ST segment

After the QRS, the trace should return rapidly to the isoelectric line.

- Does the isoelectric line return between the S and the T?

Ventricular conduction abnormalities can cause ST segments to be depressed or raised. Elevation, with chest pain, indicates infarction – ST elevation myocardial infarction (STEMI). Depression is often caused by ischaemia, but can have other causes.

If not, is it:

- elevated
- depressed?

T wave

This represents ventricular repolarisation. Slightly asymmetrical, T waves are normally larger than P waves. T wave abnormalities are 'non-specific', but common causes are

- high Ts = high serum potassium
- low Ts = low serum potassium
- inversion = ischaemia.

However, hyperkalaemia does not always cause ECG changes (Montague *et al.*, 2008).

- Does the T wave look normal?

QT interval

From the start of the Q to the end of the T should be less than half the distance between the preceding two R waves. Prolonged QT intervals mean the ventricles are depolarised (electrically active) for an excessive proportion of the cycle, and so risk of ventricular tachycardia and sudden cardiac death is increased (Straus *et al.*, 2006). Most monitors and ECG machines calculate QTc – QT time corrected to what it would have been in heart rate were 60 bpm. Normal QTc is less than 0.4 seconds. A few people are genetically prone to long QT syndrome, but crises can be provoked by drugs (e.g. vancomycin), especially ones containing sodium, so seek pharmacist advice about which drugs are safe to give.

Abnormalities

Abnormal ECGs only need treating if causing, or likely to cause, problems. Frequently seen dysrhythmias are identified below. Acute dysrhythmias may be triggered by myocardial hypoxia; if hypoxic, oxygen should be given. Underlying causes/triggers for dysrhythmias should be resolved if possible; for example, blood chemistry (especially potassium and calcium, both used for cardiac conduction) should be normalised. Optimal serum potassium for cardiac conduction is above 4 mmol/litre, slightly higher than normal physiological levels. Optimal serum total calcium is 2.2–2.6 mmol/litre; NB arterial blood gas analysers usually measure *ionised* calcium (see Chapter 8).

Artefact

Electrocardiographs record any electrical activity detected. All muscle conduction uses electricity, so skeletal muscle activity, such as shivering or tremors, may be detected. External electrical activity, such as electrical equipment, may also be recorded. Artefact usually creates constant interference ('fuzz'). If artefact appears:

- check the filter is switched on
- reposition electrodes of affected leads.

Sinus rhythms

Sinus rhythm means the rhythm originates from the sinoatrial node. A normal rate for sinus rhythm in adults is 60–100 bpm.

Sinus arrhythmia

(See Figure 14.4)
This is where two rates alternate with breathing. Some young, usually athletic, adults normally have sinus arrhythmia. It is rare in hospitalised patients, but may occur with respiratory distress. Sinus arrhythmia should not be treated, although any respiratory distress should.

Sinus bradycardia

This is sinus rhythm below 60 bpm. Very slow (<40) sinus bradycardia is usually caused by a block, so positive chronotropes (e.g. atropine) may be given to increase rate. Underlying causes (e.g. hypothermia) should be resolved.

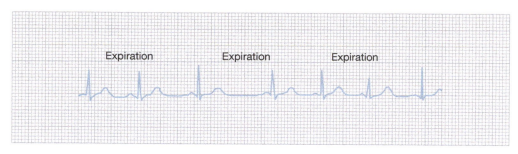

Figure 14.4 Sinus arrhythmia

Sinus tachycardia/supraventricular tachycardia

This is sinus rhythm above 100 bpm. Check the tachycardia is not ventricular:

- narrow (QRS) complex tachycardia = supraventicular
- broad (QRS) complex tachycardias = (potentially) ventricular.

Tachycardias reduce diastolic time, so reducing myocardial oxygenation while increasing myocardial oxygen consumption. Very fast rates (especially >140, usually called *supraventricular tachycardia* – SVT) can be slowed by drugs:

- adenosine (if regular)
- beta-blocker, digoxin or amiodarone (if irregular – see Resuscitation Council Tachycardia algorithm).

Atrial kick

Most bloodflow into ventricles is passive, but atrial contraction preceding ventricular contraction adds active filling, optimising ventricular volume to create a good-volume pulse. Any rhythm lacking atrial ventricular synchrony reduces stroke volume by between 5 and 15% (Task Force, 2010), causing either hypotension or provoking compensatory tachycardia. Most rhythms below lack atrial kick.

Ectopics

These are isolated beats from abnormal pacemakers, making complexes differ from underlying rhythms. They can occur in almost any rhythm. Their origin may be

- atrial
- junctional *or*
- ventricular.

Atrial ectopics have abnormal P waves and possibly different PR intervals, but normal QRS complexes (see Figure 14.5). Junctional impulses usually have no visible P waves, but normal QRS. Ventricular impulses have no P wave, but broad and bizarre QRS complexes. If all ventricular ectopics have the same shape, they are from the same focus ('unifocal'). If shapes vary, each shape is from a different focus ('multifocal') (see Figure 14.6).

Ectopics are

■ premature

if they occur before the expected complex, and

■ escape

if they appear after a missing expected complex, the ectopic 'escaping' into the gap. Premature ectopics indicate over-excitability (the problem). Escape ectopics indicate conduction failure, so the problem is failed conduction, not the ectopic. Isolated ectopics are not usually treated, but may indicate underlying problems, such as hypokalaemia, which require treatment.

Dysrhythmias and ectopics may be caused by electrolyte imbalances, especially potassium – see Chapter 2 for treatments.

Supraventricular dysrhythmias

Atrial fibrillation (AF)

(See Figure 14.7)
This is the most common dysrhythmia, especially in older people, with incidence increasing worldwide (Chugh *et al.*, 2013). Atrial rate is very rapid – typically 350–600 fibrillation waves/minute (McDonough, 2009), causing characteristically chaotic wavy baselines to ECG of 'coarse' AF, although with fine AF usually only ventricular activity (QRS complex, T wave) is seen. The AV node cannot conduct more than about 230 beats per minute (Barrett *et al.*, 2010), but ventricular rates are usually tachycardic (typically

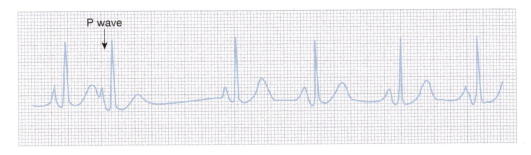

Figure 14.5 **Atrial ectopic**

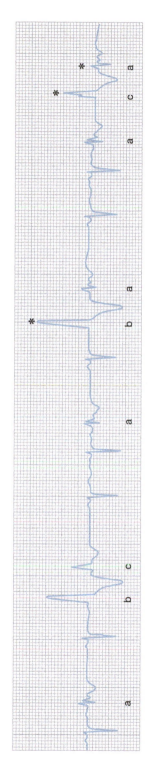

Figure 14.6 Ventricular ectopics

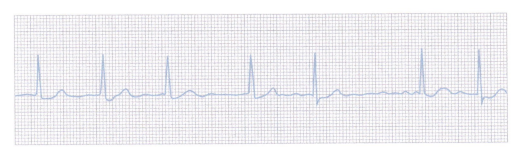

Figure 14.7 **Atrial fibrillation**

160–180) if untreated (McDonough, 2009) with 'irregularly irregular' rates. Ventricular conduction is normal (normal QRS). Irregularly irregular ECGs are usually AF, although other possibilities are:

■ multiple dysrhythmias superseding each other
■ multiple ectopics
■ intermittent AV block.

Atrial fibrillation is classified into five stages:

■ first diagnosed (regardless of duration or symptoms);
■ paroxysmal: spontaneous termination, usually within 48 hours, can persist 7 days;
■ persistent: not self-terminating;
■ long-standing: >1 year;
■ permanent ('accepted'): no cardioversion attempted.

(Task Force, 2010b)

The first four types may be considered *acute*, where the aim of treatment is to cure (remove) the AF. Permanent AF is *chronic*, so as AF cannot be cured, it should be controlled:

■ rate <110 bpm (Task Force, 2010b)
■ anticoagulation: target INR 2.5 (Keeling *et al.*, 2011).

Acute AF may be triggered by disease, treatments or other factors. But within weeks to months electrical 'remodelling' occurs (Saliba and Wazni, 2011).

Management of acute AF aims to restore sinus (or original) rhythm, whereas permanent AF cannot be reversed, but does need to be controlled. Treatable underlying causes should be reversed – patients should be normovolaemic, with electrolyte and other blood chemistry optimised. Acute AF causing life-threatening hypotension should be treated by urgent electrical cardioversion or drugs such as intravenous amiodarone (Saliba and Wazni, 2011). AF often recurs despite anti-dysrhythmic drugs (Saliba and Wazni, 2011). Catheter ablation has a higher success rate (Viles-Gonzalez *et al.*, 2011), so should be considered early if drugs fail to cure AF (Camm *et al.*, 2012).

Passive atrial bloodflow during fibrillation may have caused thrombi, so thrombotic events (e.g. stroke, pulmonary embolus). AF increases stroke risk up to fivefold (Task Force, 2010). Electrical cardioversion while cardioactive drugs (e.g. digoxin, beta-blockers) remain in circulation may cause asystole.

Permanent (chronic) atrial fibrillation should not prevent people living relatively healthy lives, provided it is controlled. Historically, digoxin was usually used to control rate, but Task Force (2010b) recommend individualising pharmacotherapy to patients, suggesting four groups of drugs:

- beta-blockers
- calcium channel antagonists
- digitalis glycosides, such as digoxin
- others, such as amiodarone.

Hypokalaemia potentiates effects of digoxin, so potassium should be checked regularly.

Anticoagulation is necessary to reduce stroke risk. Warfarin, traditionally the mainstay anticoagulant for AF, is increasingly being replaced by anticoagulation with less narrow therapeutic ranges, such as:

- dabigatran (thrombin inhibitor)
- rivaroxaban, apixaban, andedoxaban (factor Xa inhibitors).

These are reviewed by Heidbuchel et al. (2013).

Rate-control drugs, such as digoxin, should only normally be given if apex rate is above 60 bpm. If peripheral (radial, brachial) rate is 60, rate-control drugs can generally be given, but if peripheral rate is below 60, apex rate should be checked over a full minute (using a stethoscope); ideally, apex-radial deficit should be measured. Significant deficits suggest poor rate control.

Atrial flutter

(See Figure 14.8)

This is caused by an ectopic atrial pacemaker firing very rapidly – typically 300 times each minute (= one flutter wave every large ECG square). This ectopic focus creates 'saw-tooth' or 'shark's tooth' *flutter* waves instead of P waves. The AV node cannot conduct 300 impulses each minute, so imposes a block, usually even-numbered (e.g. 2:1, 4:1, 8:1). Normal ventricular conduction pathway makes QRS complexes and T waves normal.

Atrial rates of 300 each minute and 4:1 AV block cause 75 ventricular responses (pulses). But AV blocks can rapidly change, usually to another even number. 4:1 blocks may suddenly become 2:1 (ventricular response 150 bpm) or 8:1 (ventricular response 35–40 bpm).

Atrial flutter is therefore sinister. If acute, rapid reversal is necessary, with

- (urgent) electrical cardioversion

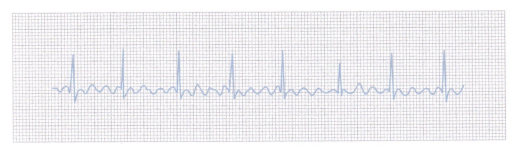

Figure 14.8 **Atrial flutter**

If this fails, chemical cardioversion may be attempted with

- amiodarone
- beta blockers
- flecainide
- calcium channel antagonists.

Radiofrequency catheter ablation is increasingly a first-line treatment (Sawhney and Feld, 2008).

Nodal/junctional rhythm

(See Figure 14.9)
This originates in or near the atrioventricular node (junction). Rates are usually 40–60 bpm, which can often be tolerated. Slower rates usually necessitate pacing. Causes for failed atrial conduction should be investigated and treated.

Blocks

These can occur anywhere in conduction pathways, but often occur at the atrioventricular junction:

- first degree block (delayed atrioventricular conduction)
- second degree block (incomplete heart block)
- third degree block (complete heart block)

or in one of the bundle branches

- bundle branch block.

A block in conduction may be caused by

- infarction
- oedema
- ischaemia.

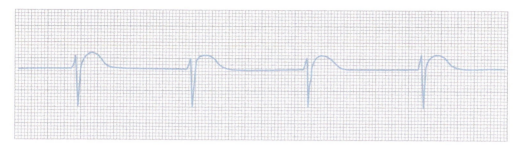

Figure 14.9 Nodal/junctional rhythm

Oedema or ischaemia can be reversed, resolving the block, but infarction usually creates permanent block.

First degree heart block

(See Figure 14.10)
This is *delay* in atrioventricular conduction, causing prolonged PR intervals (>5 small squares) and sometimes bradycardia. First degree block is usually caused either by

- age-related thickening of the AV node *or*
- by anti-hypertensive or other cardiac drugs (e.g. digoxin, beta-blockers, calcium channel blockers).

Provided cardiac output and blood pressure remain adequate, first degree blocks are not usually treated, although underlying causes should be reversed if possible. Symptomatic bradycardia may necessitate treatment (e.g. pacing).

Second degree heart block

This is *incomplete heart block*, where at regular intervals P waves are not conducted (= regularly missing pulses). The block is regular (e.g. 5:1 = 5 P waves conducted,

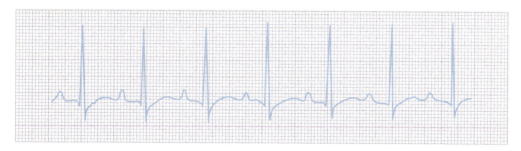

Figure 14.10 First degree block

1 unconducted), so ECGs have a pattern (*regularly irregular*). There are two types of second degree heart block:

- type 1 (Wenkebach phenomenon; Mobitz type 1): PR intervals progressively lengthen until a P wave remains unconducted (see Figure 14.11)
- type 2 (Mobitz or Mobitz type 2): PR intervals remain constant.

Second degree heart block type 1 occurs more frequently, is usually asymptomatic and resolves spontaneously. Type 2 is more serious, so more likely to require treatment:

- oxygen
- atropine
- pacing if unresponsive.

Figure 14.12 is probably second degree heart block type 2, although without consecutive PR intervals type 1 could not be excluded.

Third degree heart block

(See Figure 14.13)
This is *complete heart block*, causing complete dissociation between atrial and ventricular activity. P waves may be present and regular, but do not initiate QRS complexes (some

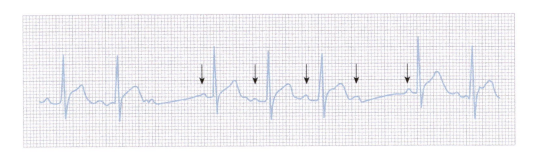

Figure 14.11 Second degree block type 1

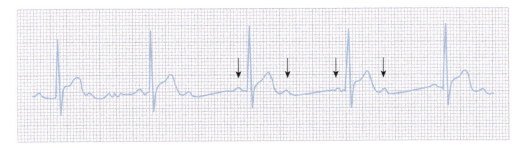

Figure 14.12 Second degree block type 2

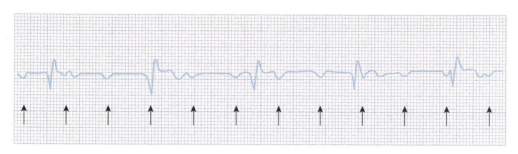

Figure 14.13 **Third degree block**

P may be 'lost' in QRS complexes or T wave). The QRS, originating in ventricular muscle, is broad and very slow (30–40 bpm), usually necessitating urgent pacing. 'First aid' is 100% oxygen and atropine. Occasionally people survive with, and adjust to, chronic third degree block.

Bundle branch block

(See Figure 14.14)

This is a block in either the left or right branch bundle. Impulses pass normally through the intact branch, creating a normal QRS. The side of the block receives the same impulse after it has crossed the septum, causing a second, broader QRS. ECGs show the two QRS complexes by a biphasic, or RSR, shape.

M or W shaped complexes are usually seen in many leads. To distinguish left from right branch bundle blocks, check chest leads. Left bundle branch blocks (LBBB) have Ws in early chest leads (C1, C2) and Ms in late chest leads (C4–6). Right bundle branch blocks (RBBB) have Ms in early chest leads (C1, C2) and sometimes Ws in late chest leads (C4–6). Bundle branch blocks may be differentiated by the mnemonics MaRRoW and WiLLiaM.

Chest pain, with a new left bundle branch block (i.e. not on the last ECG) indicates *STEMI* (see Chapter 12), necessitating urgent revascularisation with primary percutaneous coronary intervention (pPCI), or if pPCI is not practical, thrombolysis.

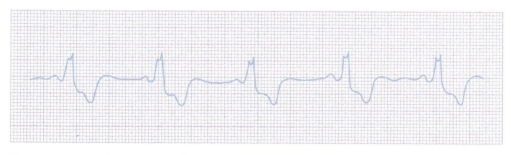

Figure 14.14 **Bundle branch block**

Ventricular dysrhythmias

Impulses originating in ventricular muscle do not use normal conduction pathways, but spread instead from muscle fibre to muscle fibre. This causes absence of P waves and broad QRS. Ventricular dysrhythmias are life-threatening, requiring urgent treatment.

Ventricular tachycardia (VT)

(See Figure 14.15)
This is a regular, but life-threatening, rhythm, showing only ventricular (broad) complexes without P waves. Cardiac output and blood pressure will be very poor. Ventricular tachycardia usually progresses rapidly to ventricular fibrillation.

Ventricular tachycardia with a pulse should be cardioverted with drugs:

- amiodarone.

Pulseless VT is a shockable cardiac arrest rhythm, treated with:

- chest compressions
- defibrillation
- drugs (e.g. adrenaline)

although there is current controversy about efficacy of adrenaline (Dumas *et al.*, 2014).

Ventricular fibrillation (VF)

(See Figure 14.16)
This is an irregularly irregular rhythm, with no cardiac output. Untreated, it is almost invariably fatal within 2–3 minutes. It is a shockable arrest rhythm. Resuscitation Council (2010) guidelines for pulseless VT and VF use the same algorithm.

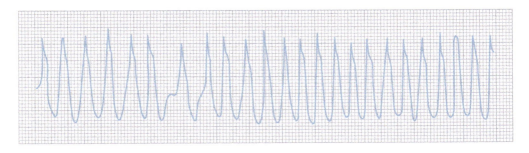

Figure 14.15 Ventricular tachycardia

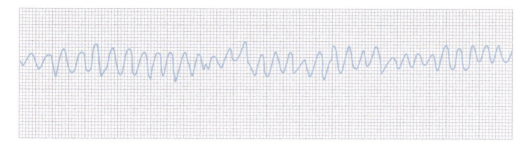

Figure 14.16 Ventricular fibrillation

Asystole

This is where there is no cardiac electrical activity, the ECG showing only an isoelectric line. If atrial, but not ventricular, activity is present, this may be termed *ventricular standstill*, which similarly produces no cardiac output. An arrest situation, it should be treated according to current resuscitation protocols. However, before putting out an arrest call, staff should look at the patient in case electrodes have become disconnected. Defibrillation is not used for asystole, as the heart is not fibrillating. Although resuscitation should normally be attempted, few patients survive asystole.

Pulseless electrical activity (PEA)

This is when there is no pulse despite complexes (usually abnormal) on the ECG. PEA is an arrest situation. Resuscitation Council (2010) list the eight reversible factors that can cause PEA in a 'consider' box below the VT/VF algorithm:

- hypoxia
- hypovolaemia
- hyper/hypokalaemia/metabolic
- hypothermia
- tension pneumothorax
- tamponade, cardiac
- toxins
- thrombosis (coronary or pulmonary).

Underlying causes of PEA should therefore be resolved as part of resuscitation.

Implications for practice

- ECGs contain much information in a small graph. Understanding normal cardiac electrophysiology and how this translates onto ECGs assists interpretation. Analyse one lead at a time, using a framework such as Table 14.1.

- Interpreting ECGs is a skill that requires practice. Take every possible opportunity to study ECGs of patients cared for, interpreting information holistically.
- Most dysrhythmias are only treated if they cause, or are likely to cause, problems.
- Underlying causes for dysrhythmias (e.g. electrolyte imbalances) should be resolved.
- Readers should be familiar with current resuscitation protocols (at the time of writing: Resuscitation Council (2010), but scheduled for revision 2015), attend annual updates, and have posters of current resuscitation algorithms displayed prominently in clinical areas.

Summary

ECGs can provide useful information for monitoring and treating acutely ill patients. However, ECG monitoring is only effective if staff have the knowledge and skill to interpret what they see. Like most skills, interpreting ECGs improves with practice, so use the framework provided here to analyse ECGs of patients you care for.

Useful website

European Society of Cardiology

Further reading

Readers should know resuscitation protocols. Hampton (2013a) and Houghton and Gray (2014) are two useful pocket-sized books on ECGs. The European Society of Cardiology provide authoritative guidelines on a range of dysrhythmias and treatments. Hampton (2013b) provides exercises for readers to test and develop interpretation skills.

Clinical exercises

1   Reflect on times you have recorded a 12-lead ECG (or observed one being recorded). What preparations were made? How was the procedure explained to patients? What anxieties did patients express or appear to have about the procedure?
2   Find a printout of an ECG from a patient whom you have cared for. Cover any printed analysis, and using the framework in Table 14.1, analyse the ECG. At the earliest opportunity, discuss your analysis with a nursing or medical colleague skilled in ECG analysis.
3   Reflecting on your experience over the last year, list the dysrhythmias you have seen. What treatments can you remember being used for each dysrhythmia? What dysrhythmias were not actively treated, and why?

Appendix: Some drugs used to treat dysrhythmias

adrenaline (epinephrine)	alpha and beta agonist: increases heart rate, stroke volume and systemic vascular resistance
amiodarone	reverses tachycardia (atrial or ventricular); must be given through a central line
atropine	positive chronotrope (increases heart rate)
calcium chloride/calcium gluconate	stabilises cardiac conduction
captopril	ACE inhibitor; reduces hypertension
digoxin	slows and strengthens atrial impulses in atrial fibrillation
diltiazim	calcium channel blocker
disopyramide	controls ventricular dysrhythmias
dobutamine	positive inotrope; beta agonist, so increases stroke volume
esmolol	beta blocker
flecainide	controls atrial tachycardias
insulin and glucose	insulin transports glucose into cell, taking potassium with it
lidocaine	controls ventricular dysrhythmias
losarten	anti-hypertensive (angiotensin receptor blocker – ARB)
nifedipine	calcium channel blocker
procainamide	controls ventricular dysrhythmias and atrial tachycardia
propanolol	beta blocker; reduces hypertension
sotalol	beta blocker; reduces hypertension
verapamil	calcium channel blocker

Chapter 15

Haemoglobinopathies

Contents

Fundamental knowledge

- Production of blood cells (see Chapter 3)
- Structure and physiology of haemoglobin

Introduction

This chapter primarily focuses on some haematological conditions that can cause or complicate acute disease:

- leukaemia
- anaemias
- sickle cell disease
- thalassaemia.

Pulmonary emboli (PE) are discussed in Chapter 4; the rare but too often fatal disseminated intravascular coagulation is discussed in the companion text *Intensive Care Nursing*. Nursing care largely centres on individual patient needs and symptoms, breathlessness and weakness being common symptoms during crises, and requirements of therapies, such as blood transfusion observations. Haemoglobinopathies, such as sickle cell disease and thalassaemia, can cause tissue hypoxia, and so organ dysfunction, as well as hypercoagulopathy (Ataga *et al.*, 2007). Lack of awareness of conditions such as sickle cell disease and thalassaemia has led to preventable deaths within healthcare (NCEPOD, 2008). This chapter describes pathophysiologies to enable readers to understand conditions of their patients. Many haemoglobinopathies are, or can be, detected in childhood, but this chapter focuses on adult care. Patients may be transferred to specialist centres, therefore priority is usually on initial management and stabilisation. Prior to transfer, advice should be sought from the receiving specialist centre.

Although not a haemoglobinopathy, thromboprophylaxis is also included, as illness and immobility predispose to thrombus formation, which may cause fatal pulmonary emboli. Thrombus risk assessment should therefore be undertaken on all patients, resulting in most being prescribed thromboprophylaxis.

1: LEUKAEMIA

Leucocytes are white blood cells; leukaemia is a group of diseases affecting white cells. Leukaemia is caused by bone marrow cancer, typically resulting is excessive production of immature (*blast*) cells (Craig *et al.*, 2010). Overproduction of blast cells can cause accumulation in bone marrow, leading to bone marrow failure, and/or accumulation elsewhere, leading to pain and organ failure. Leukaemia may be primary, or acquired, typically through chemotherapy or radiotherapy. Leukaemia may be acute (more common in children) or chronic (more common in older people). This chapter focuses on acute leukaemia in adults. The two main acute leukaemia are

- acute myeloid leukaemia (AML), which primarily affects adults;
- acute lymphoblastic leukaemia (ALL), which primarily affects children (Craig *et al.*, 2010);

depending on which type of leukocyte is predominant. Although diagnostically distinct, nursing care for both is similar.

Symptoms

Common symptoms may include

- aplastic anaemia, if bone marrow failure results in insufficient or immature erythrocytes; anaemia typically causes pallor, lethargy and dyspnoea;
- neutropeaenia, making the person susceptible to opportunistic infection;
- thrombocytopaenia, causing bruising and coagulopathies.

Although any organs may be affected, liver, spleen and lymph nodes are often painfully enlarged. High counts of circulating blast cells increase blood viscosity, often causing neurological symptoms such as headaches, nausea, vomiting, blurred vision, diplopia, confusion, fitting and coma (Treleaven and Meller, 2000).

Care

Untreated leukaemias are almost invariably fatal, death usually resulting from either massive internal haemorrhage or overwhelming infection. However, bone marrow transplants, chemotherapy and radiotherapy have markedly improved prognosis in recent decades.

Treatment for leukaemia is usually managed in specialist (oncology or haematology) centres, so staff working elsewhere may gain limited experience of leukaemias. But other treatments, or emergencies, may bring people with leukaemia into other wards and departments, possibly after recent chemotherapy or other treatments.

Many chemotherapy agents cause hyperkalaemia, so potassium should be monitored closely. Transfusions, especially of platelets and clotting factors, are often needed. Most hospitals have various support services, such as oncology departments, clinical nurse specialists and counsellors, so if nurses lack specialist knowledge and skills, they should involve appropriate resources.

Low white cell count exposes people with leukaemia to high risks of opportunist infection – infection from organisms that would be resisted by most people. Infection control is therefore especially important. Some hospitals have policies of protective isolation, also called reverse barrier nursing, for patients with leucocytes, or more often granulocytes (see Chapter 3), below certain thresholds; in the absence of specific policies, nurses should undertake individual risk assessments and ensure a high standard of infection control practice.

2: ANAEMIA

The World Health Organization (1968) defines normal haemoglobin levels as 140–180 grams/litre for men and 115–165 grams/litre for women. Anaemia (low haemoglobin – see Chapter 3) reduces oxygen carriage, and is a relatively common problem, occurring in one fifth of older men, and one eighth of older women (Mukhopadhyay and Mohanaruban, 2002). There are many types of anaemia, including

- *microcytic*: erythrocytes (red cells) are small due to chronic blood loss resulting in insufficient iron for haemoglobin synthesis. As well as being small, red cell count is often low;
- *aplastic*: red cell production is low due to lack of functioning bone marrow, typically caused by radiotherapy or chemotherapy;
- *megaoblostaic*: erythrocytes are large but abnormally shaped, due to insufficient vitamin B12 (cyanocobalamin), folic acid or intrinsic factor (an enzyme produced by the stomach that enables absorption of vitamin B12; NB there are other 'intrinsic factors' in the body);

■ *haemolytic*: erythrocytes are destroyed prematurely. This can be a hereditary condition, but frequently occurs with major illness.

In acute illness, sudden reduction in haemoglobin is often caused either by bleeding or by haemodiltution from fluid resuscitation.

As identified in Chapter 10, survival from major illness is generally highest if haemoglobin is 70–90 grams per litre (Hebert *et al.*, 1999), so blood transfusions are rarely used with mild anaemia.

3: SICKLE CELL DISEASE

The haemoglobin molecule consists of four chains. Six months after birth, foetal haemoglobin (HbF) is usually replaced by adult haemoglobin (HbA) (Thomas and Lumb, 2012), which normally has two alpha (α) and two beta (β) chains. However, some people have other forms of haemoglobin, which can negatively affect oxygen carriage. HbF occasionally persists. The most prevalent other type of haemoglobin is sickle (HbS), where glumanic acid in β chains is replaced by valine residue (Barrett *et al.*, 2010). This change provides some protection against malaria (Weatherall, 2010), so the sickle cell gene is mainly found in people whose ethnic origin is from regions where malaria is prevalent. People with one sickle gene (HbS HbA) are 'sickle cell carriers', previously called 'sickle trait' while people with both have 'sickle cell disease'. However, carriers can still develop crises. Further subtyping is used in specialist areas.

Sickle cells haemolyse prematurely, typically at 16–20 days (Sickle Cell Society, 2008), causing anaemia. Endothelial damage reduces nitric oxide production, resulting in many of the vascular diseases associated with sickle cell disease (Sickle Cell Society, 2008), such as strokes and pulmonary hypertension, while microvascular occlusion often causes renal disease, retinopathy and degeneration of hips (Sickle Cell Society, 2008).

In hypoxic conditions, which may include anaesthesia, sickle cells change shape from the usual 'doughnut' erythrocyte shape to a sickle shape. These typically occlude small blood vessels, depriving mosquitoes of their food (human blood), but also causing ischaemia, pain (De, 2008; Rees *et al.*, 2010; Anie and Green, 2015), and potential tissue damage and organ failure (Gardner *et al.*, 2010). Patients whose ethnic origin is from areas where HbS is prevalent should therefore be tested before anaesthesia (Ryan *et al.*, 2010).

During acute crises priorities are

■ analgesia, usually opioid
■ high concentration oxygen
■ fluid resuscitation

and often

■ blood transfusion (to reduce the proportion of sickle cells).

Poorly managed pain can become chronic (Yawn *et al.*, 2014).

4: THALASSAEMIA

Thalassaemia (literally 'sea blood', previously called Cooley's anaemia) is a recessive autosomal inherited condition (Peters *et al.*, 2012) causing defects in globin genes which result in premature destruction and so deficiency of numbers of red blood cells (few islands in the sea). Like sickle cells, thalassaemia provides some protection against malaria (Wetherall, 2010). There are two main variants:

- alpha (α)
- beta (β)

depending on the gene affected, although as with sickle cells, further subtyping is used in specialist areas; differences between types are not significant for general nursing care. Alpha thalassaemia occurs mainly in people of eastern Asian and eastern Mediterranean ethnic origins, while beta thalassaemia can occur in people of most ethnicities except Northern Europeans (Ryan *et al.*, 2010). It may also be classified as

- major
- intermedia *and*
- minor,

minor usually being carriers who suffer few or no complications (Peters *et al.*, 2012).

Thalassaemia can be cured through stem cell transplant or gene therapy (Taher *et al.*, 2011; Peters *et al.*, 2012). It can be treated through blood transfusion, although repeated transfusions can cause iron overload, necessitating chelation therapy (Porter, 2009; Taher *et al.*, 2011), such as with desferrioamine, to prevent liver failure (Peters *et al.*, 2012). The United Kingdom Thalassaemia Society (2008) recommends transfusion to maintain haemoglobin above 95–100 grams/litre.

5: THROMBOPROPHYLAXIS

Worldwide, most hospitalised patients are at risk of venous thromboembolism (VTE) (Cohen *et al.*, 2008). Risk increases with venous stasis, hypercoagulability and immobility. Thrombi can form anywhere, but deep vein thrombosis (DVT) occurs most often in leg veins, partly due to the presence of valves in those veins. DVTs are the most common cause of pulmonary emboli (Hyers, 2003). Less than half of fatal pulmonary emboli have been suspected before death (Meyer *et al.*, 2010). All patients should therefore be risk assessed for VTE, and unless contra-indicated surgical patients should be offered both mechanical compression (thromboembolytic deterrent stockings – TEDS) and pharmacological prophylaxis (usually subcutaneous heparin) (NICE 2012b). In practice, these precautions are extended to most or all patients. Staff should be familiar with contraindications.

Implications for practice

- Leukaemia exposes patients to high risk of acquiring infection, so follow local infection control protocols, and in the absence of other guidance risk-assess each aspect of nursing care.
- Sickle cell disease is most likely to occur in people whose ethnic origin is from the malarial belt of the world.
- Sickle cell crises are usually triggered by hypoxia and/or dehydration.
- Sickle cell causes vascular complications; in addition to chronic diseases, vascular occlusion usually causes severe pain.
- Thalassaemia can occur in almost any ethnicity except northern European, but is most prevalent in eastern Mediterranean and eastern Asian ethnicity.
- If haemoglobinopathies are suspected, they should be tested for before any high-risk procedures, such as surgery.
- All patients should be risk assessed for venous thromboembolism, and where indicated given prophylaxis (TEDS and subcutaneous heparin).
- TEDS should be removed twice daily, and remeasured before replacing.

Summary

Distribution of sickle cell disease and thalassaemia varies widely within the UK; where these conditions are relatively frequently seen, there will often be reasonable levels of awareness about them, but elsewhere they may not be considered until avoidable complications have occurred. Leukaemia is less geographically confined, but usually managed in specialist centres. With all three conditions, staff unfamiliar with managing them should seek specialist advice. In contrast, risk of DVT is present in most hospitalised patients, so all patients should be risk assessed, and thromboprophylaxis initiated when appropriate.

Support groups

Anthony Nolan Trust (for leukaemia)
The Sickle Cell Society
UK Thalassaemia Society.

Further reading

There is a surprising lack of guidelines for adult care with all haemoglobinopathies discussed in this chapter. NCEPOD (2008) is one of the few major reports that is significant for acute care. Because haemoglobinopathies are chronic conditions, reports such as Sickle Cell Society (2008), United Kingdom Thalassaemia Society (2008) and Anie and Green (2015) focus mainly on chronic care, although provide useful overviews of the conditions. NICE (2012b) provide guidance on thromboprophylaxis. Yawn *et al.'s* (2014) USA guidelines for sickle cell disease provide a comprehensive review of evidence which, as they identify, is limited.

Clinical scenario

Ms Katie Jeffries, a 19-year-old student, collapsed while running in a sponsored marathon in hot weather. She is brought into A&E by ambulance. She is known to have sickle cell disease.

1   You are the nurse caring for Ms Jeffries at the time of her admission. Using A-B-C-D-E assessment, identify your immediate priorities. List likely medical priorities.
2   Identify local resources in your workplace to support care of people with sickle cell disease and thalassaemia.
3   When you transfer Ms Jeffries to the medical admissions ward for overnight observation, the receiving nurse does not appear to be familiar with sickle cell disease. What information would you give about the condition to ensure safe care for your patient?

Chapter 16

Vascular access

Contents

Fundamental knowledge

- Venous anatomy – basilic, cephalic, median, central

Introduction

Sicker patients almost invariably require vascular access devices for treatments. Variety of available devices has increased significantly in recent years (Jackson *et al.*, 2013). Like any treatment, vascular access devices may benefit patients, but also expose patients to risks. Nurses inserting devices should therefore choose whichever device is most beneficial with fewest risks (Jackson *et al.*, 2013). Nursing care of patients includes being aware of, and monitoring for, risks, deciding when devices should be removed, and identifying need for any replacement of devices.

This chapter describes the more widely used devices:

- peripheral cannula
- midline
- peripherally inserted central catheter (PICC)
- short-term central venous catheter (CVC; central line)
- tunnelled (Hickman®/Groshong®)
- implanted port (e.g. Port-a-Cath®)

together with

- intra-osseus access (IO)

and refers to relevant anatomical structures – if unsure of their situation, refer to an anatomy resource.

Device selection may be determined by factors such as

- patient consent and compliance;
- treatments – veins/routes determined by risks from specific drugs or fluids;
- how long access is likely to be needed;
- limitations caused by difficult cannulation or urgency.

1: PERIPHERAL CANNULAE

The most widely used vascular devices are peripheral cannulae. For acute, short-term use, these have the benefit of being easy to insert, and are suitable for most drugs and fluids. Ideally, peripheral cannulae should be inserted in dorsal (lower arm) veins, as limb movement is less likely to dislodge veins cannulae. To reduce risks of infiltration, sites used should not be below recent cannulae sites (Morris, 2011). If possible, soft, resilient, large and straight veins should be selected for insertion. The smallest cannula that will deliver necessary drugs/fluids should be selected. Small cannulae are less uncomfortable and traumatic for patients, and also allow greater bloodflow around the cannula which will reduce phlebitis risks (see Figure 16.1).

Table 16.1 summarises common indications for sizes.

Equipment needed for inserting peripheral cannulae includes

- sterile cannulation pack
- equipment for cleaning skin (see local policy)
- sharps bin
- sterile saline and 10 ml syringe for flushing line once inserted
- blood bottles and equipment for taking samples.

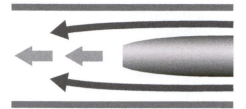 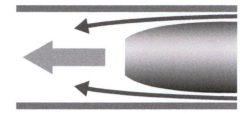

Figure 16.1 Selecting smaller cannulae improves bloodflow around devices, reducing risks of phlebitis

Table 16.1 Sizes and properties of peripheral cannulae

Colour	Common indications	Flow rate ml/min
Orange 14 g	Rapid infusion needed, especially of blood or viscous fluids	265
Grey 16 g	Rapid infusion needed, especially of blood or viscous fluids	170
White 17 g	Rapid infusion needed, especially of blood or viscous fluids	135
Green 18 g	Blood transfusion, parenteral nutrition, stem cell harvesting and cell separation, large volume fluids resuscitation	90
Pink 20 g	Blood transfusions, maintenance fluid therapy, long-term medication	55
Blue 22 g	Oncology, patients with small veins or needing longer-term medication	25
Yellow 24 g	Most drugs, short-term infusions, patients with fragile veins	24

Traditionally, equipment has included tourniquets; although these make it easier to obtain blood, prolonged tourniquet use can damage the sample, resulting in inaccuracies (Mäkitalo and Liikanen, 2013). Any skin emollients in the area should be removed, and skin disinfected according to local policy. Once inserted, blood should be drawn back through the line, and samples may be taken then if required. Blood samples should not be taken from peripheral lines at any time other than on insertion.

Complications

Although a suitable vein should be identified before insertion, potential complications both during insertion and throughout the time the cannula is in place include

- transfixation on insertion (going through vein)
- infection
- excessive pain
- bruising (ecchymosis)
- nerve injury
- infiltration/extravasation ('tissueing')

■   haematoma/embolism
■   phlebitis.

Many of these complications also apply to other vascular devices described later.

Vein walls are relatively resistant, so if cannulae are advanced, but the metal needle withdrawn once blood is seen, they usually remain in veins. But it is possible to puncture through both sides of the vein, inserting the cannula into tissue spaces. Taking blood through cannulae on insertion has the benefit of confirming that the device is where it should be. If in doubt whether a cannula is in a vein or not, no drugs should be given into it, as they may cause tissue damage. Saline injected into a cannula in tissues usually causes obvious local swelling. It is possible, although rare, to cannulate an artery. If this occurs, blood will usually be bright red. If in doubt, a sample could be sent for gas analysis. Arterial cannulation usually causes pulsatile blood flow; removal of a cannula from an artery usually causes pulsatile, high-pressure bleeds typically requiring at least five minutes of firm pressure to stop.

If cannulation has not be successful, usually due to transfixation, repeated attempts are unlikely to be successful, so generally after two failed attempts the task should be escalated to someone more experienced.

If cannulation is difficult, placing the patient's arm below their heart level can help increase volume in the vein by impeding return to the heart. Application of local heat can be useful to venodilate. Veins can be visualised through ultrasound, or a variety of other commercial products.

Vascular devices are responsible for most blood stream infections (Loveday *et al.*, 2014). Insertion, and all equipment used, should therefore be sterile. Skin should be cleaned, according to local policy. Skin should be cleaned with 2% chlorhexidine (Bishop *et al.*, 2007). Once inserted, the cannula should be stabilised and covered with a suitable sterile dressing. Any vascular device however exposes patients to risk of infection (Loveday *et al.*, 2014); traditionally, cannulae have usually been replaced every three or four days, depending on manufacturers' instructions, but Loveday *et al.* (2014) recommend replacing only when clinically indicated. Nurses should however be aware of any time limits required by local policies and manufacturers' instructions, and monitor devices at least every shift for signs of infection. Any unnecessary cannulae, or cannulae whose sites appear infected, should be removed.

Bruising, from subcutaneous bleeding, may occur at any time. Once inserted, securing the cannula reduces risks (Morris, 2011), but if bruising occurs while in place, reasons should be investigated. On removal, pressure should be maintained on the site until risk of bleeding is slight; depending on individual patients' vascular health and clotting status, sometimes bruising is unavoidable.

Cannulation is usually painful, but with peripheral cannulae pain caused by injecting local anaesthetics usually exceeds pain from cannulation. With children, topical local anaesthetics are usually used, but while EMLA (eutectic mixture of local anaesthetics) is sometimes used with adults, it is not common practice (Moore, 2009). Extreme pain radiating down the arm on insertion may indicate nerve injury, so the cannula should be removed and doctor informed (Morris, 2011).

Infiltration is when non-vesicant solutions or drugs are administered unintentionally into surrounding tissues, whereas extravasation is vesicant substances being administered accidentally into tissues (Morris, 2011). Extravasation is more likely to occur with chemotherapy. As the cannula is, by definition, not in the vein, it should be removed. With extravasation, medical staff should be informed (Morris, 2011).

Phlebitis (inflammation of veins) may be

- chemical (from drugs infused)
- mechanical (from the vascular device)
- thrombotic
- septic (from infection).

Infused chemicals that are very acidic, alkaline or hyperosmolar (see Chapter 23) may cause inflammatory responses of endothelium. It is generally recommended, although not often practised, that drugs outside pH range of 7–9 should not be given through peripheral cannulae to reduce risk of chemical phlebitis.

In newly inserted devices, mechanical irritation is the most likely cause of phlebitis, although this can occur at any time by traumatic movement of devices in veins. Traumatic movement can be reduced by firm external fixation and avoiding cannulation near bony prominences (Morris, 2011). There are many commercial products to secure devices; most Trusts have policies recommending specific products.

Thrombi are less likely to occur with narrower devices.

2: MIDLINES

Midlines, normally inserted into the antecubital fossa, are up to 25 cm long, so normally the tip is in the axillary vein. Being a large, although not central, vein, the axillary vein is suitable for infusion of many drugs which cannot be given peripherally. Midlines are also useful where longer-term access will be needed; many manufacturers advertise products as being usable for up to one year, although practice in many Trusts is to replace them after six weeks due to significant increased risks after then of mechanical phlebitis. Users should check local policies for use, frequency of flushes, and recommended dressings.

3: PICC

Peripherally inserted central lines are usually inserted into the cephalic, basilic or median cubital veins (RCN, 2010), but end in the superior vena cava. The two central veins (superior and inferior vena cava) return blood to the heart, so have the largest bloodflow of all veins. This makes them least likely to develop phlebitis. Compared with non-tunnelled CVCs, PICCs have substantially lower infection risk (Loveday et al., 2014), and can be used for up to two years.

Ideally, the tip of PICCs and CVCs should be in the superior vena cava, but may enter the right atrium, other veins (such as jugular) or extravascular tissues. PICCs are more often malpositioned than CVCs (Pilwer et al., 2012). Position should therefore be confirmed before use. Traditionally, this was by chest X-ray, although various commercial devices can also confirm position, such as using P waves on ECGs (e.g. Nautilus™) (Lee *et al.*, 2009).

PICCs are often the preferred device for long-term use, or where infusions have high risk of causing phlebitis. However, Chopra *et al.* (2013) suggest they have a higher risk of venous thromboembolism than CVCs.

4: CENTRAL VENOUS CATHETERS (CVCS)

Like PICCs, CVCs are inserted into one of the two central veins, usually the superior vena (Peris *et al.*, 2010). Subclavian insertion has the lowest infection risks (O'Grady *et al.*, 2011; Loveday *et al.*, 2014), and subclavian lines are more comfortable for patients than internal jugular (Waldmann and Barnes, 2004). However, subclavian insertion has greater risk of pneumothorax, so internal jugular is more often used for short-term access. Being shorter than PICCs, they are more suitable for rapid infusion. Multi-lumen CVCs are often used in critical care units due to likely need to infuse a variety of potent drugs for a number of days.

Non-tunnelled CVCs are the most common cause of septic phlebitis from vascular devices (DOH, 2007; Curtis, 2009), so their use is discouraged in most areas, and they should be removed as soon as it is reasonable to do so. Routine tunnelling of short-term CVCs is not recommended (Loveday *et al.*, 2014). Femoral insertion of PICCs and central lines is associated with high infection risk (Loveday *et al.*, 2014), so should be avoided unless emergency access is needed and preferred sites are impractical (O'Grady *et al.*, 2011).

Central venous pressure monitoring is discussed in *Intensive Care Nursing.*

5: TUNNELLED CVCS (HICKMAN'S®, GROSHONG®)

Long-term central venous access may use either PICCs or tunnelled CVCs, a skin tunnel being formed over the catheter. A cuff within the skin tunnel provokes fibrosis (Bishop *et al.*, 2007), creating a further barrier against infection.

One third to two thirds of patients with long-term CVCs and PICCs develop thrombi, so should be prophylactically treated with heparin (Loveday *et al.*, 2014).

Parenteral nutrition

Parenteral nutrition (PN), often called total parenteral nutrition (TPN) is manufactured in a variety of formulae, often numbered after the grams of nitrogen contained (typically 5, 9, 11 and 14). The high glucose content, and sometimes other contents, make PN potentially irritant. Nine gram PN was originally manufactured for peripheral infusion, although it often does cause phlebitis through this route. Most trusts have policies for which type of device to use for different strengths.

As parenteral nutrition is food that normally hangs for 24 hours in room temperature, risks of infection are especially high. Ideally, a dedicated lumen should be used for PN (Baker and Harbottle, 2014; Loveday *et al.*, 2014) – a lumen that has not been previously used. However, neither Baker and Harbottle (2014) nor Loveday *et al.* (2014) absolutely preclude use of a non-dedicated lumen, and USA guidelines (O'Grady *et al.*, 2011) identify need for dedicated lumens as an unresolved issue.

6: IMPLANTED PORTS (PORT-A-CATH®)

These are similar to tunnelled CVCs, except that the catheter is positioned fully within the patient, with a subcutaneous injectable port. This provides even greater defence against infection, although does expose patients to discomfort from needle insertion (Lebeaux *et al.*, 2014; Loveday *et al.*, 2014). A special ('non-coring') needle should be used to access the port; standard syringe needles should not be used, as this will damage the device.

7: INTRA-OSSEUS

Bone has a rich blood supply, so in emergency situations large bones such as the tibia and femur provide easy and relatively safe access for drugs and infusions. However, intra-osseus devices should be restricted to emergency situations or when no other access is available (RCN, 2010; Resuscitation Council, 2010). Intra-osseus devices should be clearly labelled, and normally removed after 24 hours. They are rarely seen in ward areas, so if encountered seek advice about care. They are usually removed by vascular specialists.

Suspected line sepsis

Peripheral lines suspected of causing sepsis should be removed. Midlines or central vein devices suspected of causing sepsis should be used for taking blood cultures from each lumen, and blood cultures should also be taken from a peripheral stab. If the device is the only vascular access, and access is difficult, giving antibiotics through an infected line is preferable to not giving antibiotics at all, so advice should be sought from vascular access specialists before removal. Before removal, check with the medical staff whether they want the tip sent for culture.

Implications for practice

- When inserting peripheral lines, if possible select a site on the lower forearm, but avoid inserting below any recently-used sites.
- Most bacteraemias are from vascular devices, so devices should be removed as soon as no longer needed.
- Insertion sites should be inspected at least every shift. If dressings are not intact, these should be replaced aseptically.
- Whenever handling any vascular device, use asepsis.
- Phlebitis in a newly-inserted PICC is probably mechanical; do not remove the line, but seek advice from vascular specialists.

Summary

Acutely ill patients usually need vascular access. But vascular devices expose patients to various risks. Type and number of devices should therefore be chosen by risk/benefit analysis, and removed as soon as no longer necessary. Hospitals almost invariably have proformas for recording insertion and on-going observation of vascular devices, but any relevant information not covered by these should be recorded in nursing notes.

Further reading

Staff giving intravenous drugs should be familiar with the NMC's (2007) *Standards for Medicines Management*. RCN (2010) is widely accepted as authoritative, and Philips *et al.* (2011) provide a useful handbook on venepuncture and cannulation. Staff should also be familiar with local policies and company literature of devices they use. Loveday *et al.* (2014) are the national infection control guidelines, giving substantial advice and evidence on vascular devices. Dougherty and Lamb (2008) provide a comprehensive textbook.

Clinical scenario

Mr Daniel Bridges, aged 58, is admitted for planned repair of a large left inguinal hernia. He is dialysis-dependant (three treatments each week), so has a shunt in his left arm. Due to extensive vascular disease, venous access is problematic.

Post-operatively he was transferred as planned to the intensive care unit, where among other treatments haemofiltration was used until today in lieu of dialysis. He has now returned to the surgical ward, but has a short-term right internal jugular central venous catheter in place.

1   What risks does his CVC pose in a surgical ward? Identify local policies related to CVCs, especially any specific to your ward.
2   You are working with a second year student nurse, who has not yet been allocated to ICU. How would you explain to the student what a CVC is, and what would you say about it, especially its risks and benefits?
3   Transfer to the renal department is planned for two days' time, following which he will still need intravenous medications. As he will remain in hospital, what alternatives for vascular access could be considered? Give rationales for your choice.

Part 4

Disability

Chapter 17

Neurological deficits

Contents

Fundamental knowledge

- Cerebrospinal fluid – production and normal physiology
- Meninges – pia mater, arachnoid mater, dura mater
- Circle of Willis

Introduction

Patients may be admitted to acute hospitals with new neurological deficits, or may develop problems during their admission for some other pathology – for example, brain injury from hypoxia, emboli, bleed or raised intracranial pressure. This chapter briefly revises aspects of physiology relevant to acute brain injury, then discusses the more common acute neurological pathologies seen in general acute hospitals:

- traumatic brain injury
- spinal cord injury
- stroke
- subarachnoid haemorrhage
- epilepsy.

There are specialist regional centres for most conditions discussed, so focus is generally on initial management and stabilisation prior to transfer.

Intracranial pressure

Space inside the skull (*intracranial*) is limited. Intracranial pressure is normally 0–10 mmHg (Bahouth and Yarbrough, 2013). In other parts of the body, increased contents (for example, from a bleed) cause tissue distension. However, brain tissue is confined by the skull. Brain tissue forms the vast majority of intracranial contents; the remainder is fluid, two thirds of the fluid normally being cerebrospinal fluid and one third blood (see Figure 17.1) (Cooper *et al.*, 2006). A rapid increase in intracranial contents (for example, from a bleed or oedema) therefore causes an increase in intracranial pressure, compressing other brain tissue (mostly brain cells), and causing mechanical damage.

Acute brain injury

Unlike capillaries elsewhere, those perfusing the brain ('the blood–brain barrier') do not have pores between epithelial cells. Movement across the blood–brain barrier is therefore by active transport, making transfer highly selective (Hickey and Kanusky, 2014).

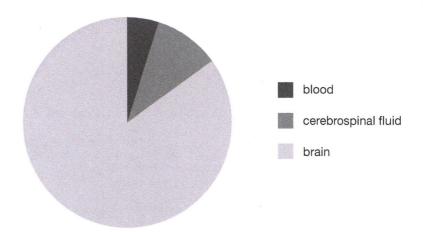

Figure 17.1 Normal distribution of intracranial contents

Metabolic waste, proteins, most drugs, some toxins are therefore kept out of brain tissue (Marieb and Hoehn, 2013). However, the blood–brain barrier is ineffective against fats and fat soluble molecules, such as alcohol, nicotine and anaesthetic drugs (Marieb and Hoehn, 2013).

Damage from acute brain injury can be divided into two stages: *primary*, which is largely irreversible, and *secondary*, which can be prevented. Just as a myocardial infarction typically has a central zone of damage and a peripheral 'at risk' area (see Chapter 12), so acute brain injury creates an 'at risk' zone where perfusion and oxygenation are poor (Treadwell *et al.*, 1994). The 'at risk' zone may either be rescued or, if not protected, damaged.

Acute brain injury causes failure of the blood–brain barrier, so plasma proteins transfer into brain tissue. As plasma proteins exert an *osmotic* pull (see Chapter 23), *vasogenic* oedema accumulates, causing brain cell damage and death. Cell trauma triggers inflammatory responses (Kuffler, 2012), increasing intracranial pressure, and potentially forcing brain-stem tissue into the spinal column – tentorial herniation, or 'coning' (Nag *et al.*, 2011).

Traditionally, neuroprotection involved

- hypothermia
- alkalinisation
- adenosine
- high dose glucocorticoids (e.g. methylprednisolone, pregabalin)

given within one hour – the 'golden hour' (Kuffler, 2012; Zamani *et al.*, 2013).

Cerebral perfusion pressure

Like tissues elsewhere in the body, capillaries will only perfuse the brain if intracapillary pressure exceeds resistance outside the capillary. Cerebral perfusion pressure is therefore the mean arterial pressure (MAP) minus the intracranial pressure. In health, the vasomotor centre (see Chapter 10) normally autoregulates cerebral perfusion pressure to about 80 mmHg (March and Hickey, 2014a). In health, therefore, a systemic MAP of 80 mmHg would ensure cerebral perfusion. However, if there are concerns of intracranial hypertension, a higher MAP is needed – 90 mmHg is generally desirable (Woodward and Waterhouse, 2009).

Intracranial hypertension

Like intra-abdominal hypertension, intracranial hypertension is a pressure greater than >20 mmHg, and causes organ injury. The most common cause of intracranial hypertension is oedema (May, 2009). Traditionally, cerebral oedema has been removed with the osmotic diuretic mannitol (Gupta *et al.*, 2010). But many neurologists now advocate hypertonic saline (see Chapter 25) (Kamel *et al.*, 2011). Patients with cerebral oedema should be nursed at angles of 15–30° to optimise drainage through the jugular veins (Bahouth and Yarbrough, 2013).

Assessment

Neurological assessment should be both informal and formal. Informal assessment includes noting any changes in behaviour – both those observed by staff and those reported by family/friends. Any concerns from informal assessment should prompt formal assessment.

Basic neurological assessment was discussed in Chapter 2:

- behaviour
- AVPU
- blood sugar.

Any AVPU score below 'Alert' should prompt further assessment, such as GCS or blood sugar. This chapter therefore includes

- Glasgow Coma Scale (GCS) scoring
- pupil reaction.

Medical (technical) assessments include

- CT scans
- intracranial pressure monitoring

not discussed in this chapter. There is no evidence routine intracranial pressure monitoring is useful (Forsyth *et al.*, 2010) and its use is largely confined to specialist centres. Computerised tomography (CT) is widely available, but it is used for medical diagnosis, not nursing management.

Glasgow Coma Scale

(See Figure 17.2)

The Glasgow Coma Scale was developed by Teasdale and Jennett in 1974 to assess level of consciousness. It combined three assessments: eye opening, best verbal response and best motor response. Best responses should be recorded, so although a new one-sided weakness should be noted and reported, the strongest (not weakest) limb movement should be scored.

Eye opening asses the brain-stem (the reticular activating system), verbal response assesses the speech centres (Broca's – expressive; Wernick's – receptive) which are both situated in the left hemisphere of the brain, and motor response assesses the cerebral cortex – see Figure 17.3. Combining these three assessments therefore scans most of the brain. Assessing responses to pain was discussed in Chapter 2.

Scores can be interpreted as:

- 15 or 14   normal
- 13   mild impairment
- 9–12   moderate impairment
- 3–8   severe impairment.

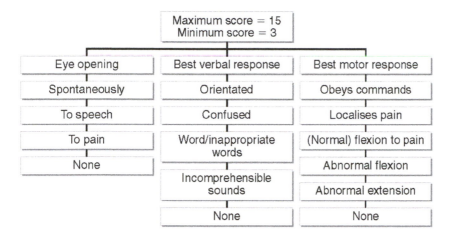

Figure 17.2 **Glasgow Coma Scale**

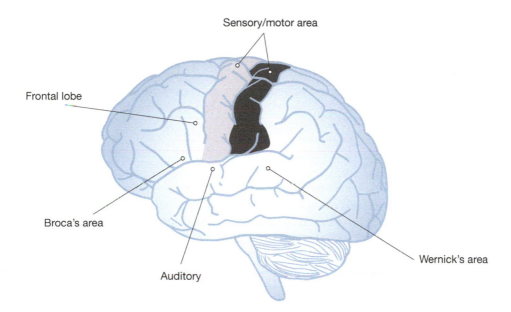

Figure 17.3 **Areas of the brain assessed by the Glasgow Coma Scale**

A genuine score of 8 or below implies such severe impairment of consciousness that the patient may not be able to protect their own airway, so should be urgently reviewed by an anaesthetist for possible intubation (Riley and de Beer, 2014). A decrease of 2 or more between assessments suggests significant deterioration, so should urgently be reported to medical staff.

Over four decades of use, the GCS has established itself as a simple and useful assessment. However, inevitably there are limitations: see table 17.1.

Table 17.1 Limitations of Glasgow Coma Scale assessment

- It combines three assessments; two patients may have identical scores for different reasons, and with different prognoses. The eye score is a poorer predictor of mortality that either the motor or verbal scores (Teoh *et al*, 2000); although aggregate scores may be recorded, charts record the three elements separately.
- Scores indicate level of consciousness only at the time of assessment, so repeat assessments should be timed to minimise risk of significant deterioration escaping notice.
- Verbal responses are problematic with dysphasia, aphasia, or intubation.
- Some elements of scoring are subjective (such as the difference between confusion and inappropriate words), resulting in potential inconsistency between different users (Green, 2011).

Pupil reaction

Not part of GCS, but usually scored on the same charts, is pupil reaction. Pupil size and response are controlled through the third cranial nerve (occulomotor), so any abnormality indicates a problem with this nerve, such as displacement of the hemispheres, or the brain-stem.

Normally, pupils dilate rapidly in darkness and constrict rapidly in light, with both pupils remaining equal in size. Pupils should be observed for

- size (in millimetres)
- equality (PE)
- reaction to light (RTL).

Dilated, fixed or unequal pupils indicate intracranial hypertension (Waterhouse, 2005), although one fifth of people normally have unequal pupils (Patil and Dowd, 2000). Pupil size and reaction may be affected by drugs, such as opioids (which constrict) and atropine (which dilates). Atropine, which may have been used to treat bradycardia from excessive vagal tone (Resuscitation Council, 2010), has a half-life of two hours.

The next stage assesses pupil response. Pupils normally constrict with light, so any bright overhead lighting should be turned off, and if sunlight is bright, curtains/blinds may need to be closed. Assessors should check lights used for testing are sufficiently bright to stimulate a reliable response. The patient's eyes should initially be covered, to allow pupils to dilate. This can often be achieved by asking patients to close their eyes, and then open them, but sometimes nurses may need to shade the patient's eyes with their hand. Once pupils have had time to dilate, the light should then be shone from the side to the centre of the open eye:

- Do the pupils react to light?
- Is reaction normal (brisk) or slow?
- Is reaction equal in both pupils?

Traumatic brain injury (TBI)

Each year, 1.4 million people are admitted to UK A&Es with head injury (NICE 2014b). It is the leading cause of death in younger (aged under 45 years) people (Messer *et al.*, 2012), and even mild injury leaves evidence of damage after four months (Ling *et al.*, 2013). All patients needing hospital admission should therefore be transferred to specialist centres (Andrews *et al.*, 2008).

With head injury, some damage may not be visually obvious, and not initially diagnosed. If the base of the skull is fractured, cerebrospinal fluid (CSF) may leak from orifices, such as the nose (*rhinorrhoea*) or ear (*otorrhoea*). CSF leak is often accompanied by blood, leaving distinct stains of a yellow ring (CSF) around blood-stains on linen – the 'halo' sign (March and Hickey, 2014b). There may also be visible bruising around the eyes ('racoon eyes' (Venkatesh, 2014)) or behind the ear ('battle sign') (March and Hickey, 2014b). If base of skull fracture is suspected, tubes such as airways or gastric tubes should be passed orally, and not nasally, as nasal insertion could pass through fractures into the brain. Base of skull fracture exposes the patient to risks of meningitis, so doctors should be informed urgently.

Possible *short-term* complications of head injury include

- pyrexia;
- hypermetabolism;
- diabetes insipidus – polyuria caused by lack of antidiuretic hormone production;
- SIADH – syndrome of inappropriate antidiuretic hormone, causing oliguria and fluid retention;
- labile blood glucose.

Longer-term complications include

- headache
- dizziness
- balance problems
- irritability
- memory loss.

(Terrio *et al.*, 2009)

While most symptoms eventually subside, irritability and memory loss often persist (Terrio *et al.*, 2009). Psychiatric problems increase risks of early mortality (Fazel *et al.*, 2014).

Spinal cord injury

Damage to spinal nerves causes actual or potential loss of function below the injury. Injury between cervical verebrae1 and thoracic 1 usually causes tetraplegia, while damage between thoracic 2 and lumbar 1 usually causes paraplegia. The main immediate risk is spinal shock, which usually occurs immediately or within hours of injury (Hoffman and Hausman, 2013) – see Chapter 13. Severe pain and spasticity are common (Harvey, 2008). Patients should therefore be transferred urgently to a spinal injuries unit.

Strokes

Strokes are the third largest cause of death and the single biggest cause of disability in the UK (Raithatha *et al.*, 2013). They are often preceded by transient ischaemic attacks (TIAs) (RCP, 2012b). Strokes are either

- ischaemic (80%)
- haemorrhagic (20%).

(Lip and Beevers, 2007; Raithatha *et al.*, 2013)

Most haemorrhagic strokes are from intracerebral bleeds, but one quarter are from sub-arachnoid haemorrhage, typically from rupture of a 'berry aneurysm' of the Circle of Willis. Most acute hospitals have on-site stroke units and teams, to whom patients should be fast-tracked. These teams will urgently arrange CT scans, to determine whether the stroke is ischaemic or haemorrhagic.

Ischaemic strokes are usually treated by *thrombolysis* with recombinant tissue plasminogen activator (rt-PA; brand name Alteplase™); tissue plasminogen activator is a thrombolytic chemical released by vascular endothelium. Thrombolysis reduces mortality (Putaala *et al.*, 2009; IST-3 Collaborative Group, 2012) and post-stroke disability (Lackland *et al.*, 2013). 2012 UK criteria for stroke thrombolysis are

- within 3 hours of stroke for any patient
- within 4.5 hours for any patient under 80 years of age
- within 6 hours, patients should be assessed on an individual basis.

(RCP, 2012b)

With haemorrhagic stroke, bleeding needs stopping, necessitating urgent intervention in, and so transfer to, a neurological centre. The preferred treatment is endovascular coiling (inserting a platinum coil into an aneurysm); alternatively, bleeding points are surgically ligated ('clipping'). With intervention, most survive a first bleed, but a second bleed has very poor prognosis. Other early complications include vasospasm and hydrocephalus. Both procedures entail risks, but ten-year survival is higher with endovascular coiling (Molyneux *et al.*, 2014).

Up to 30% of patients may rebleed within ten days, rebleed mortality being about 70% (Buckley and Hickey, 2014); during this time the patient may be transferred back to the primary hospital. Systolic blood pressure should be maintained consistently below 140 mmHg (Manning *et al.*, 2014), so for the first 21 days following neurosurgery patients should be prescribed *nimodipine*, a calcium channel blocker which crosses the blood–brain barrier, unless there are specific contraindications (RCP, 2012b). As nimodipine is given to prevent cerebral vasospasm, it should be given even if the patient is not systemically hypertensive.

One third of people with strokes suffer depression, anxiety, fatigue and apathy (Hackett *et al.*, 2013), so nursing care and psychological support can significantly improve outcome. Subarachnoid haemorrhage has especially poor outcomes, with one half of people suffering long-term physical and cognitive deficits (RCP, 2012b), and only one third returning to work (NCEPOD, 2013).

Epilepsy

Epilepsy may present in various ways (see Table 17.2). Patients may experience an 'aura', and be able to forewarn staff of impending fits, and from previous experience, patients or carers may alert staff to likely effects of fits. Otherwise, progression of fits is unpredictable, so help should be summoned. Priority is to ensure safety and privacy – are they at risk from harming themselves during the fit either by falling or from hard/sharp surfaces? Fits may cause apnoea and/or loss of gag reflex, so the airway should be kept clear – excessive saliva and any vomit should be removed; if the patient is not fully conscious, insert a guedel airway if it is safe to do so. High concentration oxygen should be given (such as 15 litres via a non-rebreathe mask). Anti-epileptic medication should be given as soon as possible. Visitors and other patients should be reassured.

Table 17.2 Classification of types of epileptic seizures

- tonic-clonic – loss of consciousness, stiffening, forced expiratory cry, rhythmic jerking, clenching of teeth and single or double incontinence
- clonic – symmetrical, bilateral semi-rhythmic jerking, possible loss of bladder/bowel control
- tonic – sudden increase in tone and forced expiration
- myoclonic – sudden brief body jerks
- atonic ('drop attacks') – sudden loss of tone, falls
- absence

(After Arbour, 2013)

Spasticity

Neurological problems can cause spasticity (Woodward and Waterhouse, 2009) so early prevention should be initiated by:

- physiotherapy and occupational therapy
- active/passive exercises
- positioning
- removing stimuli which reduce muscle tone (e.g. constipation).

Neglect during the acute phase may prolong or limit rehabilitation.

Prognosis

Recovery from neurological problems can be long, and too often incomplete (Klein *et al.*, 2013). This can prove frustrating for both patients and their families, so much psychological support will be needed. Patient and family motivation improves outcome (Langhorne *et al.*, 2011), so discharge planning should begin on admission, with early discussion about prognosis. During recovery, and if it remains incomplete, family often become carers, so involving them in care enables them to develop skills they may need later. Once patients are sufficiently stable, they should be transferred to specialist units.

Primary damage is largely irreversible, but much secondary damage may be preventable. Nursing care, together with input from professions allied to medicine, can make significant differences to outcome. For the future, animal studies suggest that in future stem cell transplants may be able to cure diseases and complications which are currently irreversible (Osanai *et al.*, 2012).

Implications for practice

- Cerebral perfusion pressure is mean arterial pressure less intracranial pressure, so in the absence of intracranial pressure monitoring, aim to keep MAP above 85 mmHg.
- Outcome is improved if patients are transferred to specialist centres, so immediate priority is stabilisation for transfer.
- Recovery is often prolonged, and too often incomplete, so planning for discharge and rehabilitation should begin on admission.
- Good nursing care, including positioning and exercises, can do much to reduce complications.

Summary

Initial care should focus of stabilisation and preventing secondary harm – primarily by ensuring oxygenation and perfusion of the brain and other vital organs. Allowing for resistance to cerebral blood flow from potentially raised intracranial pressure, target mean atrial pressure target should initially be 85–90 mmHg. Early discharge planning, with patient and family involvement, improves outcome.

Support groups

There are support groups for most neurological pathologies, including

- Headway
- Stroke Association

Further reading

Hickey (2014) remains the key text for neurological nursing. National guidelines include RCP (2012b, scheduled for review 2016) and NICE (2014b). NCEPOD (2013) provides a succinct overview of subarachnoid haemorrhage. Woodward and Waterhouse (2009) is a useful handbook.

Clinical scenario

Barbara Jackson, 82 year of age, collapsed 4 hours ago with a suspected stroke. She has a past medical history of hypertension and has recently experienced 'dizzy spells'. On admission to A&E her vital signs are

HR 54 bpm
RR 23 bpm
T 35.4°C
BP 105/82 (MAP 90) mmHg
SpO_2 100%

An ECG shows first degree heart block. Her speech is incoherent, but she opens her eyes to sounds. She has been incontinent of a large amount of urine, which does not smell offensive. Her next of kin is her younger, and only, sister, with whom she lives; her sister does not accompany Mrs Jackson.

1   You are caring for Mrs Jackson in A&E. Using A-B-C-D-E assessment, identify your five main concerns. What nursing care would you plan to meet these needs?
2   Analyse her haemodynamic status. What do you think may be the reason for her first degree heart block? Is it significant at present? Do you have any other concerns about her haemodynamic status? If so, why?
3   What medical interventions and investigations would you expect the doctors to initiate?

Chapter 18

Psychological needs

Contents

Introduction

Chapter 1 identified links between physiology and psychology, via the stress response. Positive psychological care is desirable not just for humanitarian reasons, but also because it can help reduce stress responses that so often complicate acute disease.

Confusion and delirium occur in many acutely ill patients, especially older people (Amador and Goodwin, 2005; Olin *et al.*, 2005; Siddiqi *et al.*, 2006; Lloyd *et al.*, 2012), increasing vulnerability, morbidity and mortality (Pandharipande *et al.*, 2013). Caring for confused patients is challenging, especially in busy acute general medical/surgical wards. This chapter explores strategies for recognising and reducing delirium, but sometimes delirium can be prevented by providing quality holistic care.

Confusion may have many causes, including physiological imbalances from hypoxia, hypotension, neurotoxins, hyper/hypo-glycaemia (Hare *et al.*, 2008; Sendelbach and Guthrie, 2009). Obvious physiological imbalances should be treated, and other possible physiological causes investigated, such as pain and bowel function (Anderson, 2005; Bienvenu *et al.*, 2012). A-B-C-D-E assessment (see Chapter 2) is recommended, which should maintain safety by identifying any immediate risks. Once safety has been ensured, and physiological causes excluded, psychological causes should be assessed. If physiological and psychological causes have been excluded, the cause is probably organic – damage to the organ of the brain, such as one of the dementias.

Psychology is a speciality in its own right; this chapter cannot hope to comprehensively analyse psychological care in acute wards. Instead, it aims to increase awareness of key problems and suggest actions that are achievable within realities of general nursing practice.

Delirium

Delirium, acute confusion, may be

- hyperactive
- hypoactive
- mixed (sometimes hyperactive, sometimes hypoactive).

Hyperactive delirium is usually fairly easy to identify – the person behaves out of character in extrovert and bizarre ways, or says bizarre things. Unfortunately most deliriums are hypoactive (Lloyd *et al.*, 2012), where the person withdraws into themselves, and is quiet and passive. Hypoactive delirium is often unrecognised (Eeles *et al.*, 2010), especially on busy wards. As well as being undesirable, delirium increases morbidity, such as progression to dementia, and mortality (Eeles *et al.*, 2010; Ehlenbach *et al.*, 2010; Witlox *et al.*, 2010; McCusker *et al.*, 2011; Pandharipande *et al.*, 2013).

Ahmed *et al.* (2014) found commonest risk factors for delirium were

- dementia
- older age
- co-morbidities
- severity of illness
- infection
- 'high-risk' medication
- diminished activities of daily living
- immobility
- sensory impairment
- urinary catheterisation
- urea and electrolyte imbalance
- malnutrition.

Not all of these are modifiable, but many modifiable aspects such as nutrition should be met by basic physiological care, and are discussed in other chapters.

Tiredness

Sleep and fatigue are worse in hospitalised patients than in healthy people (Ünsal and Demir, 2012). While some causes, such as disease, are unavoidable, modifiable reasons may include

- noise
- pain
- fear
- strange environments
- excessive ambient light.

Sleep deprivation can impair immunity, exacerbate disease and increase mortality (Bollinger *et al.*, 2010). Nightingale (1859/1960 p.5) described unnecessary noise as 'the most cruel absence of care'. Noise contributes to disturbed sleep and cardiovascular disease (Basner *et al.*, 2014). Duty of care often conflicts with facilitating sleep (Eyres *et al.*, 2012), but unnecessary noise should be removed, and necessary noise should be minimised – for example, telephone volume should be turned down. Devices such as earplugs (Richardson *et al.*, 2007) and eyemasks (Daneshmandi *et al.*, 2012) can help reduce disturbing sensory inputs. Many patients need night sedation to help them sleep in hospitals; as with all medicines, effectiveness of night sedation should be assessed, including through discussion with the patient.

Managing confusion

A commonly cited nursing approach to managing confusion is reality orientation (Marques *et al.*, 2014), such as orientating patients to time and place. As well as verbal orientation, these may be achieved environmentally through clear and large signs and clocks, or though decorations. At the right time and in the right quantity reality orientation is beneficial (Marques *et al.*, 2014). But it would be both naive and dangerous to treat every patient admitted to your ward with furosemide; to adopt identical psychological strategies of care is equally illogical. Reality orientation can cause distress, increasing risk of coronary heart disease (Todaro *et al.*, 2003).

Many strategies used in mental healthcare can be time-consuming and impractical for general wards. But understanding patient experiences and perspectives can help develop empathy. One way to achieve this is through transactional analysis – literally analysing transactions (or interaction) between people. Transactional analysis identifies three main roles each person can take in an interaction:

- parent
- adult
- child.

Some roles have further sub-classifications, but broadly the parent tells or commands, adults share and discuss but ultimately make up their own minds and respect others' rights to differ, while the child obeys. In most healthcare situations adult to adult relationships are promoted; for example, nurses may provide patients with information about options, accepting that patients have the right to choose options they would not choose for themselves. However, in some situations parent/child relationships become preferable: for example, during a cardiac arrest someone needs to take overall charge, directing actions of the rest of the team. Whichever is desirable for the situation, adult/adult and parent/child are both stable. Other interactions are unstable, either resolving into one of the two stable interactions, or provoking conflict.

Time out 18.1

In an environment outside your workplace, observe how two people, or two groups of people, interact. Note what roles they adopt, and how effective those roles are. How might other roles have been adopted, and what result do you think they might have had?

Repeat this exercise in your work area.

The value of transactional analysis is that it helps us understand subsequent responses and behaviour – people respond to the way they are treated. You have probably heard someone say 'if they treat me like a child, I'll behave like a child'. Parsons (1951) identified how acceptance of the 'sick role' by patients can contribute to progression of diseases; similarly, Kitwood (1997, p.46) suggested 'malignant social psychology' is 'deeply damaging to personhood . . . undermining physical well being', or as Seligman (1975) observed people treated as helpless learn to become helpless. Approaching patients through adult to adult relationships, respecting them as individuals in their own right, therefore empowers their independence and promotes recovery.

Isolation

Some diseases necessitate physical isolation, either to protect the patient who is isolated (e.g. neutropenia) or to protect other patients from contagion. Isolation may also be social – reflect on the last patient you nursed who had head lice, and how you and other people felt about the patient.

Isolation (barrier nursing) may be necessary to reduce infection risks, but it also reduces social interaction (Maben, 2009), and can result in avoidable physiological harm, such as falls (Maben, 2009).

Sensory balance

Our cerebral cortex makes sense of our environment through information from our five senses (sight, hearing, touch, taste, smell).

Time out 18.2

As soon as you have read this exercise, close your eyes and focus on what you can hear, feel and smell. After a few minutes, open your eyes, and list sensory inputs.

At an early opportunity, repeat this exercise in your work area, having positioned yourself safely out of harm's way. It should only take a few minutes to compile a reasonable list of workplace sensory inputs. Note any phrases you hear colleagues use that might confuse patients. At leisure, compare the two lists.

If rubbish is fed into a computer, it is likely to produce rubbish; similarly, disordered sensory inputs to the cerebral cortex are likely to produce delirium. Disordered inputs may be due to physiological impairment (for example acute hearing loss caused by absence of hearing aids or ototoxic drugs, such as intravenous furosemide or gentamicin being given too quickly), or psychological factors (such as unfamiliar environments or loss of status).

Disordered sensory input can have harmful effects, provoking stress responses. But senses can be used positively. For example, Henricson *et al.* (2008) found that caring touch, such as a reassuring holding of hands, reduces sympathetic nervous system activity (stress responses). However, what one person finds comforting, another may find threatening (Davidhizer and Giger, 1997). Touch, or use of other senses, should therefore be individualised to each person.

Sensory information is processed by the reticular activating system, part of the medulla oblongata in the brain-stem. This filters stimuli, blocking nearly all inputs to prevent sensory overload and maintains sanity (Marieb and Hoehn, 2013). Reticular activating system function may be impaired by:

- reduced sensory input
- repetitive stimulation
- relevance deprivation
- unconsciousness.

(O'Shea, 1997)

Hallucinogenic drugs, such as LSD, also impair the reticular activating system (Marieb and Hoehn, 2013).

Awareness of potential psychological problems is an important first step, enabling nurses to observe for signs of stressors. But major barriers to person-centred care are lack of time (West *et al.*, 2005) and inadequate staffing (Williams and Irurita, 2004; McHugh and Chenjuan, 2013). Optimising sensory input and reassuring human contact should be part of care (Bienvenu *et al.*, 2012), and every bed area should receive natural daylight (DOH, 2013). Delirium may be caused by withdrawal from alcohol, nicotine or illicit drugs; these causes can be treated pharamacologicly.

While drugs should not be the first-choice therapy for delirium, they may be necessary to prevent harm (NICE, 2010d). Haloperidol is the most widely used drug to manage acute agitation (Borthwick *et al.*, 2006), although it only modifies behaviour, not the duration of delirium (Page *et al.*, 2013).

Relatives

Relatives and significant others are part of the team. Bergbom and Askwall (2000) found presence of relatives gave patients the courage to struggle for survival. They can also provide some simple aspects of care that nurses may not have time to give, such as helping patients with meals (check local policies before allowing relatives to assume tasks).

RIGHTS

Confused people have the same rights as other patients, but may be vulnerable if not able to assert their rights. Three illustrations are included here:

- consent
- restraint
- children.

Consent

In law, no-one else has the right to give consent for a mentally competent adult (DOH, 2009). However, impaired consciousness or other factors may prevent patients being able to make decisions. The NMC (2015) expects nurses to act in patients' best interests at all times, and that nurses must get properly informed consent before carrying out any action. Legal expectations are clarified by the five key principles of the Mental Capacity Act (Parliament, 2005):

- Staff must presume patients have the capacity to make decisions until proven otherwise.
- Staff must support people to make their own decisions using 'all practical means'.
- Staff must not treat people as lacking capacity to make decisions because their decision is unwise.
- Patients' best interests are paramount.
- Decisions by others must interfere least with rights and freedom of action of those lacking capacity.

Restraint

Safety is fundamental. If force is used against a patient, it must be proportional to the likelihood and seriousness of harm (Musters, 2010). Unreasonable force could result in loss of registration, and actions in both criminal and civil courts. Cotsides may be viewed as restraints if patients have not consented to their use. If used with confused patients, cotsides may be perceived as imprisonment, provoking an urge to escape, and so increasing risks of falls (Tzeng and Yin, 2012). There are times restraint is necessary to maintain safety, but restraint should be a last resort (RCN, 2008c). Sedatives, such as haloperidol, are chemical restraint (BACCN, 2004).

Children

The Children's Act (1989) and the Fraser Guidelines of 1982–5 which followed the Gillick civil case established the principle that children generally have the right to make their own decisions if they have mental competence to do so (Dimond, 2011). This can cause complex dilemmas. In areas such as A&E adult care nurses are sometimes expected to care for children even though they are not qualified in paediatric care. There are however resources they can use: some colleagues may have paediatric qualifications; most hospitals have paediatric units; and most Trusts employ a legal department. So if faced with dilemmas about rights (or other aspects) of children, seek advice.

Implications for practice

- Good psychological care promotes physiological health.
- Good psychological care is patient-centred care.
- Optimise positive sensory input, especially (caring) touch.
- An important role of night nursing is to facilitate sleep.
- Relatives are usually a valuable support for patients, and should be supported to facilitate this role.
- Confused patients have the same rights as orientated ones, but may need advocates.

Summary

Acute wards are busy places, and nurses have to prioritise their workload, often having to sacrifice aspects of care that take lower priority. Too often psychological care is relegated to low priority. Nurses however have significant control over the ward environment, and can proactively optimise this to meet both physiological and psychological needs. Some aspects of psychological care, such as reassuring touch, can easily be incorporated into daily care without consuming significantly more time.

Further reading

Much has been written about psychology, often from specialist aspects. For acute care, Ouldred and Bryant (2011) review delirium, and NICE (2010d) have published guidance. Pritchard (2009) discusses preoperative assessment of anxiety.

Clinical scenario

Mr Albert Lloyd, aged 74, is admitted to your ward with community-acquired pneumonia. A widower, he lives independently in his own home, supported by frequent visits from his son and daughter. By day 4, blood results indicate he is responding well to antibiotics. However, since admission he has developed diarrhoea, so has been moved into a sideroom. He has become increasingly distressed, and on day 2 asked his family to stop visiting, although they continue to telephone the ward daily. He now appears to have developed a hypoactive delirium.

1   Assess Mr Lloyd's risk factors for delirium. How might these have been avoided or minimised if identified earlier?
2   Identify and list local resources to support care of patients with delirium.
3   Devise a care plan for Mr Lloyd's problem of delirium.

Chapter 19

Thermoregulation

Contents

Introduction

Pyrexia, and less often hypothermia, can be problems exacerbating, or even causing, disease. Hypothermia is also used therapeutically. Despite the frequency of these problems in many patients over many centuries, management of pyrexia, and often knowledge about it, remains suboptimal. This chapter focuses mainly on managing pyrexia, but also includes hypothermia (accidental and therapeutic). As with other chapters in this book, discussion assumes acutely ill adults. Management of pyrexia in children can differ; readers working in areas where children are admitted should read National Collaborating Centre for Women's and Children's Health (2013).

Normal temperature

Management of pyrexia remains strongly ritualistic (Scrase and Tranter, 2011). Pyrexia may have different causes, so it is illogical to treat all pyrexias in the same way. But even if causes are the same, costs to the individual patient may vary. So when managing pyrexia, the

Time out 19.1

1 Your patient has a temperature of 37.8°C. List actions you would initiate as a nurse, and any actions you would request other staff to initiate.
2 Think of the last time you had flu. List what you did for yourself.
3 Compare the two lists. There are probably very few similarities; if so, consider why you treat your patients differently from how you treat yourself.

- cause *and*
- cost

should be considered.

Normal temperature varies in different parts of the body. For example, the liver is normally the 'hot spot', as a major function of the liver is metabolism (see Chapter 26), and metabolism releases heat. Normal ranges for temperature therefore differ depending on site of measurement. Crawford *et al.* (2005) in a report for the DOH suggest normal ranges are:

- rectal 34.4–37.8°C
- axilla 35.5–37.0°C
- ear 35.6–37.4°C
- oral 36.0–37.6°C
- forehead 36.1–37.3°C
- core 36.8–37.9°C.

Extremes of temperature can be fatal. The hypothalamus, in the brain-stem, regulates body temperature, balancing heat gain and heat loss to maintain homeostasis. Brain-stem temperature is almost constant, normally varying no more than 0.5 °C (Faulds and Meekings, 2013). Body temperature is measured by thermoreceptors, specialised nerve endings that sense heat, located in most parts of the body, including the brain-stem; thermoreceptors in our skin make us sentitive to ambient temperature. If more heat is needed, the hypothalamus initiates heat-conservation and heat-production mechanisms:

- peripheral vasoconstriction
- shivering (muscle work produces heat)
- arrector pili (hairs rise on skin trapping heat in air pockets – 'goosebumps').

If heat loss is needed

- peripheries vasodilate (more heat reaches skin surfaces)
- sweat glands are activated

and so heat is lost through evaporation. In addition, the cerebral cortex initiates behavioural responses, such as putting on more clothing if cold. The hypothalamus primarily ensures brain-stem temperature remains constant, and therefore temperatures elsewhere, especially skin temperature, can vary significantly.

Thermometers

Many types of thermometer are commercially available; most clinical thermometers are reliable (Sessler, 2008). The ideal temperature site would be the hypothalamus, but as this is impractical, any site used is an approximation to brain-stem temperature. Like other equipment, thermometers can malfunction; any suspected of inaccuracy should be tested by the hospital's medical engineers. Suspect readings may also be due to user error, so staff should be familiar with how to use equipment, and remeasure if inaccuracy is suspected.

Pyrexia (hyperthermia)

The two common causes of pyrexia in hospitalised patients are

- metabolism *and*
- infection.

A less common possibility is

- hypothalamic damage (e.g. from head injury or intracranial pathology).

All cells need energy, which they produce through metabolism, normally glycolysis. Metabolism produces heat, which is transported by blood. Increased cell work increases heat production – exercising skeletal muscle can increase metabolic rate twentyfold (Marieb and Hoehn, 2013). Tissue repair increases metabolic rate, so post-operative pyrexias commonly occur (Barone, 2009), usually low-grade (<38.3°C). Similarly, blood transfusions commonly cause low-grade (metabolic) pyrexia.

Infection normally triggers defensive inflammatory responses. Activation of T cells (lymphocytes, a sub-group of white cells) releases pyrogenic cytokines, especially tumour necrosis alpha (TNFa) and pro-inflammatory interleukins (IL-1, 6, 8 and 10). These pro-inflammatory mediators stimulate prostaglandin production, and prostaglandin resets the hypothalamus (Bleeker-Rovers *et al.*, 2009). The reset hypothalamus attempts to achieve a higher body temperature (Faulds and Meekings, 2013), which is why infections make us feel cold and shiver. Peripheral cooling, by removing blankets and using fans, is likely to distress the pyrexial patient who feels cold and shivery, inducing a stress response, with all its negative sequelae; but peripheral cooling is also likely to stimulate heat production, needing more energy (glucose and oxygen) and producing more waste (carbon dioxide, metabolic acids, water). If the person is malnourished, or has respiratory or renal limitations, the increased cost from cooling is likely to worsen their condition.

So with metabolic pyrexia we feel hot and want to cool ourselves down, with infective pyrexia we feel cold and want to be warmer. Not all pyrexias are caused by infection.

However, infective pyrexias are mediated through inflammatory responses, and if the immune system is impaired through age (Woodford, 2010), drugs or disease (Varghese *et al.*, 2010), pyrexia may not occur with infection. Generally, metabolic pyrexias are below 38.3°C, whereas infective pyrexias are high, which is why the American Society of Critical Care Medicine considers a clinically significant temperature to be above 38.3°C (Isaac and Taylor, 2003; Dellinger *et al.*, 2013).

As the hypothalamus regulates temperature, hypothalamic damage (e.g. from head injury) usually disrupts thermoregulation, typically causing extreme, and sometimes fatal, pyrexia.

Pyrexia itself has both benefits and burdens. It accelerates chemical reactions, increasing antibody production, assisting cell repair, and destroying bacteria (Scrase and Tranter, 2011). But increased metabolism brings the costs of needing more nutrients, oxygen and waste clearance. And while heat damages rapidly replicating bacterial protein, it also damages the body's own protein, which in malnourished patients may cause significant muscle wasting. Each rise of 1°C increases chemical reactions by 10% (Marieb and Hoehn, 2013).

Pyrexia is an adaptive response, not an illness. The cause of pyrexia should be investigated, and the cost considered. If burdens exceed benefits, then the pyrexia should be reversed. Infective pyrexias are caused by prostaglandin changing the hypothalamic setting. Central cooling, halting prostaglandin synthesis, can usually be achieved with paracetamol, aspirin, or non-steroidal anti-inflammatory drugs (NSAIDs – see Chapter 20) (Malaise *et al.*, 2007; Barrett *et al.*, 2010).

Infective pyrexia may be due to sepsis; is sepsis is suspected, blood cultures should be taken within 45 minutes, and broad-spectrum antibiotics given within one hour (Dellinger *et al.*, 2013). In your list from Time out 19.1, you probably gave yourself drinks, but not your patient. Perspiration from pyrexia, and tachypnoea, increase fluid loss, so drinks or intravenous fluids will be needed, unless a fluid restriction order is in place. There may also be electrolyte imbalances and metabolic acidosis, so the patient should be medically reviewed.

Hyperpyrexia (>40°C) can damage the protein of the central nervous system – the brain. As thermoregulation fails, pyrexia becomes fatal at about 43°C (Marieb and Hoehn, 2013). Hyperpyrexia is a medical emergency, and help should be summoned urgently.

Pyrexia may therefore be staged

- 37.0–38.3°C: low grade, probably metabolic;
- 38.4–39.9°C: high grade, probably from infection, especially sepsis;
- 40.0°C and above: hyperpyrexia, a life-threatening medical emergency.

Hypothermia

Hypothermia is a temperature below 36°C (American Society of PeriAnesthetic Nurses, 2001). It is sometimes classified into

- mild: 32–36°C
- moderate: 28–31.9°C
- severe: <28°C.

Like pyrexia, hypothermia has both benefits and burdens. Each reduction of one degree reduces cerebral metabolic rate 6–7% (Bernard and Buist, 2003), so may be neuroprotective in potentially hypoxic situations. It also reduces production of the toxic radical hydrogen peroxide (H_2O_2) (Kuffler, 2012). Therapeutic hypothermia (target 32°C–34°C) has been recommended for cardiac arrest (NICE, 2011b; Nunnally et al., 2011) on the basis of studies which showed improved survival. However, Nielsen et al. (2013) found no improvement in survival, and the value of therapeutic hypothermia is now questioned.

Burdens of hypothermia include vasoconstriction, causing metabolic acidosis, and with temperatures below 30°C a high risk of cardiac dysrhythmias (Bourdages et al., 2010). Hypothermia with traumatic brain injury can cause damage detectable after four months (Ling et al., 2013). Therapeutic hypothermia with bacterial meningitis increases mortality (Mourvillier et al., 2013).

Implications for practice

- Treat the patient, not the thermometer (Marik, 2000).
- Managing pyrexia needs individual assessment (cause, cost).
- Not all pyrexias are caused by infection; not all infections cause pyrexia.
- Use peripheral cooling (e.g. fans) only if patients find it comfortable.
- Infection needs antibiotics (after blood cultures if sepsis is suspected).
- The use of therapeutic hypothermia is controversial; readers should check local policies.

Summary

In health, the hypothalamus autoregulates body temperature to maintain homeostasis. In ill-health, autoregulation may become disordered, exposing the body to pyrexias which may be beneficial or harmful. Traditional approaches to pyrexia, and hypothermia, have been largely rooted in ritualistic practice. The cause, and cost, of each should be individually assessed to enable delivery of evidence-based care.

Further reading

Physiology of thermoregulation can be reviewed from anatomy and physiology texts. Many nursing articles over many years have highlighted the same ritualistic practice; Scrase and Tranter (2011) is a recent, and useful, review. Readers should be familiar with NICE (2011b), but also the more recent conflicting evidence of Nielsen et al. (2013).

Clinical scenario

Mr Bruce Maddox, aged 52, had a laproscopic cholecystectomy yesterday. He had no significant medical history apart from recent vomiting and colicky pain. Post-operatively, his temperature has been consistently about 37.4°C. Other vital signs were within normal limits yesterday, but he had now developed a tachycardia of 118 beats per minute (regular).

1   List possible reasons for (a) a metabolic and (b) an infective pyrexia. Compare your lists; which do you think caused his pyrexia? What actions would you take, and why?
2   Today's bloods show a fall in haemoglobin, from115 grams/litre to 75. He did not received significant volumes of intravenous fluids, and is now drinking. He is prescribed two units of blood over two hours each, but by the time of the second unit his temperature has risen to 38.2°C. What actions would you take now, and why?
3   How would you explain to a junior member of staff, or a student, your actions in each of the situations above?

Chapter 20

Acute pain management

Contents

Fundamental knowledge

- Nerve conduction (including A and C fibres)
- Gate Control theory (Melzack and Wall)
- The meaning of 'half life'

Introduction

Acute pain may be caused by disease or treatments. Pain is undesirable for obvious humanitarian reasons. But pain also impairs recovery, increasing morbidity and, potentially, mortality. Detrimental effects of pain can include

- insomnia (Pasero and Stannard, 2012)
- anxiety and depression
- reluctance to mobilise
- reluctance to breathe deeply
- stress responses, which has many undesirable physiological effects, including delaying healing.

Effective pain management is essential to achieve and maintain patient comfort and good clinical outcomes (Pasero and McCaffery, 2011), and is therefore a core aspect of nursing. Yet acute pain is often under-recognised and under-treated (Bell and Duffy, 2009; Hartog *et al.*, 2010; Wu and Raja, 2011).

Pain is often divided between acute and chronic. This chapter describes acute pain management. While there are many differences, there is inevitably some overlap, and patients with acute pain problems may also suffer chronic pain. This chapter focuses on pathophysiology of acute pain, although includes some discussion of more commonly used analgesics for acute pain management. It can neither discuss all options, nor every aspect of drugs mentioned. Most Trusts have pain management services, so problems beyond the skills and knowledge of ward staff should be escalated to appropriate services.

What is pain?

For nurses, the most familiar definition of pain is likely to be Pasero and McCaffery's (2011) description of pain being whatever the patient says it is. While this usefully emphasises the individual nature of each person's pain, and the importance of listening to what they say, it approaches being a non-definition. The International Association for the Study of Pain (1986) define pain as 'An unpleasant sensory and emotional experience associated with actual or potential tissue damage, or described in terms of such damage'. This emphasises physiological origin and value of pain as a defence mechanism. Acute tissue damage, or inflammatory responses, create pressure on nociceptors, the nerve endings that sense pain. Acute pain therefore should resolve once the injury has healed. But the IASP definition is problematic for chronic pain: unless tissue damage can be identified and reversed, chronic pain has no clear function. With acute pain, analgesics are often commenced at relatively high doses, which should be able to be titrated down as pain resolves; chronic pain usually persists, and so doses are commenced relatively low and titrated slowly up until effective (or abandoned).

Types of pain

Nociceptive pain occurs when signals travel from tissues through afferent pain-conducting nerves (*nociceptors*) to the brain. Such pain is generally a warning sign of tissue damage.

Neuropathic pain is caused by damage to central or peripheral nerves, but has little protective/warning function. Nerve damage may not be at the site of acute injury. It is often described as

- shooting
- tingling
- stabbing
- numb
- burning
- freezing
- throbbing
- aching
- stiff.

Neuropathic is relatively common, can occur quickly (within hours), may remain undiagnosed, and so inadequately treated. It occurs in up to 3% of patients seen by acute pain service (Hayes *et al.*, 2002), and nearly one fifth of trauma patients (Crombie *et al.*, 1998). When usual analgesics fail to relieve acute pain, neuropathic pain is involved. Analgesics such as pregabalin, gabapentin and amitryptaline are often useful (Joffe *et al.*, 2013). Doses are usually commenced low, and increased incrementally. Low-dose ketamine may be useful if pain persists despite more commonly used opioids (Visser and Schug, 2006; Chumbley, 2011).

Somatic pain from skin, muscles and joints often causes especially sharp pain, these tissues being rich in the A delta (Aδ) nerve fibres sending rapid signals to the brain. These nerve fibres usually localise the pain clearly, enabling patients to identify where pain originates. Somatic pain causes sharp responses, such as crying, screaming or cringing.

Visceral pain, from deeper tissues, is usually transmitted more slowly, and less specifically, through C fibres. Visceral pain usually persists longer, often causing guarding or defensive responses.

Referred pain occurs when nerve pathways remaining from embryo development transmit pain, which is sensed as originating from somewhere other than the damaged areas. Common, but not inevitable, examples of referred pain are

- liver → thoracic cavity
- gall bladder → shoulder
- bladder → back of legs
- cardiac → left side of jaw/left arm.

Phantom pain has long been recognised, but is sometimes too easily dismissed. Most limb amputees suffer pain 'in' the amputated limb (Richardson, 2008). Causes of phantom pain are debated; there may be psychological aspects, but nerve fibres to the amputated limb remain intact above the stump. Unfortunately, phantom limb pain seldom responds to treatment (Richardson, 2008), but neuropathic analgesics may help.

A psychological phenomenon

Pain signals travel to the cerebral cortex of the brain, which interprets them in contexts of previous experiences. Pain is the interpretation of these signals, not the signals themselves. So if signals can be interrupted before reaching the cerebral cortex, pain will not exist. Equally, if the cerebral cortex interprets other signals as painful, then pain exists. Melzack and Wall's (1988) Gate Control Theory suggests that low-grade stimulation of A delta (Aδ) signals in the dorsal horn of the spinal cord can relieve pain by blocking the 'gate' to C fibre signals. It is probable that scratching an itch, or using Transcutaneous Electrical Nerve Stimulation (TENS) relieves pain through this mechanism.

Assessing pain

Because pain is individual to each patient, each patient should be asked about their pain. Patients may not report pain because they

- do not want to appear 'weak'
- think busy staff have higher priorities
- expect to suffer pain
- have not been fully informed about ways to relieve pain.

(Pasero and McCaffery, 2011)

Many assessment tools are available, but most acute wards use tools based on numerical scales (such as 0–3 or 0–10, see Figures 20.1 and 20.2), where the lowest figure represents no pain, and the highest figure represents the worst pain imaginable. An advantage of the 0–3 scale is that it follows the WHO 'analgesia ladder' (see Figure 20.3).

This 'ladder' provides a simple step-by-step guide to increase, or decrease, analgesics.

The mnemonic SOCRATES has been developed to trigger assessors' memory of what to ask:

- **S**ite (where is the pain?)
- **O**nset (when did it start? how long ago?)
- **C**haracter (ask the patient of describe the pain)
- **R**adiation (where does it go?)
- **A**ssociations (how does the pain affect their lives: social, emotional, family, financial)
- **T**ime (does the pain follow a pattern over the day or longer period of time?)
- **E**xacerbating/relieving factors (does anything relieve the pain?)
- **S**everity score (ask how bad the pain is – see scales).

Whether such a lengthy and tenuous mnemonic is helpful will vary between users; the questions reflect those that should however be asked whenever assessing pain.

Alternative assessments for patients who cannot use verbal or visual rating scales include the Behaviour Pain Scale Tool (Young *et al.*, 2006); which uses such visual signs

0 = none at rest or on movement
1 = none at rest, slight on movement
2 = intermittent on rest, moderate on movement
3 = continuous at rest, severe on movement

Movement: ask patient to cough, observe facial expression and/or ask patient to try to touch the opposite side of the bed.

Figure 20.1 **0–3 pain score**

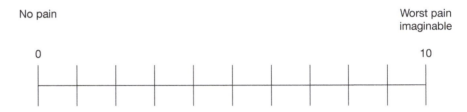

Figure 20.2 **0–10 scale**

as facial expression and position. Although not ideal assessments, other nonverbal signs may indicate pain:

- sudden hypertension and/or tachycardia
- position and other body language (e.g. immobility, guarding)
- interaction with, or information from, visitors.

(Murdoch and Larsen, 2004)

However, while acute pain typically stimulates the sympathetic nervous system to cause tachycardia and hypertension, sympathetic stimulation wanes with time, to be replaced by parasympathetic stimulation, which causes bradycardia and hypotension. Prolonged pain may therefore produce the opposite nonverbal signs to those usually expected. Nonverbal assessments, reviewed by Gelinas *et al.* (2013), can be useful, but bring dangers of imposing others' subjectivity to patient experiences.

Analgesics

Drugs are the main, although not only, means for relieving acute pain. Acute care nurses should therefore have reasonable knowledge about options available, including side effects and interactions, so they can request prescriptions of specific drugs (including drugs to alleviate side effects), and choose the most appropriate analgesic prescribed. Patients should be informed about benefits and side effects of drugs.

Many analgesics can be given through a variety of routes; the best route will be the one that achieves most effective analgesia with fewest risks/complications. Rapid analgesia

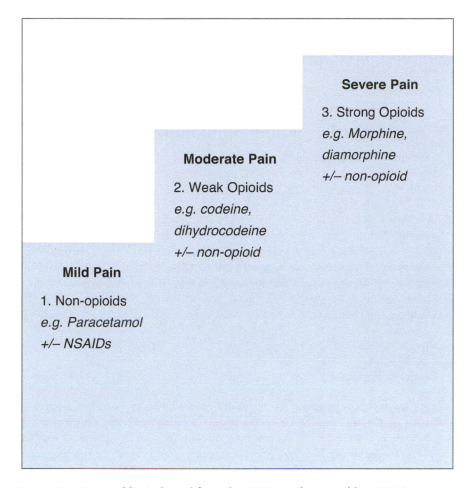

Figure 20.3 **Pain Ladder (adapted from the WHO Analgesic Ladder, 1996)**

can be achieved intravenously, but clearance (metabolism) and adverse effects are also more rapid. Potential respiratory depression from opioids usually restricts intravenous use to specialist, well-staffed areas. Transcutaneous patches take time to be absorbed (many are 24 hours, but time varies between drugs), so are not useful for acute pain. Multimodal pain relief is more effective (American Society of Anesthesiologists Task Force on Acute Pain Management, 2012), so many patients will be prescribed a number of different analgesics.

Opioids

Opioids act on specific receptors, mainly in the brain and spinal cord, which cause side effects such as

■ nausea (the most common)
■ constipation

- respiratory depression
- hypotension
- sedation
- urinary retention
- pruritis.

(Macintyre and Schug, 2007)

When opioids are prescribed

- reversal agents (e.g. naloxone)
- anti-emetics
- laxatives

should be routinely prescribed 'PRN'.

Naloxone (Narcan™) reverses opioids such as morphine, diamorphine, fentanyl and pethidine. While naloxone reverses serious side effects such as respiratory depression, it also reverses analgesia, so it should be given incrementally, and pain reassessed. Naloxone has a shorter half-life than opioids, so further doses may be needed to prevent return of serious side effects.

As well as being unpleasant, nausea and vomiting can cause

- stress responses
- dehydration
- electrolyte imbalance.

Although opioids reduce gut motility, opioid-induced nausea is mainly caused by stimulation of the vomiting centre in the brain (Golembiewski and O'Brien, 2002). So anti-emetics which primarily increase gut motility (e.g. metoclopramide) may not provide relief (Wigfull and Welchew, 2001). Anti-emetics which target the vomiting centre (e.g. ondansteron, prochlorperazine, cyclizine) are more effective, and may be given in combination with each other.

While opioids are potentially addictive, likelihood of developing addiction from short-term use for acute pain is remote. Generally, patients should be given the analgesia they need, without doses being withheld for fear of addiction.

Morphine remains the 'gold standard' opioid. Long-acting oral preparations (e.g. Zomorph®, OxyContin®) provide good background analgesia, while short-acting use ones (e.g. Oramorph®, OxyNorm®) are useful for breakthrough pain.

Diamorphine (heroin), a morphine-derivative that readily crosses the blood–brain barrier and so is more powerful, is rarely used in acute care in the UK.

Fentanyl is widely used for epidurals, and for transcutaneous patches. Viscusi *et al.* (2007) suggest that fentanyl patches are as effective as intravenous morphine, although can take up to 24 hours to become fully effective. Patches should remain in place for 72 hours. Compared with morphine, benefits include:

- reduced histamine release, so less pruritis (itching)
- less likely to cause hypotension
- less sedative.

Intravenous fentanyl, and fentanyl derivatives such as alfentanil, sufentanil and remi-fentanil, are used in surgery and critical care units where mechanical ventilation removes risks from respiratory depression.

Pethidine is generally less useful than other opioids as it

- is shorter acting (half-life 2–3 hours);
- produces the long-lasting neurotoxic metabolite norpethidine (Pasero and McCaffery, 2011);
- is highly addictive;
- provides no better pain relief than morphine (McQuay and Moore, 1998).

However, when other opioids prove problematic or ineffective, it may be worth considering.

Codeine is converted into morphine, although one fifth of Caucasians lack receptors to achieve this. Oral codeine phosphate (30 mg, 60 mg) is useful for moderate pain. It is also used to stop diarrhoea. Drugs such as co-codamol and co-dydramol contain some codeine, so nurses should be aware how much opioid drugs contain and be careful not to exceed maximum dose if mixing opioid-containing drugs.

Non-opioids

Although weaker than opioids, non-opioids have important roles in acute pain management. The World Health Organization (1996) recommends paracetamol for mild pain, and paracetamol combined with other non-steroidal anti-inflammatory drugs (NSAIDs) and/or opioids for moderate to severe pain.

Paracetamol

Paracetamol and NSAIDs are 'opioid sparing' (Maund *et al.*, 2011; American Society of Anesthesiologists Task Force on Acute Pain Management, 2012), reducing the amount of opioid needed for effective pain relief, and so reducing opioid-related side effects. Although a mild analgesic, regular paracetamol (1 gram, 6 hourly) should generally be prescribed whenever opioids are given. Some compound moderate analgesics, such as co-codamol, contain paracetamol, so paracetamol prescriptions should be adjusted to account for this. Although usually prescribed as maximum 4 grams daily, doses should be weight-related if patients weigh under 50 kg.

Non-steroidal anti-inflammatory drugs (NSAIDs)

Conventional NSAIDs (e.g. ibuprofen) may cause

- **G**astric ulceration/bleeding
- **R**enal impairment
- **A**sthma in up to one fifth of aspirin-sensitive asthmatics
- **B**leeding

Pregabalin, gabapentine, amitryptaline

These drugs are useful analgesics for neuropathic pain, but can also help reduce opioid need, and so reduce opioid side effects such as vomiting (Zhang *et al.*, 2011; Mishriky *et al.*, 2015). Pregabalin can cause visual disturbances (Zhang *et al.*, 2011).

Patient-controlled analgesia (PCA)

Intravenous, or subcutaneous, analgesics can be administered by patients themselves through PCA pumps. Giving patients control within maximum (dose, preset lock-out) limits, usually achieves better analgesia (Taylor, 2010). Morphine is the most widely used PCA opioid, although any injectable analgesic can be used. Typical regimes are 1 mg doses with 5 minutes lock-out.

PCA analgesia does not suit everybody. About 12% of patients find them difficult to use (Mackintosh, 2007). If patients are frightened to use PCA analgesia, encouragement is needed, with reassurance that overdose is almost impossible, as drowsiness from morphine would prevent them activating further doses. Neither staff nor relatives should ever activate delivery.

Patients receiving PCA analgesia should be closely monitored for:

- vital signs (respirations, oxygen saturation, pulse, blood pressure)
- level of consciousness
- nausea
- pain
- dose used.

Usually, observations should be made hourly. Many hospitals have specific charts and protocols for PCA analgesia. If possible, it is best not to nurse patients using PCAs in side rooms.

PCA analgesia may be needed for a few days. Infusions should be changed according to local protocols. When discontinued, suitable step-down analgesics should be prescribed – usually medium strength analgesics, with PRN opioid.

Epidurals

Epidural analgesia is usually the best way to relieve severe pain (Marret *et al.*, 2007), so often used following major surgery (Mackintosh, 2007). Epidurals usually mix opioids (morphine or fentanyl) with local anaesthetics (usually bupivacaine). Unfortunately one quarter of epidural catheters are misplaced (Ballantyne *et al.*, 2003); catheters can also migrate, especially if patients are mobile. This causes either insufficient block, or necessitates increased doses with increased risk of side effects. Epidurals usually run continuously, so overdose can occur. Patients receiving epidural analgesia should therefore be closely observed by staff familiar with epidural care.

Local anaesthetics can be neurotoxic and cause cardiovascular collapse/arrest. Signs of local anaesthetic toxicity include

- numbness around mouth/tongue
- light-headedness
- ringing in ears (tinnitus)
- slurring of speech
- muscle twitching
- drowsiness
- convulsions
- respiratory depression
- bradycardia, cardiac arrest.

If toxicity is suspected, an anaesthetist should be summoned urgently. There is no reversal agent for bupivacaine.

As with PCAs, most hospitals provide courses and protocols for managing epidurals. Observations (usually hourly) should include

- vital signs (respirations, oxygen saturation, pulse, blood pressure)
- level of consciousness
- nausea
- pain
- dose delivered
- level of block (usually tested by cold spray)
- checking the dressing is intact, not leaking (no wet sheets) and no signs of haematoma.

If epidurals cause hypotension, patients should not be placed head down, as this would cause drugs to flow down to the brain, with probably fatal results. Epidurals should be stopped if the block is too high, as it may cause respiratory failure:

- numb nipples = 4th thoracic vertebra (T4) block
- arm numbness or weakness = T1 block
- difficulty breathing = 5th cervical vertebra block.

Epidurals often cause hypotension (Weetman and Allison, 2006), which may need additional intravenous fluids. Hypotension and possible weakness/numbness make it advisable to use hoists the first time patients transfer from bed post-operatively. Initial mobilisation will usually be by physiotherapists. Epidural lines are incompatible with vascular devices, but catheters, lines and equipment must be clearly labelled to ensure drugs are not given into incorrect routes (NPSA, 2007b).

Most Trusts provide special training for epidurals, which readers caring for patients with epidurals should attend, as well as being familiar with local policies. Epidural use is usually limited to a maximum of four days, as infection risks rise significantly after this time. Insertion site haematoma, a rare complication, can cause fatal sepsis or meningitis (Darouiche, 2006). Prophylactic heparin should therefore not be given before and after removal of catheters; most hospitals have protocols for heparin omission. Catheter tips usually have distinctly-coloured tips (e.g. blue) – when removing the catheter check the tip is intact, and if in any doubt, inform the anaesthetist.

Non-pharmacological approaches

Analgesics, especially opioids, are the mainstay of acute pain management. But some pain may be relieved or reduced by simple comfort measures, such as

- smoothing creases in sheets
- relieving prolonged pressure
- turning pillows over
- placing limbs in a comfortable, well-supported position
- reducing noise and light
- touch, explanations, reassurance and empowerment strategies.

Patients with chronic pain may have developed strategies to ease it. Transcutaneous Electrical Nerve Stimulation (TENS), other complementary therapies (e.g. hot/cold pads, aromatherapy) and relieving anxieties (reassurance, relaxation, distraction) may help reduce discomfort. Hence the significance of asking patients what relieves pain.

Implications for practice

- Pain is a complex phenomenon involving both physiological transmission of pain signals and cognitive interpretation.
- Pain is individual to each person, so should be assessed individually.
- Promoting comfort and alleviating/minimising pain is fundamental to nursing care.
- Acute pain management often necessitates opioid drugs.
- Regular paracetamol should be prescribed with regular opioids.
- With NSAIDs, remember G-R-A-B.
- Consider also non-opioid and non-pharmacological ways to relieve pain.
- Evaluate effectiveness of pain relief, and observe for side effects.
- Causes of pain should be investigated.

Summary

Pain is unpleasant, but also has detrimental physiological effects, such as delaying healing, so pain should be relieved for both humanitarian and physiological reasons. Stoic endurance of pain is detrimental to health. Acute pain is frequently experienced by acutely ill patients, usually needing large initial doses which can be reduced as acute causes subside. Nurses should assess each patient's pain frequently, have sufficient working knowledge of commonly used analgesics to select the most appropriate pain relief, and know common side effects of analgesics. Readers should access local resources such as pain specialists and courses.

Acute pain often needs opioids, although non-opioid drugs can provide useful synergy with opioids, and non-pharmacological approaches should be considered. Patients with acute pain may have concurrent chronic pain, which may necessitate different management. Evaluating and documenting effectiveness of pain relief helps optimise its effect and minimise its complications.

Further reading

Classic texts on pain management that have recently been updated include Pasero and McCaffery (2011) and McMahon *et al.* (2013). There are many handbooks on acute pain management, such as Argoff and McCleane (2009); your local nursing library should stock a selection.

Clinical scenario

Mr Michael Newberg, aged 73, had an elective Hartmann's procedure (major bowel surgery) two days ago. Due to insufficient staffing levels, his fentanyl and bupivicaine epidural infusion was discontinued and the catheter removed overnight; he was prescribed regular codeine 60 mg with paracetamol 1 gram at 6 hourly intervals with as required intramuscular morphine 10 mg. On the morning ward round he admitted feeling pain, and was given a morphine injection. He also identified shoulder pain, for which he has since been given a heat pad. Now, two hours following the morphine injection, his respiration rate is only ten breaths per minute.

1 How would you assess Mr Newberg's pain? Identify the strengths and limitations of your preferred methods of assessment.
2 Evaluate the likely benefits and adverse effects of the various post-operative analgesics provided so far for Mr Newberg.
3 Identify changes for managing Mr Newberg's pain, together with the reasons for your recommendations and how you would evaluate their effectiveness.

Chapter 21

End-of-life care

Contents

Introduction

Acute care aims to provide treatments and cures for people with potentially life-threatening illness. But inevitably not all patients will survive. Hospice care is often viewed as optimal for the terminally ill, yet most people die in acute hospitals (NCEPOD, 2009a; Clark *et al.*, 2014), where preoccupations with treatment can too often result in terminal care we would not wish for ourselves or our loved one (Willard and Luker, 2006). This chapter explores three main themes surrounding death in acute hospitals:

1   Attitudes of nurses and other staff towards death. Some staff need support following death of patients. While patients may not be admitted for terminal care, life-saving treatment can become futile, unethical and unkind.

2   Treatment, including:
   - when and how such decisions should be made
   - what should be withdrawn and what should remain or be provided as part of palliative care.
3   Needs of patients, family and friends during and after terminal care.

Death in acute wards may be sudden, leaving people little time to adjust to impending loss. This creates unique needs that cannot always be met by theory and practice drawn from areas specialising in palliative care. Many issues and needs discussed do not significantly change, so although much literature cited is relatively old, it remains largely relevant.

A century ago, people were usually exposed to death at an early age; life expectancy was generally lower, people usually died at home, and dead bodies would usually remain at home until the funeral. Western societies have sanitised death. It is largely a taboo subject, few people being willing to discuss it, or face their own mortality. Most professional courses devote scant time to bereavement. When recovery becomes unlikely, prolonging life (or death) with futile heroics may become cruel.

Many researchers are understandably cautious about approaching bereaved families in case they increase or revive distress. Research-based evidence is therefore limited both in quantity and sample sizes, making findings more than usually tentative.

Death - a medical failure?

Prolonging life, rather than allowing patients to die, sometimes becomes the unreasonable option. However when to change from life-sustaining to life-withdrawing treatment is debatable, value-laden and fraught with ethical moral and sometimes legal dilemmas. Death has traditionally been viewed as a medical failure (Stringer, 2007). Medical and nursing values have traditionally been contrasted as cure versus care. While potentially over-simplistic, nurses may consider prolonging a person's life is immoral/unethical, and consider that their own status and professionalism are undermined if their views are ignored or over-ridden.

The patient . . .

For some, death is the beginning of an afterlife. But for many, death may bring psychological and/or spiritual pain and regrets that many staff may feel uncomfortable discussing. Palliative care teams and chaplains are usually more experienced in supporting people facing death than most nurses on general wards. Some patients wish to sort out their affairs before dying, such as making their will; it is unwise for nurses to witness patients' wills, and most employers discourage this.

Where possible, patients should be informed of their prognosis, and participate in discussion about end-of-life care (Leadership Alliance, 2014). Advance directives ('living wills') indicate patients' wishes, but advance directives are often either not made or not obviously available. Patients have a right to dignified care; they do not however have a right to futile treatment.

Unfortunately, acute illnesses causing terminal conditions may prevent people understanding explanations, or being able to make decisions. Where patients cannot be involved in decision making, requirements of the Mental Capacity Act (see Chapter 18) must be observed. In Scotland, the Adults with Incapacity Act (Parliament, 2000) has similar requirements.

Withdrawing treatment

When further life-prolonging treatment becomes inappropriate, comfort and dignity should become the focus of care. Decisions to withdraw life-prolonging treatment should be made by a team, ideally including the patient. The decision not to resuscitate ultimately rests with the most senior clinician currently in charge of the patient's care, but all staff caring for the patient should where reasonably possible contribute to the decision. Nurses therefore need sufficient knowledge and confidence to participate appropriately. Decisions to withdraw treatment involve individual values, morals and ethics.

Practices of withdrawing treatment vary greatly (Azoulay *et al.*, 2009; Leadership Alliance, 2014). Nurse advocacy requires nurses to ensure that decisions in which patients cannot (or do not) participate are in the patient's best interests and reflect the patient's, rather than someone else's, values.

Time out 21.1

Image you are acutely ill. You have been diagnosed as having life-threatening illness. Your doctor informs you that you have only a 20% chance of survival.

Would you wish life-prolonging treatment to be given?

At what point would life change from being acceptable to unacceptable? Identify an appropriate percentage figure.

List any factors that might alter your decision.

Discuss this exercise with some colleagues at work and compare differing values.

Science cannot ultimately *know* chances in each individual case. Assuming life is worse than death is also value-laden, as no-one knows what death is like (Aksoy, 2000).

Withdrawing life-prolonging treatment does not mean withdrawing care. Treatments that provide comfort should be continued, and are often escalated. The person must be supported to eat and drink as long as they wish to (Leadership Alliance, 2014).

Pain

A good death is usually described as pain-free (Stringer, 2007). Pain is the main reason euthanasia is requested (Emmanuel *et al.*, 2000). Pain, and other symptom relief, is emphasised as a priority by Leadership Alliance (2014). However, nurses' assessment and management of pain is often poor (see Chapter 20), and many bereaved families consider analgesia needs of their loved one could have been improved (Danis, 1998). Pain relief often necessitates opioids, which can cause nausea, so anti-emetics should be given. Opioid doses may be larger than those prescribed for most patients. This is not to hasten their death, which would be both illegal and unethical; as long as the primary intention remains to relieve pain and not hasten death, opioids may morally be given in whatever quantities are needed to relieve pain. There is however a significant difference between being pain-free and lacking consciousness, so use of sedatives creates ethical dilemmas (Gallagher and Wainwright, 2007; Leadership Alliance, 2014).

Depression

One quarter of patients receiving palliative care are depressed, a figure likely to apply to palliative care in acute hospitals (Taylor and Ashelford, 2008). Depression is not a normal part of grief, so should be alleviated. Although drugs may be needed for this, psychological support should be attempted first – palliative care specialists may be able to offer advice and resources.

Not for resuscitation

Where death is likely, or successful resuscitation would be unlikely, attempting resuscitation would be cruel. Yet too often futile resuscitations are attempted, sometimes through lack of foresight but more often through fear of instigating DNR CPR (do not resuscitate with cardiopulmonary resuscitation). This should be a team decision, although currently the final order has to be signed by a medical consultant. Decisions not to resuscitate should be clearly recorded, following local policies. Most hospitals have proformas for 'do not attempt cardiopulmonary resuscitation' orders.

Spiritual care

Patients' spiritual values should be considered at all times, but spiritual values often become especially important when facing death. Most hospitals have chaplains, but also have access to information on faiths likely to be followed by their patients. Responses to death may be affected by cultural influences, such as religion. Nurses should therefore be sensitive to cultural and religious needs of patients and their families. There are hundreds of different faiths, so staff cannot be expected to be familiar with all, and covering all possibilities would require a book by itself. For example, Buddhist families may wish to stay with their departed for prolonged lengths of time, while Hindus often prefer to perform last offices themselves, keeping jewellery or 'sacred threads' on the body, and Muslims often wish to die facing Mecca. Unfortunately, assessment and recording of spiritual needs in nursing records are often poor (Swift *et al.*, 2007).

... The family ...

Whatever the personal beliefs and values of each nurse, death of patients is an inevitable part of nursing in almost any speciality. Family and friends of each patient are unlikely to have seen as many people die, but would have known the patient longer and more intimately, than the nurse. So however caring nurses are, experiencing bereavement is likely to be unique to family in a way it cannot be to the nurse. This almost inevitably places nurses outside the intimate circle of grieving.

Breaking bad news, and other sensitive interviews, should occur away from the bedside, preferably in a comfortable room where you will not be disturbed – hang a notice on the door; if possible, switch off any telephones. Do not obstruct the door, in case relatives unable to handle the situation need to rush out. Offering tea and other comforts can help to humanise an inevitably distressing situation.

Breaking bad news and witnessing suffering can cause stress (Wright, 1996; Farrell, 1999), so understandably many staff are uncomfortable doing this. Doctors' communication with families is often inconsistent (Ravenscroft and Bell, 2000) and could be improved (Danis, 1998). Nurses' communication is probably similarly variable. Staff should therefore try and find out what the family have already been told, both to avoid inconsistencies, and to try and ensure families are given sufficient information to meet their needs. Staff trained in counselling skills are more likely to be able to support family more effectively. However family often trust particular members of staff, and may value that member of staff speaking with them – for families, interpersonal skills are more important than their professional rank (Finlay and Dallimore, 1991).

Guilt is probably the most painful aspect of grief (Kubler-Ross, 1970). Bereaved families often seek reasons for the death. However irrational, they often blame themselves for causing or contributing to the death. Nurses can profoundly affect how families respond to bereavement (Coolican, 1994). Whenever possible, families should be informed honestly and clearly about impending death of their loved one so that they may begin grieving (Eastland, 2001).

Sudden death makes relatives feel helpless (Wright, 1991). Suddenly bereaved families may need more support, but often receive less (Yates *et al.*, 1990). Nurses should therefore help families to regain control and power while giving them the freedom to express their feelings and face the pain of death (Wright, 1991). The time immediately surrounding sudden death is crucial in determining families' ability to accept death and deal with the crisis (Lindermann, 1994), partly because disbelief can be very strong (Jackson, 1996). Families need both practical advice/information, such as how to make funeral arrangements, and someone to talk to (Hall and Hall, 1994). Providing printed information can be particularly helpful, as grieving families may not remember everything they are told. Many hospitals provide information booklets giving details such as local places to register the death.

Anticipating events, or imaging what happened if not present, is often worse than reality (Kent and McDowell, 2004). Because reactions are unpredictable, it is usually best to inform relatives of sudden death after they have arrived in the hospital (Kent and McDowell, 2004). Viewing the body after death helps grieving (Chapple and Ziebland, 2010), providing an opportunity to 'say goodbye'. Families may feel 'cheated' if they are not allowed to see and touch their loved one (Ellison, 1992). Unfortunately the busyness of acute hospitals may undermine opportunities to support bereaved relatives. Up to half of people contacting a branch of CRUSE (a voluntary group for bereaved families) did so because of feelings of anxiety and anger towards hospitals, doctors and nurses (Ewins and Bryant, 1992).

Grief is a process, families needing continuing support. Bereaved families usually value being contacted by nurses who cared for their loved one (Jackson, 1998), and some nurses may wish to attend funerals of those they have cared for, although a significant minority do not (Jackson, 1998). Many wards have bereavement programmes, such as sending condolence cards (Burke and Seeley, 1994), ideally sent 2–6 weeks after the death (Kubler-Ross, 1991; Wright, 1991; Jackson, 1996).

... And the nurse

Few nurses can avoid witnessing death. Death of patients can be distressing to nursing staff as well as families (Stringer, 2007; Valiee *et al.*, 2012), reviving unresolved grief from personal losses, or reviving fears about their own mortality. Many healthcare staff dislike being with dying people (Ellershaw and Ward, 2003).

Being with people in emotional pain is distressing, but the pain is caused by death, not the nurse. Nurses have the opportunity to help ease the pain by providing quality end-of-life care. Emotions are often raw, but nurses should not try and hide their tears – most families find it comforting to see staff are also upset (Finlay and Dallimore, 1991).

Peer support could be informal, or structured through debriefing or reflective sessions. Peer support should be mutual – offer support to others when they are caring for dying patients. End-of-life care is often included in pre- and post-registration courses, although being an emotionally fraught topic, can be difficult to facilitate and participate in. Many hospitals and other organisations also offer study days on bereavement.

Implications for clinical practice

- Nurses should be actively involved in decisions about whether to prolong or withdraw active treatment.
- Whenever possible, patients should be involved with decision-making.
- Withdrawing active treatment does not mean withdrawing care; terminal care should provide comfort and maintain dignity.
- Dying people often need much psychological, social and spiritual support; these aspects are often challenging for acute wards to offer, but may be available through outside resources; involve palliative care specialists.
- During and following death, the family, friends and often staff, need support, individualised to each person's needs.
- Families value follow-up support from wards where their loved one died.
- A system should be maintained for contacting families 2–6 weeks following bereavement.
- Peer and team support is valuable at what can be an emotionally distressing time for staff as well as relatives.

Summary

Acute hospitals are designed to provide life-supporting treatments, but not all patients survive. Death is not a medical failure, but the inevitable end of each person's life. Nurses should strive to meet the needs of patients and their families. Nurses should actively participate in decisions about prolonging or withdrawing active treatment. Once active treatment is withdrawn care should focus on comfort and dignity.

Bereavement is likely to be traumatic for family, friends and sometimes staff. Nurses should therefore provide support to families during bereavement, including practical information and space to express their emotions. Families value being able to see the body of their loved one. Needs of staff should also be supported.

Quality bereavement care can ease the trauma, but not remove it. Families usually need prolonged support, which hospitals can often initiate. Because reactions to loss are individual, any of the supports identified in this chapter may be valuable for both staff and families. The Leadership Alliance (2014) emphasises the importance of developing individualised careplans, whenever possible involving the patient and family.

Further reading

Leadership Alliance for the Care of Dying People (2014) provide national guidance on terminal care, although this reads as part provision, ahead of NICE guidance promised for 2015. The GMC (2010) provides authoritative guidelines for doctors about withholding and withdrawing treatment. The Marie Curie website (www.mcpcil.org.uk/) has useful resources. Classic texts about bereavement include Kubler-Ross (1970), Buckman (1988) Parkes (1996) and Wright (1996). Articles frequently appear in the medical and nursing press, such as Chapple and Ziebland (2010).

Clinical scenario

Mr Albert Jones was admitted following a myocardial infarction and thrombolysis in A&E. Since taking early retirement three years ago at the age of 58, he and his wife have been able to travel more, including visits to their only son and his family, who live 350 miles away.

Mr Jones' condition has stabilised sufficiently to return to a medical ward. However, his cardiac function is poor, and he becomes very breathless on exertion. His chances of survival to discharge are estimated at best to be 10–20%. The medical team have suggested withdrawing treatment.

1 Identify your role as nurse advocate for Mr Jones. What factors would influence your views of whether treatment should be withdrawn?
2 Consider the likely needs of Mr Jones' family up to the time of his death.
3 Reflect on follow-up facilities available in your ward, hospital, and local area. How far do these meet the needs suggested by evidence-based practice?

Chapter 22

Tissue donation

 Contents

Introduction

Any patient that dies is a potential tissue donor. There is however a gross lack of awareness about this possibility among both healthcare staff and the public (Rodríguez-Villar *et al.*, 2009). The opportunity to donate is therefore often missed (Magraph and Boulstridge, 2005), denying the patient who has died something that they might have wished, as well as denying potential recipients opportunities for improved quality of life.

During the twentieth century, organ donation became an increasingly practical treatment for end-stage organ failure. However, organ donation relies on organs being perfused while the patient is dead – this traditionally required diagnosis of brain-stem death, although more recently donation after circulatory death (DCD) has also been accepted. In practice, brain-stem death and DCD confine organ donation largely to ventilated patients on intensive care units. In contrast, tissue donation can occur in the mortuary, and so is possible for patients who die elsewhere.

This chapter focuses on tissue donation rather than organ donation. However, tissue donation has developed largely in the wake of organ donation, and most literature is about organ rather than tissue donation. Organ donation is therefore necessarily discussed, as it creates the context within which tissue services operate.

Last wishes

DOH (2008b) found that three quarters of the UK population favour donation, but only one quarter were registered donors (numbers have increased slightly since). In 2005 NHS Blood and Transplant (NHSBT) was formed, to co-ordinate blood transfusion and transplant services. NHSBT manage the national organ donor register, although some people may have expressed their wishes through other means (e.g. a section on driving licences now includes donation wishes). Although called 'organ donor register', there is a reasonable assumption that people wishing to donate organs would also wish to donate tissues.

DOH (2008b) identified that Spain had the highest rate of organ donation in Europe, largely due to having a transplant co-ordinator in each hospital. The DOH therefore recommended that the UK should do the same. NHSBT funds a senior nurse for organ donation (SNOD) for each UK Trust. SNODs will normally facilitate tissue, as well as organ, donation.

Donating tissues

Many tissues can be donated, including

- skin
- bone
- tendons
- corneas
- heart valves
- (femoral arteries)
- meniscus.

Due to the extent of tissues that may be donated, one donor can potentially help up to 50 recipients. There are however age limits and other exclusion criteria. Transplants may transfer disease to recipients (Pruss *et al.*, 2010), so diseases known to be potentially transferrable, those suspected of being potentially transferable, and those of unknown aetiology will almost invariably be excluded. Whereas organs can save lives, tissues generally improve quality, rather than increase quantity, of life. Therefore there are more stringent criteria for tissue than for organ donation. Specific criteria are not identified in this chapter, as they change with evidence and practice. Tissue services co-ordinators involved in the donation process will advise what may be considered for donation, but will also request any required tests.

To optimise condition of tissues, the body should be in the mortuary within six hours, and retrieval will normally occur within 2 hours of death. The option of donation should therefore be offered to relatives as early as possible.

Relatives may decline donation due to not wishing to 'sacrifice' the body (Sque *et al.*, 2008), but where donation is potentially disfiguring, tissues will be replaced with prostheses (eyes, bones) to avoid distress to relatives viewing the body.

Skin

A thin film of skin is removed, not the whole skin layer. This necessitates donation from large skin surface areas, such as the back and legs. Although these areas are not normally exposed in the mortuary, if seen they typically look like sunburn.

Skin is used as a dressing, typically for severe burns. Grafted skin provides a surface for the patient's own skin to granulate against, after which donated skin dies, leaving a better cosmetic result than artificial dressings. Although usually cosmetic rather than life-saving, donated skin arguably did save lives after the July 2007 London bombings.

Bone

Donated bone may be used for replacement of major bones or spinal fusion, but is more often used as a base for revision of joint surgery, ground bone creating a new acetabulum for the prosthesis. One donation can therefore help many people.

Tendons

Tendon injury is painful, and can take months or years for recovery to occur. Achilles tendons and patellae from younger donors can supply many tendon grafts. Repairing knee ligaments is especially useful for sporting injuries.

Eyes

Corneas were the first tissues to be transplanted, and have restored the sight of many people. Although corneal grafts are likely to be the most useful aspect, the whole eye is removed, and replaced with a prosthesis. Glaucoma can damage the sclera of eye, so sceral transplants can also restore sight.

Heart valves

Severe heart valve disease, such as mitral incompetence, necessitates replacement. The three options available are:

- mechanical valves
- xenotransplantation (animal valves, usually from pigs)
- human valves.

Mechanical valves have proved problematic, and condemn the recipient to lifelong anticoagulation therapy. Animal valves are better, but human valves are ideal. Valves are not part of the myocardium, so myocardial infarction is not an exclusion criterion.

Meniscus

Menisci are fibrous cartilage connected to the tibia, which act as shock absorbers (Mickiewicz *et al.*, 2013). Loss of menisci is a major cause of osteoarthritis (McNicholas *et al.*, 2000).

Other tissues

If people wish, they may leave their bodies to medical science, although this is not an option available for relatives to choose after death. Other tissues, such as brain and spinal cord tissue, may be offered for research purposes, but currently would not be transplanted into a recipient. Tissue for research purposes would only be excluded if potential diseases expose laboratory staff to significant risk, such as hepatitis. Research into currently irreversible degenerative diseases, such as Parkinson's disease, may one day provide cures.

Consent

Under the Human Tissue Act of 2004 the wishes of patients are paramount. However, this has not been, and is unlikely to be, tested in court, so the former practice of seeking consent from the next of kin remains. The UK, like most countries, has traditionally had an opt-in system – people choose actively to donate. However, since 1999 the British Medical Association (BMA) has supported changing to an opt-out (presumed consent) system. In 2013 the Welsh Assembly passed the Human Transplantation Wales Bill, and at the time of writing it seems that Scotland, and possibly other UK countries, will follow. There is however little evidence that changing to an opt-out system will increase donor rates (Coppen *et al.*, 2006).

Contacts

Local Senior Nurses for Organ Donation (SNODs) are part of a regional team, one of whom is always on call 24 hours a day. The hospital switchboard will have the pager number for the on-call SNOD.

Although patients may have identified their wish to donate through other means, healthcare professionals can find out if their patient is on the national donor register by calling 01179 757580.

Staff telephoning this number will need to leave details (their name, the patient's name and details, the hospital, the hospital switchboard number and the ward extension; NB direct line numbers for wards should not be used).

There will also be various regional contacts for tissue services, which may be available locally and can be supplied by the regional co-ordinator.

Approaching families

Families are grieving at the time they need to be approached about donation. However, knowing that their loved one has helped other people is usually a comfort. In the stress of bereavement, families are unlikely to think about donation, but may think about it later, perhaps when media report a story about donation. By the time this occurs, the opportunity to donate is almost invariably lost, adding further to their grief. Asking about donation is very unlikely to make their grief worse, but to deny the opportunity may increase later distress.

Donation should be routinely considered with end-of-life care, both for the benefit of the majority who wish to be donors, and those who can benefit from donated tissue. When initially approaching families, it is useful to know whether the patient was on the organ donor register. But as most people are not on the register, the patient's wishes can often be identified by questions such as

- 'Did you ever talk about donation as a family?'
- 'Do you know if . . . carried a donor card?'
- 'What would . . . have wished about tissue donation?'

No religions prohibit donation (Randhawa, 2012).

SNODs, and people employed by transplant services, are skilled at discussing issues with families, but initial approaches from nurses are valuable both because nurses are immediately present, and because family will often have developed a rapport with the nursing staff.

Implications for practice

- The majority of people would wish to be donors, but only a minority have recorded this wish on the national donor register.
- Not to offer donation denies choice; asking should be the norm, and be a routine part of end-of-life care.
- Bereaved relatives are unlikely to think about donation.
- The body should be in mortuary within six hours.
- Tissues can be retrieved in the mortuary within 24 hours following death.
- Refer early – time is tissue.

Summary

Tissue donation improves quality of life for recipients, but can also fulfil patients' wishes and bring comfort to relatives. However, gross lack of awareness by both healthcare professionals and the public results in many opportunities being missed, which may increase future distress for bereaved families. Recent changes in Welsh law may be extended to other UK countries, but whether opt-in or opt-out systems are in place, nurses caring for dying patients and their families have a valuable role in initiating conversation and contacting specialist services.

Further reading

Although focusing on organ donation, DOH (2008b) is the key national document in relation to transplants, and created much of the context within which tissue services operate. Hadingham (1997) is an old article, but skills for talking with bereaved relatives remain unchanged. Gumbley and Pearson (2006) provide one of the few nursing articles about tissue donation.

Clinical scenario

Mr Patrick Jones, aged 52, was admitted following a road traffic accident. He was found to have sustained a subarachnoid haemorrhage, and was transferred to a centre for neurosurgery. One week later he was transferred back to the initial hospital, with a GCS of 7. Although breathing for himself, through a tracheostomy, there was no significant improvement in this condition. One month later palliative care was initiated, and Mr Jones died on the ward, surrounded by his family.

1   What previous exposure (theory or practice) have you had to tissue donation? Is there any information about it on your ward for staff, patients or relatives? Does your ward have contact details for donation services? Discuss with your colleagues what they know about tissue donation.
2   Contact your Trust's SNOD, or any other local services, to find out what is available.
3   Reflecting on your experiences of breaking bad news, how might you raise the possibility of donation with Mr Jones' family? What aspects might you wish to raise (it may help to think of families of patients you are currently caring for)?

Part 5

Environment (internal)

Chapter 23

Fluid balance

Contents

Introduction

Sixty to eighty per cent of bodyweight is from water (Marieb and Hoehn, 2013). The proportion of water to other components varies between individuals. In health, the single most important difference is caused by build: muscular people have proportionately more water (muscle holds water), whereas people with more fat have proportionately less water (fat repels water). In ill health, the most significant factors affecting fluid balance are usually:

- ability to obtain fluid
- ability to excrete fluid (renal function).

Insensible loss

On an average day, an average-build adult may have a fluid turnover of 2–3 litres. Most fluid that enters the body will do so as liquid (drinks), with a small amount entering in food. Most fluid loss will be in urine, but a small amount is lost 'insensibly':

- perspiration
- respiration
- defecation.

In health, insensible loss may be about 500 ml/day (Thomas *et al.*, 2008). But profuse sweating, tachypnoea or loose stools may double insensible loss, while hypothermia, bradypnoea or constipation will significantly reduce insensible loss. As insensible loss forms a significant proportion of fluid lost from the body, it should be considered when calculating fluid balance – either by actually including it in calculated balance, or allowing for it when planning target daily aims.

Fluid compartments

While most of the body is water, the water is contained in distinct compartments:

- intravascular
- interstitial
- intracellular.

Intravascular fluid is blood. A 70 kg healthy person has approximately 5 litres of blood, of which about 2 litres are cells (mainly red cells, which are mostly haemoglobin) and 3 litres are plasma. Plasma is mostly (about 90%) water. Interstitial fluid, fluid between the blood vessels and tissue cells, forms just under one third of body water (12 litres in the healthy 70 kg adult). Nearly two thirds of body water is inside cells – intracellular fluid. Typical healthy balance between these three compartments is illustrated in Figure 23.1

Many anatomy texts describe intravascular and interstitial fluid together, naming it *extracellular* fluid. However, acute illness often causes hypovolaemia (lack of blood volume) together with excessive interstitial fluid. It is therefore useful to view these as distinct compartments. Anatomy texts describing only two main fluid compartments often

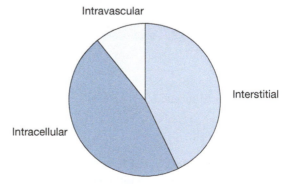

Total body water

Figure 23.1 Typical healthy balance between different fluid compartments

refer to 'third spaces', better thought of as 'potential' spaces – small fluid compartments in such spaces as the pericardium (normally 10–20 ml, see Chapter 13) and pleura (normally 2–5 ml, see Chapter 7). Although physiologically useful, and actual rather than potential spaces, these are normally insignificant for fluid balance.

Fluid shifts

Although diagrams such as Figure 23.1 identify distinct fluid compartments, fluid constantly shifts between them.

Whereas most of the cardiovascular system has three layers, capillaries' walls are a single layer of cells. Capillary cells are *squaemous* epithelium – 'scale-like' cells that are thin, overlapping each other like fish scales. This creates gaps between cell walls, which fluid can cross. Movement of water between capillaries and interstitial (extravascular) spaces is regulated by pressures:

- hydrostatic
- osmotic.

At the arteriole end of capillaries, pressure inside capillaries is higher than pressure outside (hydrostatic pressure). Average capillary pressure is often cited as 32/28 mmHg (see Chapter 10); average interstitial pressure is 0–10 mmHg (Singh *et al.*, 2004). Water and solutes are therefore forced from plasma into interstitial spaces. Glucose and electrolyte levels are therefore similar in the two compartments, hence physiologists often referring to the two together as extracellular fluid. Only substances above 35 kilodaltons (kDa), essentially blood cells and plasma proteins, do not normally extravase (Doherty and Buggy, 2012). Molecular weights are discussed further in Chapter 25.

As volume moves out of capillaries, intracapillary pressure falls. As this happens, osmotic pressures become predominant. Osmotic pressure is about 'pull', holding water in the compartment, and potentially attracting more water towards it. Osmotic pressure is perhaps best illustrated by the poorly controlled diabetic, who due to hyperglycaemia has glycosuria. Sugar exerts an osmotic pull; the sugar in urine therefore holds onto water, causing polyuria. Similarly, sodium has a high osmotic pressure ('where salt goes, water follows'). While blood contains both glucose and sodium, both molecules are small enough to cross capillary walls, and therefore interstitial and intravascular concentrations are similar. Therefore neither sodium nor glucose normally have significant roles in the balance between vascular and interstitial volume. Osmotic pressure of blood is therefore created primarily by chemicals that do not normally extravase – plasma proteins, especially albumin. Average healthy colloid osmotic pressure, from plasma proteins, is approximately 28 mmHg (Hall, 2011). So, once hydrostatic pressure falls below this level, colloid osmotic pressure pulls water and solutes into the capillary. This normally occurs near the venule end, to bring waste products of metabolism (carbon dioxide, acids) into the bloodstream, for disposal. Sicker patients usually have low serum albumin levels (see Chapter 3), contributing to oedema formation.

Fluid homeostasis, as described above, is largely based on the work of Starling (1896), which influenced fluid therapy for much of the twentieth century (the 'colloid versus crystalloid' debate). Starling reported animal experiments; in health, his findings remain largely valid. But increasing evidence from recent decades suggests that normal mechanisms, and therefore traditional approaches to intravenous fluids, often fail acutely ill patients (see Chapter 25).

Acute illness often causes, or is accentuated by, inflammation (see Chapter 1). Inflammation causes release of various chemical mediators into blood, including leukotrienes. Leukotrienes increase capillary leak, a homeostatic mechanism to facilitate transfer of white blood cells into tissues where infection is present. However, excessive inflammation causes excessive capillary leak.

Another possible explanation of changes in ill health is *glycocalyx*, also called 'endothelial surface layer'. Glycocalyx is a 'slime' coating that some cells possess, which assists function of the cells, and sometimes surrounding tissue. Vascular glycocalyx helps regulate clotting, capillary bloodflow and capillary permeability (leak) (Reitsma *et al.*, 2007). It is therefore possible that illness causes dysfunction of glycocalyx, or perhaps some as yet unidentified homeostatic mechanism. Fluid overload impairs glycocalyx function, predisposing to oedema (Marik and Lemson, 2014).

Oedema, excess interstitial fluid, can be caused by:

- increased hydrostatic pressure (venous congestion)
- increased capillary permeability
- decreased osmotic pull.

However caused, oedema is not only unsightly, and increases risk of pressure ulceration, it also impairs diffusion of oxygen from blood to cells. Extensive oedema therefore increases risk of cell necrosis.

Some movement across cell membranes is passive, but most is active. Various 'gates', 'channels' and 'pumps' regulate what does, and does not, cross cell membranes, maintaining a very different biochemical environment inside cells. One of the most important of these mechanisms is the sodium-potassium pump, which repels sodium in exchange for potassium (Barrett *et al.*, 2010). Sodium is mostly extracellular, whereas most potassium is inside cells:

Normal levels	Plasma (and interstitial)	Intracellular
Sodium (mmol/litre)	133–146	Approximately 10 (Hall, 2011)
Potassium (mmol/litre)	3.5–5.3	Approximately 150 (Greenlee *et al.*, 2009)

Cells unable to make sufficient energy (ATP) start to fail. As the sodium-potassium pump fails, sodium moves into cells. Where salt goes, water follows. Cells therefore start to swell – Chapter 10 likened necrosis to an explosion – causing further cell and tissue damage.

Dehydration

Many patients are dehydrated on admission to hospital (Cunningham and McWilliam, 2006), and more become dehydrated while in hospital (Wakefield *et al.*, 2009).

Dehydration increases mortality (Wakefield *et al.*, 2009; Ruxton, 2012; El-Sharkawy *et al.*, 2014). Common causes of fluid imbalance include:

- diseases (e.g. heart failure, kidney failure)
- inflammation
- treatments (e.g. diuretics, intravenous fluids).

Fluid balance can be assessed by:

- patient history (cause of admission, risk factors);
- fluid balance charts;
- urine output (remembering effects of diuretic therapy and osmotic diuresis);
- vital signs (e.g. compensatory tachycardia);
- daily weight; recent gain/loss;
- gut function (bowels, vomiting);
- wounds and drains (including nasogastric and wound exudates);
- 'Third Space' loss (e.g. peritonitis, plaster casts);
- blood results;
- physical examination.

Blood results (see Chapter 3) may indicate:

- renal insufficiency (raised creatinine and urea, low GFR);
- dehydration (haemoconcentration of many results, especially hypernatraemia);
- water overload (haemodilution);
- inflammation (raised CRP), and so likely capillary leak;
- decreased osmotic pull (low plasma protein, especially albumin).

Signs of dehydration from *physical examination* are listed in Table 23.1.

Table 23.1 (Some) physical signs of dehydration

Signs	Approximate fluid deficit
Thirsty	Less than 5%
Dry tongue, concentrated urine	5%
Oliguria	10%
Poor circulation (peripherally cold)	15%
Hypotensive	20%

Fluid overload may necessitate fluid restriction and/or diuretic therapy, although fluid overload may be accompanied by arterial hypovolaemia and/or oedema, which further impair perfusion and tissue oxygenation.

Rehydration

In health, the thirst reflex prompts us to drink to maintain normal fluid balance. In the absence of diseases such as heart or renal failure, hypervolaemia increases diuresis. If patients are able to drink, oral rehydration is usually best (Thomas *et al.*, 2008). However, some patients may be unable to drink, due to problems such as dysphagia, impaired consciousness, or imminent treatments such as surgery; all of these create risks of aspiration. The thirst response is often blunted with age (El-Sharkawy *et al.*, 2014), making older people especially prone to dehydration. If patients are breathless, tachypnoea leaves little time between breaths in which to drink. If patients have mobility problems they may not be able to reach or hold drink. Jugs of water that have been standing for some time in the typically warm temperature of most wards are seldom appetising. Significant fluid deficits may necessitate using other routes, usually intravenous. Intravenous fluids are discussed in Chapter 25.

Implications for practice

- Fluid imbalances are common in hospital, especially in sicker patients.
- Ill-health often causes imbalances between fluid compartments, with capillary leak causing hypovolaemia and oedema, both of which are problematic.
- Dehydration increases morbidity and mortality.
- Assessing fluid balance is therefore part of nursing care.
- Fluid imbalances should trigger fluid balance monitoring.
- Where possible, oral rehydration is usually best, but severe deficits often need intravenous resuscitation.

Summary

The body contains more water than everything else put together. Fluid balance is therefore vital to health. Fluid imbalances frequently occur in ill health and, if not resolved promptly, increase mortality and morbidity. Early identification of fluid balance problems, together with early and effective treatment, is therefore a key role of all clinical staff.

Although intravascular fluid is necessary for perfusion, it is the smallest of the three main fluid compartments; most body water is inside cells. Water constantly moves between intravascular, interstitial and intracellular compartments, and is affected by various factors, most of which are compromised by ill-health.

Further reading

A physiology book is useful for understanding normal distribution and balance of body fluid. Ruxton (2012) provides a useful nursing review.

Clinical scenario

Mrs Joan Henderson, an 85-year-old widow, is admitted from home, where she was found collapsed on the floor in a very drowsy and disorientated state. There are multiple bruises, especially on her left arm and leg. Her skin looks dry, and she appears very emaciated. A CT scan has excluded any visible neurological injury. She is to be transferred from A&E to a medical ward. She has not yet passed urine since admission. An infusion of 500 ml gelatin is prescribed 'stat'.

1   List signs that might indicate dehydration.
2   List problems that might be caused by (a) aggressive intravenous rehydration; and (b) inadequate rehydration.
3   List concerns, in order of priority, that you would hand over to the ward nurse.

Chapter 24

Acute kidney injury

Contents

Fundamental knowledge

■ Renal anatomy and physiology

Introduction

Renal disease may cause admission, but for most hospitalised patients acute kidney injury (AKI; previously called 'acute renal failure') is a common and often preventable complication of acute illness, occurring in 13–18% of hospitalised patients (NICE, 2013a). It significantly increases morbidity and mortality. This chapter outlines pathophysiology, focusing on monitoring renal function and preventing injury where possible, and managing and treating injury when it does occur. Chronic kidney disease (CKD) is mentioned, but not discussed, as this is a large topic, a speciality in its own right, and not an acute problem.

Functions

The most obvious function of the kidney is to produce urine. Urine removes most metabolic waste products, and in health maintains fluid, electrolyte and (metabolic) acid–base balance. The kidney also has endocrine functions: erythropoietin, which stimulates production of red blood cells in bone marrow, and renin (see Chapter 10) are the main, but not only, hormones it produces. It also has a role in vitamin D synthesis, and therefore contributes to health of bones and teeth. Renal disease therefore affects many systems. Endocrine and vitamin D functions are significant with CKD, but with acute diseases problems are almost solely confined to urinary dysfunction and its effects.

Urine is produced in the nephron. Each kidney has about one million nephrons (Eckardt *et al.*, 2013) which filter fluid from blood at the glomerular bed and process it into urine in the tubules (see Figure 24.1).

The kidney's ability to autoregulate means that volume filtered by glomeruli can reduce by three quarters before causing detectable changes (raised serum creatinine, oliguria). Healthy glomerular filtration rate (GFR) exceeds 90 ml/min/1.73 m^2 (Murphy and

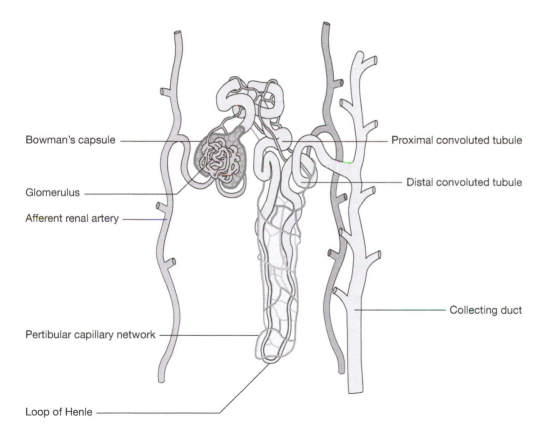

Figure 24.1 **A nephron (diagrammatic)**

Robinson 2006); levels below 50 usually necessitate review of drug dosages to prevent toxicity. Currently, it is only practical to estimate glomerular filtration rate from serum creatinine.

End-stage renal failure

The end-stage of chronic kidney disease, end-stage renal failure (ESRF), means that kidneys can no longer support life. ESRF is fatal unless either a kidney transplant or frequent dialysis is available. ESFR occurs when GFR is below 15 ml/min/1.73m² (Marieb and Hoehn, 2013). AKI is a significant risk factor for developing chronic kidney disease (Coca et al., 2012). First signs of AKI occur with 75% non-function; this leaves a very narrow margin between the first signs of acute kidney injury and a potentially fatal condition. Acute kidney injury should therefore be prevented if possible, and identified and treated early if it does occur.

Defining AKI

Creatinine is the best marker of renal dysfunction (Brochard et al., 2010), as unlike urea it is not reabsorbed by the renal tubule. Stage 1 acute kidney injury (the earliest stage) is one of

- serum creatinine increased by 0.3 mg/dl or more (≥26.5 mmol/litre) within 48 hours;
- serum creatinine increased by 1.5 times baseline or more (known or presumed to have occurred within prior 7 days);
- urine volume less than 0.5 ml/kilogram/hour for six hours.

(KDIGO, 2012)

Oligura (less than 0.5 ml/kilogram/hour) may be

- volume-responsive
- intrinsic
- post-renal.

The most frequent cause of oliguria in acute illness is volume-responsive – the kidney does not receive sufficient blood to make enough urine, usually because of systemic hypovolaemia. The treatment for volume-responsive oliguria is to give volume.

Inadequate renal perfusion causes both oliguria and ischaemic damage (Perazella, 2012); inflammatory responses cause oedema, which compresses tubules, causing acute tubular necrosis (ATN), the most common cause of intrinsic acute kidney injury (Stevens, 2007). Intrinsic acute kidney injury, damage to renal tissue itself, can also be caused by nephrotoxic drugs, such as non-steroidal anti-inflammatories (NSAIDs), ACE-inhibitors, metformin, and (most) intravenous dyes. Whereas recovery from volume-responsive acute kidney injury follows quickly from giving volume, recovery from intrinsic acute kidney injury can only occur once oedema subsides, or cells regenerate; this usually takes 7–21 days (Hussein et al., 2009), although may take longer, or progress to CKD.

Post-renal problems are caused by obstruction to urine flow. Common causes are cancers of the kidney or bladder, stones in the kidney or bladder, and enlarged prostate. While relatively common problems in the community, they are unlikely to develop during acute hospitalisation. They may however be present on admission, and complicate recovery. If obstruction is suspected, a bladder scanner can indicate whether urine is reaching the bladder.

Managing AKI

Kidneys often fully recover from acute insults, provided the patient survives. Mortality from AKI is typically 25–30% (NICE, 2013a), but acutely ill patients usually develop AKI as a complication of cardiovascular (perfusion) failure, so mortality in this context is about 50% (Ympa *et al.*, 2005). Prevention, early identification and treatment therefore reduce mortality and morbidity.

If not promptly resolved, volume responsive AKI usually progresses into intrinsic failure. Timing of onset of hypotension therefore gives a clue about whether the injury may still be volume-responsive. Concentrated urine (specific gravity >1.018) indicates volume-responsive AKI (Rahman and Treacher, 2002). But the best indicator is usually to give a fluid challenge and see if the kidney responds by producing urine.

NCEPOD (2009b) found that one fifth of AKIs occurring in hospitals were both predictable and preventable. Nurses should therefore assess risk factors, perform admission urinalysis, and monitor fluid balance when there are any concerns. Nurses may also identify problems from medical tests such as blood results and scans. Any concerns should be escalated urgently, before volume-responsive AKI progresses to intrinsic. Diuretics should be avoided with known or suspected volume-response AKI (Davenport and Stevens, 2008) as they increase mortality and progression to chronic kidney disease (Mehta *et al.*, 2002).

Urinalysis

Ward urinalysis is probably the most frequent urological investigation in hospitals. It can provide useful screening, but is also useful for monitoring renal function. Except for specific gravity and pH, normal levels for tests are below zero/negative. Tests available vary slightly between test-strip manufacturers, but usually include the following.

Appearance

Visual appearance can indicate likely causes, although there can also be less likely causes for many aspects:

- dark ('*golden syrup*') – concentrated (dehydration)
- rusty – rhabdomyolysis
- cloudy – infection
- frothy – protein.

Drugs can also affect urine colour; for example, rifampicin creates an orange tint.

Blood/leukocytes

Blood cells are not normally filtered by the glomerulus. Inflammatory disease may allow cells to pass into urine, or trauma to the urinary tract (e.g. stones, cancers, catheterisation) may cause bleeding. If blood is present, so is protein. Leukocytes (white blood cells) are part of the immune system, and are usually only found in urine if infection is present (urinary tract infection – UTI).

Nitrite

Bacteria convert the nitrate, which is normally in urine, to nitrite (Steggall, 2007), so nitrite is only found if urine is infected. However, absence of nitrite cannot exclude urinary tract infection, as some bacteria do not convert nitrate (Steggall, 2007).

Urobilinogen/bilirubin

Bilirubinuria only occurs with raised blood bilirubin levels. Bilirubin is a waste-product of erythrocyte metabolism (see Chapter 3). Normally converted by the liver into bile which flows to the gall bladder, gall-bladder disease causes bilirubin loss in urine (Wilson, 2005). While a positive dipstick test may raise concerns, it is insufficient to screen for disease (Walthour and Dassow, 2014). Bilirubinuria usually causes urine to look dark.

Protein

Protein is not normally filtered by the glomerulus (Bertuccio, 2011), so proteinuria usually indicates an inflammatory response (disease, such as infection) in the kidney that has enabled it to pass through the glomerulus (Steggall, 2007). Proteinuria is the single most important indicator of kidney injury (Barratt, 2007).

pH (normal: 5–6)

Urine is made from blood, which normally has pH around 7.4. Renal excretion of hydrogen ions (an essential chemical for acids) is therefore important for metabolic acid/base balance (see Chapter 8). Thus urinary pH varies according to physiological needs, but is almost always acidic. Provided renal function is reasonable, high pH may reflect alkalaemia, while low pH may reflect acidaemia.

Specific gravity (normal: 1.002–1.035)

Urine is mainly water, which (if pure) has a specific gravity of 1.0. High specific gravity suggests increased water reabsorption by the kidney, usually in response to dehydration – i.e. volume responsive AKI. Low specific gravity (watery urine) often means excessive water in urine, suggesting hypervolaemia, but other causes include

- age-related decline in ability to concentrate urine in older people (Wilson, 2005);
- osmotic diuresis, such as from glycosuria with poorly-controlled diabetes;

■ intrinsic and post-renal failure impairing ability of renal tubules to concentrate urine (Barratt, 2007).

Polyuria can cause various electrolyte imbalances, especially excessive loss of potassium, magnesium and phosphate.

Ketones

Ketones are waste products of fat metabolism. Blood sugar, not fat, is normally the main source of cell energy, so ketones in blood (and urine) indicate lack of availability of blood sugar. The two main reasons for this are

■ lack of insulin (diabetic ketoacidosis – see Chapter 27)
■ starvation (including some extreme diets).

As well as indicating problems, ketones may form acids, hence the metabolic acidosis found with diabetic ketoacidosis.

Glucose

The kidney filters blood sugar, but normally reabsorbs it all provided blood sugar is below 11 mmol/litre (Gerich, 2010). Glycosuria therefore usually indicates hyperglycaemia. Glucose has a high osmotic pressure, reducing water reabsorption, causing polyuria and dilute urine (low specific gravity). Diabetes is often initially detected from routine urinalysis. Acute illness and many drugs (especially cardiac) can cause transient hyperglycaemia.

Implications for practice

■ Acute kidney injury is a common complication of acute illness, incidence increasing with acuity of other diseases.
■ AKI increases morbidity and mortality.
■ The kidney is often the 'innocent bystander' of acute illness.
■ Urine output should be assessed, and when there are concerns about oliguria (<0.5 ml/kg/h), fluid balance should be monitored.
■ Untreated (or poorly treated) volume-responsive AKI is likely to progress to intrinsic injury, which delays recovery and increases mortality risk.

Summary

Outside renal and urological services, most renal problems are a complication of perfusion failure caused by underlying disease. Acute kidney injury is therefore potentially both predictable and preventable. Renal perfusion should be optimised by ensuring adequate hydration. Concerns about renal function should be urgently escalated.

Useful website

www.kidney-international.org

Further reading

KDIGO have a user-friendly website with many guidelines and other documents; although most are for chronic kidney disease, their AKI guidelines (2009) is useful. National guidelines include NICE (2013a) and NCEPOD (2009b). The key textbook for renal nursing is Thomas (2014).

Clinical scenario

Mr Graham Reading, aged 79, has had a left total hip replacement under general anaesthesia. He has a past medical history of diabetes type 2 (well controlled with metformin) and heart failure. There is no history of renal impairment, and pre-operative blood results caused no special concerns. His admission weight was 86.4 kg. His operation lasted just over two hours. On return to the ward his vital signs are

RR 18 bpm
HR 112 bpm
BP 95/63 (MAP 78) mmHg
T   34.6°C

He is drowsy, but responds appropriately to voice. An intravenous infusion of Hartman's (CSL) is running at 83 ml/h.

1 Identify Mr Reading's risk factors for developing acute kidney injury.
2 Mr Reading was catheterised on induction. On return to the ward 300 ml was emptied from the bag. In the first hour he only passes 25 ml. How much urine should Mr Graham have passed? What nursing and/or medical interventions (if any) should be taken in regard to his urine output?
3 Urinalysis reveals

pH   4.0
SG   1.030
glucose   ++
ketones   trace

There are no other abnormalities. Identify likely causes for these results.

Chapter 25

Fluid management

Contents

Fundamental knowledge

- Normal fluid balance
- Factors affecting fluid balance in acutely ill patients (see Chapter 23)
- Osmolality (see Chapter 23)

Introduction

Many sicker patients are acutely dehydrated, or have fluid imbalances, necessitating active fluid management – usually supplements. For most sicker patients, this necessitates intravenous fluids.

All intravenous fluids are primarily water. However, dissolved or suspended in the water are various substances which affect where the fluid will, or will not, move to. Traditionally, evidence about different types of fluids was based largely on animal studies, clinical observations and opinions. This generated much controversy. Publication of conflicting, and often weak, evidence and opinions has increased exponentially in recent years. This chapter explores contents of, and differences between, commonly used intravenous fluids:

- 0.9% saline
- 5% glucose
- compound sodium lactate (Hartmann's)
- gelatins
- albumin.

Properties of fluids are explored largely through 'time out' exercises; unless stated otherwise, normal serum ranges can be found in Chapter 3. Variants of these fluids (hypertonic saline, stronger strengths of glucose, glucose/saline) are briefly included. Continuing debates and flux in fluid management necessitate any conclusions being tentative.

Historical perspective

With widespread availability of intravenous fluids during the twentieth century, early philosophies of replacing blood with blood (whole blood, from blood donors) and replacing water with water (0.9% saline or 5% glucose) evolved into the crystalloid versus colloid debate. This drew significantly on Starling's (1896) work (see Chapter 23), suggesting that water-based fluids quickly extravased, whereas blood largely remained in the vascular space. Debate was complicated by development of more options, including artificial colloids which replaced use of whole blood for volume resuscitation. As identified in Chapter 23, Starling's findings remain largely true in health, but less applicable in ill-health.

In very recent years, major concerns have been raised about artificial colloids, although much evidence can be disputed. Currently the colloid versus crystalloid debate appears to have been largely replaced by a saline versus balanced solutions debate. For structure, this chapter adopts a crystalloid/colloid divide. However, individual responses and pathophysiologies mean that the same fluid may act differently in different patients.

Key issues

Rather than naively assume that crystalloids extravase and colloids do not, three key issues should be considered with each fluid:

- pH
- osmolality
- properties of solutes.

Most acute illnesses cause acidosis: respiratory, metabolic or mixed. Most IVIs are also acidic. Infusing acid into patients whose blood is already too acidic is illogical and potentially dangerous.

Normal serum osmolality is 275–295 (see Chapter 23). Increasing serum osmolality is likely to draw interstitial fluid into blood, while giving hypo-osmolar fluids is likely to cause more fluid to accumulate in tissues.

Molecular weight

Molecules are measured by weight, weight increasing as size increases. Table 25.1 lists typical molecular weights of many substances in intravenous fluids.

Table 25.1 Typical molecular weights

Water (H_2O)	18
Sodium (Na^+)	23
Chloride (Cl^-)	35
Potassium (K^+)	39
Calcium (Ca^{++})	40
Glucose ($C_6H_{12}O_6$)	180

Although glucose is significantly heavier (larger) than the electrolytes listed, it is still considered a small molecule, extravasing rapidly (glucose is the normal energy source for cells – see Chapter 28). For comparison, albumin (the main plasma protein) weighs about 66,500. Capillary pore size varies in different parts of the body, the leakiest normally being in renal glomeruli, the least leaky normally being in the blood–brain barrier (see Chapters 17 and 24). Renal threshold, the maximum size of substances which can be filtered, is normally about 69,000. Albumin is just small enough to be filtered by kidneys, but being negatively charged, is repelled by other negatively charged proteins (sialoproteins) in glomerular beds (Betruccio, 2011), just as two negative magnets' poles repel each other.

Maintenance or resuscitation?

As Chapter 23 identified, sicker patients often have fluid imbalances. Inflammatory responses, as well as diseases, often cause hypovolaemia, threatening tissue perfusion. Fluid resuscitation therefore involves giving large volumes of fluid quickly to restore circulating volume (blood pressure and perfusion, often indicated by urine output). Once blood volume has been resuscitated, fluid management should switch to maintenance, replacing volume lost to maintain euvolaemia. NICE (2013b) suggests indications for fluid resuscitation are

■ systolic blood pressure <100 mmHg;
■ heart rate >90 beats per minute;
■ capillary refill time >2 seconds or peripheries are cold to touch;
■ respiratory rate >20 breaths per minute;
■ ViEWS 5 or more.

For fluid resuscitation, NICE (2013b) recommends using 500 ml of a fluid containing 130–154 mmol/litre sodium (i.e. 0.9% saline or compound sodium lactate) over 15 minutes.

In health, increasing venous return in hypovolaemia should increase stroke volume, and so blood pressure. However, cardiac function of many hospitalised patients is often limited, and only about half of patients will respond to volume resuscitation (Marik and Lemson, 2014). Maitland *et al.'s* (2011) study found that any fluid bolus increased mortality. In first-aid situations, or to test likely effectiveness, fluid resuscitation may be achieved by lifting up one leg (Marik and Lemson, 2014), which returns about one unit of blood to the heart.

CRYSTALLOIDS

Crystalloids are water that contains dissolved crystals, such as salt or sugar. There are three main crystalloids:

■ 0.9% saline
■ 5% glucose
■ compound sodium lactate (CSL, often called 'Hartmann's').

Solutes in these fluids have low molecular weights, enabling rapid extravasation. As most body water is outside the bloodstream, crystalloids are useful for whole-body hydration. Whether they are ideal for acutely hypovolaemic, hypotensive patients is more debateable.

0.9% sodium chloride w/v

Where fluid (or drug) concentration is given as a percentage, the number is grams per hundred ml. So 0.9% sodium chloride is 0.9 grams of salt per 100 ml, or 9 grams per litre; 'w/v' indicates weight to volume: salt is measured by weight, water by volume.

Time out 25.1

Find a one litre bag of 0.9% sodium chloride.

1   What is its pH?
2   The fluid will usually be infused into veins. What is the normal pH of venous blood? (see Chapter 8)
3   How many mmol of sodium (Na⁺) are in the litre?
4   What is the normal serum sodium range?
5   How many mmol of chloride (Cl⁻) is contained in the litre?
6   What is the normal serum chloride range? (see Chapter 8)
7   What is its osmolality (mOsm/L – milliosmoles per litre)?

The acidity is caused by the excessive chloride ions. With sodium concentrations being similar to serum, free chloride ions are released. Being negatively charged, they seek positively charged ions to bind with. This is most likely to be hydrogen (H⁺), from the most common chemical in both the blood and body – water (H₂O). HCl is hydrochloric acid. Saline infusions can therefore cause hyperchloraemic acidosis (Ochola and Venkatesh, 2009). Hyperchloraemia can also provoke acute kidney injury (Yunos *et al.*, 2012), Smorenberg *et al.* (2013) suggest saline is proinflammatory; if so, this will exacerbate most acute illnesses.

Saline has relatively high osmolality ('where salt goes, water follows'). This may be advantageous, but as saline readily extravases, saline accumulation in interstitial spaces exerts an osmotic pull that may accelerate oedema formation, which is why salt intake is often restricted with heart failure.

With saline, most volume infused will extravase – Ochola and Venkatesh (2009) suggest only one quarter remains in the blood. Sodium is repelled by sodium-potassium pumps in cell membranes (see Chapter 23), so salt water mostly stays in interstitial spaces (Leach, 2010).

0.9% saline is often called (and prescribed as) 'normal'. It is not normal, and the term 'normal saline' should not be used (BNF, 2014). Reasons for its popularity are largely historical (there were fewer alternatives in the distant past) and cost – it is the cheapest of the intravenous fluids.

There are hypertonic (e.g. 2.7%) and hypotonic (e.g. 0.45%) variants of saline. Hypertonic exerts a high osmotic pull, so is useful for removing cerebral oedema (Kamel *et al.*, 2011) (see Chapter 17). Historically, hypotonic saline was often given if patients were hyponatraemic, but giving any salt with hypernatraemia is arguably illogical, and use of hypotonic saline may cause hyponatraemia (Wang *et al.*, 2014).

5% glucose w/v

This contains 5 grams of glucose in every 100 ml (= 50 grams glucose per litre).

Time out 25.2

Find a one litre bag of 5% glucose.

1   What is its pH?
2   What is the normal pH of venous blood?
3   Does packaging indicate how many kilojoules (kJ) of energy each litre provides? (Many manufacturer's no longer state this, but in the past 836 kJ was a typical energy content.)
4   On a standard chocolate bar, find out how many kilojoules the bar contains (NB the whole bar, not equivalent for 100 grams).
5   What is the osmolality of 5% glucose?

Five percent glucose (=5% dextrose) is sometimes described as 'free water'; this distinguishes it from salt water. Like saline, glucose rapidly extravases, but not being repelled by sodium-potassium pumps of cells, glucose water passes freely into cells. It is therefore a useful fluid for cell hydration (approximately two thirds of body water is inside cells). But the free movement of glucose water can be dangerous with raised intracranial pressure, so glucose solutions should generally be avoided with neurological injury (Haddad and Arabi, 2012).

There is relatively little energy in 5% glucose, so it should not be viewed as a nutritional replacement.

Glucose/saline

Traditional intravenous fluid maintenance for nil by mouth patients was one litre of 0.9% saline and two litres of 5% glucose. This was viewed as providing a small volume for intravascular fluid, nearly one third for interstitial spaces, and nearly two thirds for cells – physiological normal proportions. Sometimes, prescribers replaced this regime with on-going 8 hourly litre bags of glucose (or dextrose) saline. However, not all bags of glucose saline have the same contents. Historically, glucose saline was usually 0.18% saline and 4% glucose:

■   30 mmol sodium/litre
■   30 mmol chloride/litre
■   40 grams glucose/litre (670 kJ).

This mixture is approximately one quarter saline and almost the full 5% glucose, and has caused fatal hyponatraemias (NPSA, 2007c; Powell-Tuck et al., 2008/2011). Some formulations are 0.9% saline and 5% glucose:

■   154 mmol sodium/litre
■   154 mmol chloride/litre

- 50 grams glucose/litre
- pH 3.5–6.5
- 585 mOsmol/litre.

Time out 25.3

If available, find a one litre bag of glucose saline.

1   What are its contents?
2   What is the pH?
3   What is its osmolality?
4   Have you seen this fluid used? If so, why?

Compound sodium lactate (CSL – Hartmann's solution)

CSL is the most complex of the crystalloids discussed in this chapter.

Time out 25.4

Find a one litre bag of compound sodium lactate.

1   What is the pH?
2   List the contents (mmol/litre); next to each item, identify normal serum levels
     (for bicarbonate, see Chapter 8).
3   What is its osmolality?

Contents are relatively similar to normal serum levels, so CSL is often called a 'balanced' solution. Usually, the most important content is the bicarbonate, as bicarbonate is the main buffer for acids in the bloodstream (see Chapter 8). CSL therefore prevents acidosis (Smorenberg *et al.*, 2013), which is why it is favoured with surgery. However, due to chemical instability, the bicarbonate of CSL is 'as lactate'. Lactate is potentially harmful, and can form lactic acid (see Chapter 8). Normally, lactate is metabolised by the liver into bicarbonate. The variable pH stated on most CSL packaging is due to the variable response by each patient, largely depending on their liver function. CSL should therefore be avoided with lactic acidosis, and usually avoided with significant liver dysfunction. Although potassium content is within normal serum range, CSL may be an unwise choice with hyperkalaemia. Being balanced, CSL should spread proportionately across the fluid compartments.

Boldt *et al.* (2009) found that lactate was anti-inflammatory, although as nearly all of Boldt's work has been retracted by publishing journals, this finding needs to be treated with caution.

Ringer's lactate was largely a forerunner of CSL, with slightly less normal physiological contents. It is almost obsolete, but if Ringer's lactate, or any other CSL variant, is used in your workplace, repeat Time out 25.4 with that fluid.

COLLOIDS

Artificial colloids were developed to replace blood transfusion for volume; blood products, including packed red cells, are now transfused only if specific blood products are needed. Traditionally, colloids were viewed as 'plasma expanders', and there were concerns that crystalloid fluid resuscitation would need large volumes (Hinds and Watson, 2008), which would cause more oedema (Norberg *et al.*, 2005; Brochard *et al.*, 2010; Powell-Tuck *et al.*, 2008/2011). However, there is no evidence that fluid resuscitation with colloids is more effective (Bayer *et al.*, 2012; Perel *et al.*, 2013), and increasing concerns about many artificial colloids (Hartog *et al.*, 2011) has reduced their use.

Artificial colloids, and some blood products such as human albumin solution (HAS), contain relatively large molecules suspended in a crystalloid solution. Properties of both the colloid molecule and the crystalloid solution therefore should be considered. A number of different artificial colloids have been marketed, but the only ones still in widespread use are the gelatins. Readers should be familiar with the natural colloid HAS from mandatory blood transfusion training, but its use as an alternative to artificial colloids will be discussed.

Gelatin

First used in 1915, and originally derived from the same gelatine of bone marrow that is used to make jelly, most commercial gelatins are now succinylated.

Time out 25.5

Find a bag of gelatin for infusion (most are 500 ml). Your Trust may stock more than one type of gelatin; if so, obtain one bag of each type, repeating the exercise for each one.

1   Is the gelatin succinylated? If not, what type is it? If it is not succinylated, use the internet or other sources to identify how the gelatine is made, and what clinical significance (if any) this may have.
2   What is the pH?
3   What is its osmolality?
4   What is the average molecule weight of the colloid molecules?
5   Which approximate type of crystalloid fluid is in the bag (contents may not match exactly the crystalloids listed above)?

As colloids have been used with sicker patients, complications are more likely to occur, and whether complications are due to underlying diseases or treatments is often debateable. For example, Bayer *et al.* (2011) found that renal function was impaired by gelatins, while Saw *et al.* (2012) found renal function was improved. Artificial gelatins are suspended in either saline or balanced solutions, and Yunos *et al.* (2011) found that hyperchloraemic fluids, including gelatins in saline, impaired renal function, so even if infusion does induce acute kidney injury the cause may be the crystalloid rather than colloid component.

Gelatin molecules are relatively small, about half of renal threshold, and therefore gelatins are lost in urine, limiting the duration of their effect to often 3–4 hours, depending on many patient-specific factors. Patients receiving gelatins therefore often need early review by medical teams.

Human albumin solution (HAS)

Albumin is the main plasma protein, and available as a blood product, usually in two strengths. Concentrated (20%, in 100 ml bottles) albumin is used for creating hypertonic pull, such as after ascitic drainage. Increasing concerns about artificial colloids have revived interest in using isotonic HAS (4.5% in 500 ml) as a plasma expander. The 1998 Cochrane review claiming that albumin increased mortality is now discredited (BNF, 2014), and Hartog *et al.* (2011) consider albumin safe. It is also anti-inflammatory (Woodcock and Woodcock, 2012), an advantage for sicker patients where inflammation almost invariably complicates their disease. However, HAS is albumin suspended in saline, and therefore being hyperchloraemic may induce acute kidney injury (Yunos *et al.*, 2012).

Implications for practice

- Intravenous fluids are frequently used with sicker patients.
- All IVIs are mainly water, providing volume; solutes and suspended molecules have additional effects.
- Fluid therapy should distinguish between resuscitation (restoring blood volume and pressure rapidly) and maintenance (maintaining the status quo).
- Evidence about each type of fluid is often conflicting.
- It is likely that debate, and conflicting evidence and fashion, will persist.
- 0.9% saline targets interstitial fluid; 5% glucose targets the cells; balanced solutions such as compound sodium lactate should spread proportionately across the fluid compartments.
- 0.9% saline is not 'normal'.
- Duration of plasma expansion from colloids is limited; gelatins are often limited to 3–4 hours (or less).

Summary

Fluid therapy is complicated by controversy, rituals and (often) lack of knowledge – fluids are commonly prescribed by junior doctors who do not know the contents of 0.9% saline (Powell-Tuck *et al.*, 2008/2011). Different crystalloids, and different colloids, have different properties (Powell-Tuck *et al.*, 2008/2011) caused by the solutes and molecules they contain ('fine-tuning'). As part of the multidisciplinary team, and the staff most often administering intravenous fluids, nurses should be aware of likely effects and concerns about fluids used.

Further reading

Powell-Tuck *et al.* (2008/2011) provide consensus guidelines on fluid management, although physicians were notably absent from bodies involved. NICE (2013b) provides guidelines for fluid resuscitation. Readers should be aware of any local fluid policies. Yunos *et al.* (2011) raise significant concerns about hyperchloraemic fluids. Many studies provide conflicting and often limited evidence, so studies should be read critically.

Clinical scenario

Mrs Jean Richardson, aged 77 weighing 82 kg, had an emergency repair of a fractured femur, following a fall in her garden. Pre- and peri operatively she suffered large blood loss. On return to the ward she is hypotensive and tachycardic; two Robinsons drains are already half full of frank blood. She has an IVI in progress of compound sodium lactate, running at 125 ml/h. You have called the surgical team, and checked her haemoglobin on a venous blood gas (115 grams/litre).

1 If Mrs Richardson is hypovolaemic, why is her haemoglobin not lower?
2 What type of fluid, and how much over what timescale, would you suggest to the surgeons? Give rationales for your decisions.
3 Identify any local guidelines that would be relevant to Mrs Richardson's fluid needs. Discuss your thoughts with nursing and medical colleagues, and ask reasons for any different choices.

Chapter 26

Gut function and failure

Contents

Fundamental knowledge

- Liver anatomy and physiology

Introduction

Unless gut failure is the cause of hospital admission, gut function is too often ignored until problems occur. The gut is a large and complex system; pancreatitis and diabetic emergencies are discussed in Chapter 27. Chapters focusing on gastrointestinal bleeds and acute liver failure are included in *Intensive Care Nursing*, so these problems are only briefly summarised. This chapter mainly focuses on liver failure, especially chronic, but concludes with a section on bowels.

Although lower gut problems are seldom immediately life-threatening, ignoring the lower gut can cause significant complications. Aspects discussed include:

- endogenous infection
- constipation
- diarrhoea.

Understanding factors that can precipitate problems enables nurses to reduce complications.

1: GASTROINTESTINAL BLEEDS

The purpose of the gut being to absorb nutrients, it is highly vascular, and therefore prone to major bleeds. Upper gastrointestinal (GI) bleeds tend to be more life-threatening, whereas lower GI bleeds tend to threaten quality of life. Major upper GI bleeds usually necessitate urgent endoscopy (Toubia and Sanyal, 2008; Barkun *et al.*, 2010). Large blood loss can cause haemorrhagic shock and necessitates fluid resuscitation to prevent further organ failure. Upper GI bleeds are discussed further in *Intensive Care Nursing*.

Lower GI bleeds tend to be more insidious and often cause chronic anaemia which necessitates frequent blood transfusions. Persistent bleeds may necessitate hemicolectomy and colostomy formation.

2: LIVER FAILURE

The liver has many functions, but these can be grouped into four main areas:

- detoxification (drugs, alcohol, hormones);
- digestive (bile formation, nutrient metabolism), including protein synthesis (albumin, clotting factors);
- infection control (macrophages, complements);
- storage (glycogen, vitamins).

Although symptoms of failure are usually relatively slow to develop, compared with other organs, effects can be widespread, and devastating. The All-Party Parliamentary Hepatology Group (APPHG, 2014) identify liver disease as one of the five biggest killer diseases in the UK, and the only one increasing, with average age of death being 59 and falling, and suggest that the main causes (alcohol, obesity and viral hepatitis) are all preventable. Aspects of care for acute and chronic failure can often be managed in general hospitals, but liver failure may need transplantation or other specialist interventions, so tertiary centres should be involved. If transplantation is not an option for end-stage liver disease, then palliation is indicated.

Acute liver failure tends to cause sudden, massive necrosis of hepatocytes, resulting in loss of liver function. If caused by paracetamol poisoning, it may be reversed with intravenous N-Acetylcystine (Parvolex™) (Patton *et al.*, 2012). Otherwise, severe acute failure usually necessitates transplant (Fontana, 2008). System support may necessitate transfer to intensive care units. Acute liver failure is discussed further in *Intensive Care Nursing*.

Chronic liver failure is caused by progressive fibrosis and scarring, which obstructs bloodflow through the liver. Symptoms are often insidious, complications usually having occurred by the time of diagnosis.

Acute or chronic failure may be

- compensated *or*
- decompensated.

As long compensation occurs, quality of life can be reasonable; but once liver failure becomes decompensated, progressive complications to multiple body systems limit quality of life and expose patients to significant mortality risks. Acute and chronic liver failure often cause similar problems, so discussion below includes both. The ultimate treatment, transplantation, is not available outside specialist centres, so is beyond the scope of this book.

Causes

Because the liver metabolises most chemicals in the body, many substances are potentially hepatotoxic. The most common cause of acute liver failure is paracetamol overdose (Rashid *et al.*, 2004); O'Shea *et al.* (2010) suggest alcohol is the most common cause of chronic failure, although LaBrecque *et al.* (2014) identify non-alcoholic fatty liver disease (NAFLD) and non-alcoholic straeto-hepatitis (NASH) as the main causes. Fatty liver predisposes to the hyperglycaemia and high triglyceride levels of metabolic syndrome (Yki-Järvinen, 2014). Viruses can cause acute and/or chronic hepatitis; besides viruses called hepatitis (A, B, C, D, E), many others including herpes simplex, varicella, cytomegalovirus and Epstein-Barr have occasionally been reported as sources (Patton *et al.*, 2012). Chronic failure from hepatitis C is increasing (Nash *et al.*, 2009).

Paracetamol metabolism varies between individuals, so small overdoses may prove fatal to some people, while others may survive significantly larger overdoses. Plasma levels usually peak within 1–2 hours after ingestion (Smith, 2007), but may take up to 4 hours to be interpretable (Bateman, 2007). Levels exceeding 200 mg/litre after 4 hours or 50 mg/litre after 12 hours are likely to cause hepatocyte damage (Higgins, 2013) and can cause renal tubular necrosis (Bateman, 2007). Initial symptoms may be limited to nausea, but damage is slow and progressive. Intravenous acetlycysteine should be given if

- blood paracetamol levels are 100 mg/litre at 4 hours
- blood paracetamol levels are 15 mg/litre at 15 hours
- the overdose was staggered *or*
- there is doubt over the time of paracetamol ingestion.

(Commission on Human Medicines, 2012)

Chronic inflammation of the liver causes fibrosis, leaving scar tissue between liver cells (*cirrhosis*), which causes obstructive liver disease. As bloodflow through the liver is obstructed, detoxification fails, creating problems identified above with obstruction. Obstructed blood flow increases pressure in the hepatic portal vein (*portal hypertension*). Cirrhosis usually progresses to chronic liver failure and can progress to cancer (Williams *et al.*, 2014).

Symptoms

Decompensated liver failure typically causes

- jaundice
- encephalopathy (confusion, drowsiness or other neurological changes)
- coagulopathy (e.g. bruising, bleeding).

Severe/chronic liver failure often causes ascites, but this is often a late complication. As the liver has multiple functions, many other complications can occur, especially nutritional deficiencies. Patients' medical and social history may suggest liver disease, although they may also deny or moderate risk factors such as alcohol. Recent foreign travel may have exposed them to viral hepatitis.

Mortality

Death from liver failure (acute or chronic) is usually caused by

- encephalopathy
- infection
- haemorrhage.

Encephalopathy

With liver failure, detoxification becomes suboptimal. Ammonia and other toxins increase blood–brain barrier permeability (Bernal *et al.*, 2010), enabling formation of cerebral oedema. Up to four fifths of people with cirrhosis develop encephalopathy (Sargent, 2007). Traditionally, regular lactulose has been given to remove toxins (Nilles and Subramanian, 2012), but currently other drugs are being assessed, such as the non-absorbable antibiotic Rifaximin (Patton *et al.*, 2012; EASL, 2014).

Depending on severity, symptoms may include

- acute confusion
- drowsiness/coma
- fitting.

(Patton *et al.*, 2012)

Nursing care should include skilful psychological support of both patient and relatives, as well as maintaining safety (e.g. airway – preventing aspiration) and providing fundamental aspects of care. Nursing staff may also need to involve other professionals for specialist support (e.g. social workers). EASL is currently developing guidelines for hepatic encephalopathy (EASL, 2014).

Infection

The liver has important roles in preventing infection. Any gut bacteria reaching the liver should be killed by liver macrophages (previously called Kuppfer cells). The liver also releases a group of chemicals which collectively form the 'membrane attack complex', adhering to micro-organisms to encourage phagocytosis. Both these mechanisms are impaired with liver failure. Four fifths of patients with acute liver failure develop bacterial infection (Fontana, 2008), especially chest infections (Gunning, 2009).

Haemorrhage

Many clotting factors are produced in the liver (see Chapter 3), so liver failure predisposes to bleeding. Three main blood vessels enter the liver. The largest is the hepatic portal vein, flowing from the gut to the liver, carrying nutrients absorbed by the gut. With liver obstruction, portal hypertension increases, causing development of collateral vessels – weak, tortuous vessels which develop to bypass obstruction. The main collateral vessels which develop from obstructive liver disease are oesophageal varices, usually around the base of the oesophagus. Being weak, these easily rupture, causing massive bleeds. Cirrhosis usually causes varices (Toubia and Sanyal, 2008); variceal bleeds are usually massive and immediately life-threatening, necessitating urgent endoscopy. For all patients with liver failure, anything that can provoke bleeding, such as wet shaving, should be avoided.

Ascites

Ascites is usually a complication of chronic failure (EASL, 2010), but can occur with acute failure. Mainly caused by hypernatraemia (EASL, 2010), it forms protein-rich fluid which exerts osmotic pressure, drawing more fluid towards it.

Ascites can cause many complications, including organ damage from intra-abdominal hypertension (see below) and splinting of the diaphragm which impairs respiratory function. Large collections are usually drained (paracentesis), with concurrent salt-poor (20%) albumin infusion. Subsequent care to reduce recurrence often includes

- fluid restriction
- salt restriction
- aldosterone antagonists (e.g. spironalactone).

(Gines and Cardenas, 2008; Hou and Sanyal, 2009)

and sometimes insertion of shunts to bypass the liver, such as trans-systemic intrahepatic portal shunt (TIPS) linking the hepatic portal vein directly with the inferior vena cava. (EASL, 2010). Alfa pumps, which drain ascites into the bladder, are currently experimental (Bellot et al., 2013) due to their complications, but may offer future hope.

Intra-abdominal pressure

Interstitial pressure inside the abdomen is normally 5–7 mmHg (De Keulenaer *et al.*, 2009). Intra-abdominal hypertension (>20 mmHg) damages organs (Malbain *et al.*, 2005). One of the simplest ways to measure intra-abdominal pressure is with a manometer attached to a urinary catheter. Causes of excessive pressure, such as ascites, should be removed if possible. Persistent intra-abdominal hypertension may necessitate decompressive laparotomy ('open abdomen') with ICU admission.

Nutrition

Patients with liver failure are often malnourished, partly because the liver metabolises most nutrients, and often partly from their lifestyle. The liver stores many nutrients, including fat-soluble vitamins (A, D, E, K) and glucose (as glycogen), so failing livers will store little even if dietary intake is adequate. Early enteral feeding should be commenced, and referral made to dieticians. With malnutrition, refeeding syndrome can occur (see Chapter 28).

Nurses should offer health promotion advice. The obvious advice for alcoholic liver disease is abstinence from alcohol. Dietary advice will usually be offered by dieticians. Other advice will depend partly on causes of the failure, and its effects.

3: BOWELS

Normal gut flora (bacteria) aid digestion, but can become pathogenic if they translocate into either the bloodstream or surrounding tissue. The gut wall secretes lysozyme and other antibacterial substances, although some bacterial translocation is probably normal (MacFie, 2013). Lack of enteral nutrition may cause gut wall atrophy and failure of defences (MacFie, 2013).

Healthy bowel function is important for eliminating solid waste from the body, yet bowel care is frequently overlooked (RCN, 2008a). Nurses should assess and monitor bowel function. Initially, this usually means asking patients, or their families, about bowel function and habit. Any recent changes in bowel function, difficulty passing stool, or blood, should be investigated further. If bleeding is suspected, a stool sample should be obtained. Social stigma may prevent some patients from reporting bowel problems. Restlessness, agitation and confusion may be symptoms of constipation, so nurses should assess restless patients by asking when they last opened their bowels. Constipation may also cause nausea and reluctance to eat.

Bowel function should be therefore assessed, and monitored if concerns are identified. Type of stool should be recorded: colour, consistency, amount. The Bristol Stool Chart, discussed in *Intensive Care Nursing*, is widely used to monitor bowel function. Contrary to widespread belief, not everyone normally opens their bowels daily, so asking what is normal for the person should be part of routine nursing assessment on admission. Nurses should also ask whether people have noticed any change in regularity or abnormalities in their stool. Abnormalities include

- constipation
- diarrhoea
- blood
- fat (streatorrhoea – pale, offensive stools that float in water).

Constipation may have various causes, including reduced mobility and dehydration, so mobilising patients is usually an important part of bowel care. But initially, constipation often necessitates laxatives (Bharucha *et al.*, 2013):

- *stimulant laxatives* (e.g. senna) increase gut peristalsis, so are often the first choice of laxative for new constipation;
- *osmotic laxatives* (e.g. lactulose) lubricate the stool, so may be useful with severe constipation, often in combination with stimulant laxatives;
- *bulk-forming laxatives* (e.g. bran) increase faecal volume, so are generally the best choice where chronic constipation is likely, such as from severely reduced mobility.

If laxatives are ineffective after a few days, suppositories, and later enemas, may be needed to evacuate bowels. Long-term use of laxatives should be discouraged. Where patients have persistent problems with constipation, dieticians can provide advice about high-fibre diets.

Bowel assessment may need digital rectal examination, and occasionally manual evacuation may be needed, but both procedures should only be performed if necessary, following individual assessment, and with patients' consent (RCN, 2008a).

Diarrhoea occurs when more fluid enters the bowels than they can absorb. Possible causes include

- excessive fluid
- rapid peristalsis
- reduced absorption (e.g. hypoalbuminaemia – see Chapter 3).

Peristalsis is increased if normal gut flora is destroyed, typically either by broad spectrum antibiotics, or by infection (e.g. *Clostridium difficile*, *Norovirus*). If caused by infection, diarrhoea is a natural way to remove pathogens from the body (but risks causing cross-infection). If caused by therapeutic antibiotics, gut motility can be slowed by drugs (e.g. loperamide, codeine phosphate). Probiotics have been advocated (Kelly and Lamont, 2008; Allen *et al.*, 2010), although a recent trial did not find them beneficial (Allen *et al.*, 2013). Severe diarrhoea can cause fluid and electrolyte imbalances, necessitating replacements.

Implications for practice

- Large bleeds need urgent fluid resuscitation and close haemodynamic monitoring.
- Liver dysfunction exposes patients to greater risks of opportunistic infections, so infection control becomes especially important.
- With liver failure, hypoglycaemia may develop rapidly, so monitor blood sugar.
- Increasing drowsiness may be a sign of encephalopathy.

- Causes of liver failure, such as alcoholism or paracetamol overdose, may cause guilt and/or anger among relatives, creating psychological needs for both them and the patient.
- Early enteral feeding helps promote gut integrity.
- Nurses should monitor bowel function, anticipating and if possible preventing possible causes of constipation or diarrhoea.

Summary

The gut has many functions. As gut failure seldom causes acute hospital admission, the system can be too easily ignored until complications occur. Preventing problems reduces mortality and morbidity. Generally, early nutrition with standard feeds promotes normal gut function and health (use it or lose it).

Useful websites

European Association for the Study of the Liver: www.easl.eu/
All-Party Parliamentary Hepatology Group: www.appghep.org.uk/

Further reading

The European Association for the Study of the Liver (EASL, 2010) guidelines for managing ascites provide an authoritative review; they have also published guidelines on encephalopathy (EASL, 2014). RCN (2008a) offers guidance on bowel care. Specialist medical journals *Gut* and *Gastroenterology* are generally useful sources for material on this topic. O'Shea *et al.*'s (2010) USA guidelines for alcoholic liver disease provide a comprehensive review of this aspect.

Clinical scenario

John Sanders, aged 28 years old, was staying in a hotel. This morning he was found in a drowsy state. In the ambulance he admitted taking a paracetamol overdose the previous evening, but would not admit how many he had taken. There were two empty packs of 32 tablets nearby. He stated that he wished to die, having recently been left by his long-term partner. A stomach washout in A&E produced only a few remains of tablets. He has been transferred to a medical assessment ward, with acetylcystine infusion already in progress. He is now less drowsy with a Glasgow Coma Score of 11.

John is self-employed. His next of kin is his windowed mother, who lives 250 miles away, has been contacted and is travelling to the hospital by train.

1   From this chapter, and any other sources available, use A-B-C-D-E assessment to identify the nursing priorities immediately following John's arrival in Medical Assessment.
2   Using this list of priorities, devise a plan for John's immediate nursing care.
3   Paracetamol levels, which were taken in A&E after the washout, are reported as being 200 mg/litre. John has been referred to the regional liver centre. Meanwhile, he is to be transferred to a general medical ward once a bed is available. What aspects of physical and psychological care should be highlighted to ward nurses?

Chapter 27

Pancreatitis and diabetic emergencies

Contents

Fundamental knowledge

- Familiarity with pathophysiology and treatment of diabetes mellitus, and differences between type 1 and type 2 diabetes

Introduction

The pancreas is both an endocrine and exocrine organ. Problems with either function can lead to, or complicate, acute illness. It produces four hormones, but the most significant is insulin. Insufficient insulin causes diabetes. Three diabetic emergencies are discussed:

- severe hypoglycaemia
- diabetic ketoacidosis (DKA)
- hyperosmolar hyperglycaemic state (HHS).

Its exocrine function is to secrete digestive juices, such as amylase, into the duodenum. Obstruction causes

- pancreatitis.

1: PANCREATITIS

Pancreatitis is a relatively common disease, and incidence continues to increase (Kingsnorth and O'Reilly, 2006; Baddeley *et al.*, 2011). Most cases remain mild, causing few problems beyond abdominal pain. But one fifth progress to severe acute pancreatitis (Rickes and Uhle, 2009). Progression is unpredictable (Tenner *et al.*, 2013), but usually rapid when it occurs. Close nursing observations and escalation of concern can therefore improve outcome if deterioration occurs. Severe pancreatitis is discussed in greater detail in *Intensive Care Nursing.*

The pancreas releases digestive enzymes ('juices') in a reflex response to acid in the duodenum. Pancreatic enzymes are alkaline (pH around 8.0 (Marieb and Hoehn, 2013)), so neutralise acid in the duodenum. Secretion therefore creates a negative feedback mechanism – acid having been neutralised, there is no further stimulus to release pancreatic enzymes. However, if the pancreatic duct transporting the enzymes is blocked, the stimulus remains; unable to flow into the duodenum, digestive juices make the pancreas engorged, inflamed, and acutely painful. Usually, pancreatitis resolves with time, medical and nursing care largely being limited to symptom control and observation.

Severe pancreatitis occurs if enzymes digest pancreatic tissue itself, provoking severe inflammatory responses. If a fistula forms into the peripancreatic fat, this fat is also digested, leaving necrotic tissue that can be a focus for infection, pancreatic abscesses and necrotising pancreatitis. Release of pro-inflammatory mediators into the bloodstream triggers a systemic inflammatory response syndrome (SIRS, distributive shock – see Chapter 13).

Serum lipase is the recommended laboratory test (UK Working Party, 2005), pancreatitis causing levels above 110 units/litre. Serum amylase (normal 30–100 units/litre) is massively increased with pancreatitis, although levels do not reflect severity of the disease (Hayden and Wyncoll, 2008). The inflammatory marker CRP (see Chapter 3) does indicate severity (UK Working Party, 2005).

Pancreatitis is usually caused by

- alcoholism
- gallstones

although a significant minority of cases are caused by other factors, including drugs such as NSAIDs and thiazide diuretics (Hughes, 2004), and about 15% of cases have no cause identified (Rickes and Uhle, 2009).

Gallstones

Salts in bile can form 'stones' which, if small enough, may pass down the bile duct only to be trapped at the ampulla of Vater, where the common bile duct enters the duodenum.

Because the common bile duct has joined the bile duct and pancreatic duct, digestive enzymes are unable to enter the duodenum. Biliary pancreatitis more often occurs in women in their fifties (Hale *et al.*, 2000).

Alcohol

Alcohol can cause damage (hardening) to many tissues in the body, including the pancreatic duct. One half of cases of pancreatitis are caused by alcohol (Lowe and Sevilla, 2012), typically in males with a median age of 51.5 years (Lowe and Sevilla, 2012). One in ten abusers of alcohol develop acute pancreatitis (Williams and Williamson, 2010). Incidence of alcohol-related pancreatitis is increasing (Williams and Williamson, 2010); chronic pancreatitis is usually due to alcohol (Hughes, 2004).

Mortality

Overall mortality from pancreatitis is about 7% (Rickes and Uhle, 2009), rising to about 30% with severe acute pancreatitis (Hayden and Wyncoll, 2008).

Complications

Pancreatitis can cause many complications, including

- pain
- cardiovascular
- respiratory
- metabolic
- nutritional.

Pain

Pain from pancreatitis is often severe. Pain usually causes nausea and (often) vomiting. Opioids, usually morphine, and anti-emetics are usually needed.

Cardiovascular

Inflammation and stress cause large shifts of fluid from the bloodstream into tissues, causing

- hypovolaemia and shock;
- ascites and oedema;
- pericardial effusions, often causing dysrhythmias and raised ST segments;
- electrolyte imbalances.

Aggressive fluid therapy should be given to prevent organ failure (UK Working Party, 2005; Tenner *et al.*, 2013). Close monitoring, including urine output (target >0.5 ml/kg/h), continuous ECG, fluid balance and central venous pressure, are usually needed.

Respiratory

Severe attacks often cause acute lung injury and pulmonary oedema. Breathing may also be compromised by

■ pain
■ diaphragmatic splinting from abdominal distension
■ pleural effusions
■ pulmonary oedema.

Supplementary oxygen is often needed. Close and frequent respiratory monitoring should include rate, depth and oxygen saturation.

Metabolic

Impaired insulin release, insulin antagonism and excessive glucagon release often cause hyperglycaemia. Insulin therapy and frequent blood glucose monitoring may be needed. Many electrolyte imbalances occur, partly from fluid shifts and partly from poor diet or impaired intake. Blood calcium, needed for cardiac conduction, clotting and cell repair, is often low (Hale *et al.*, 2000). Biochemistry (U+Es) should be checked and stabilised.

Medical treatment

Historically, the treatment for pancreatitis was surgery, hence patients are usually admitted under surgical teams. However, surgery is only beneficial if there is an abscess of drain, or necrotic tissue to debride. Infected pancreatic necrosis necessitates early surgical debridement (Nathens *et al.*, 2004; Malangoni and Martin, 2005). Gallstones may be removed using endoscopic retrograde colangio-pancreatography (ERCP) or lithotripsy. Cholecystectomy may be performed to prevent recurrence (Mitchell *et al.*, 2003). Otherwise, medical treatments are largely supportive.

Nutrition

Patients may be malnourished or reluctant to eat due to pain or precipitating causes. Early enteral nutrition improves outcome (UK Working Party, 2005; Meier *et al.*, 2006; Tenner *et al.*, 2013). Any precipitating causes for pancreatitis (alcoholism or fatty diet) should be identified and health promotion offered.

2: DIABETES MELLITUS

Diabetes means 'fountain-like', from the early observation of polydipsia and polyuria. Subsequently two different diseases were identified: diabetes inspidus, caused by lack of antidiuretic hormone (see Chapter 17) and diabetes mellitus, caused by insulin deficiency. Diabetes without any suffix refers to diabetes mellitus.

Diabetes is one of the most common disease, causing many potential complications, including cardiovascular disease (Tocci *et al.*, 2011), blindness (Watkins, 2003), chronic kidney disease (Sego, 2007) and neuropathy (Yagihashi, 2011). There are two types of diabetes mellitus: type 1 and type 2. Type 1 typically manifests in childhood (Lambert and Bingley, 2002), and is caused by autoimmune destruction of producing insulin-beta cells in pancreas (Walltmahmed, 2006; Hex *et al.*, 2012). With little insulin produced, and often high insulin resistance, type 1 diabetes usually necessitates life-long insulin therapy. Type 2 diabetes typically develops with increasing age, especially in obese people, although there is a worrying increase in children who are type 2 diabetics (Haines *et al.*, 2007). A total of 85–90% of diabetics are type 2 (Hex *et al.*, 2012), and although initially usually managed by diet and later oral hypoglycaemics, around half will eventually need insulin (Walltmahmed, 2006).

Type 2 diabetes is often preceded by the 'metabolic syndrome'. Criteria for this syndrome vary, but Achike *et al.* (2011) cite a World Health Organization definition:

- presence of diabetes mellitus, impaired glucose tolerance, impaired fasting glucose or insulin resistance and any two of
    - hypertension (140/90 mmHg or more)
    - dyslipidaemia (raised triglyceride and/or high-density lipoprotein–cholesterol)
    - obesity
    - microalbuminuria.

Identifying risk factors enables earlier health promotion (Kramer *et al.*, 2013), so although diagnosing metabolic syndrome is more useful for primary care, the term may be encountered in hospital practice.

Diabetes may be co-incidental to the cause of hospital admission. Initially, previous diabetic management will be maintained, but blood sugar should be closely monitored, as stress responses from disease may exacerbate hyperglycaemia, necessitating more aggressive management. Diabetes is often initially diagnosed from routine admission urinalysis, or symptoms that have necessitated admission. Suspected, newly-diagnosed, or unstable diabetics should be referred urgently to diabetic specialists. Nurses should identify any activity of living deficits, and provide appropriate help and support where necessary.

Diabetic emergencies

Severe hypoglycaemia

This is usually caused by insulin overdose or severe malnutrition, but can by iatrogenic. It should be reversed by giving glucose, usually intravenously.

Iatrogenic hypoglycaemia can be caused by insulin, or other hypoglycaemics, being given without sufficient glucose or carbohydrate, and with insufficient monitoring of blood glucose. In sicker patients, it is therefore safer to maintain mildly elevated levels of 7.8–10.0 (NICE-SUGAR Study investigators, 2009; Preise *et al.*, 2009; Krinsley and Keegan, 2010).

Diabetic ketoacidosis

This usually occurs in type 1 diabetics. It causes

- ketonaemia ≥3 mmol/litre (×10 normal); more than ++ on standard urine dipsticks; > 6 mmol/litre = severe DKA;
- blood glucose >11 mmol/litre;
- metabolic acidosis: bicarbonate <15 mmol/litre and/or venous pH <7.3.

(JBDS, 2013)

Lack of insulin deprives mitochondria of glucose. Energy is therefore produced from fat, which releases ketones. Ketones diffuse into blood, forming ketoacids, hence the metabolic acidosis. Serum ketones and glucose exceed renal reabsorption thresholds, resulting in ketonuria and glycosuria, both of which cause osmotic diuresis (Keays, 2014). Gross polyuria causes severe dehydration. JBDS (2013) identify priorities as

- point of care ketone monitoring;
- reducing blood glucose with fixed rate intravenous insulin infusion (FRIII);
- monitoring venous pH;
- fluid resuscitation.

Their metabolic treatment targets are listed in Table 27.1.

Table 27.1 JBDS (2013) metabolic targets for managing diabetic ketoacidosis

- reduce blood ketones by 0.5 mmol/litre
- increase venous bicarbonate by 3.0 mmol/litre
- reduce capillary blood glucose by 3.0 mmol/litre
- maintain serum potassium 4.0–5.5 mmol/litre

Hyperosmolar hyperglycaemic state

This is rare, but usually occurs with type 2 diabetes (Keays, 2014). Caused by insulin insufficiency rather than total lack, it develops more insidiously. The body therefore has time to compensate for hypovolaemia by transferring cell water into the bloodstream. Once patients present to acute hospitals, they are whole-body dehydrated, rather than just hypovolaemic. They also tend to be older, with more co-morbidities. Mortality is therefore higher than with DKA (Keays, 2014). Hyperglycaemia usually resolves with rehydration, so insulin should only be given if ketosis is present, and even then at low doses (0.05 units/kg/h) (JBDS, 2010).

Implications for practice

- Pancreatitis causes acute pain, often needing opioid analgesia and often anti-emetics.
- Hyperglycaemia may occur with pancreatitis, so blood sugar should be assessed. Insulin may be needed.

- Early enteral nutrition generally speeds recovery from pancreatitis.
- Diabetes is a common disease which can cause significant complications.
- Stress responses from acute illness can complicate glycaemic control.
- Diabetic emergencies can be life-threatening, necessitating urgent stabilisation.

Summary

Pancreatitis often requires urgent intervention. Most cases of pancreatitis remain mild, but an unpredictable minority progress rapidly to acute severe pancreatitis, with significant mortality. Medical treatment of severe acute pancreatitis is difficult and remains largely limited to supporting failing systems. Nursing care focuses around providing relief from pain and nausea, providing other care that patients need, and close observation and monitoring so that any deterioration can be reported and treated promptly.

Diabetes is a common disease, which may be co-incidental to acute hospital admission, be stable and well-managed, and so existing care should be maintained. But it may be newly suspected/diagnosed or unstable, necessitating urgent investigation and stabilisation. Diabetes may be destabilised by illness, and may proceed to or present as a diabetic crisis. Most acute hospitals have specialist diabetic nurses, who should be informed of any problems with diabetes.

Useful websites

Joint British Diabetes Societies
DiabetesUK

Further reading

The Joint British Diabetes Society (JBDS 2010, 2013) provide guidelines for diabetic management and emergencies. Current UK guidelines on pancreatitis date from 2005 (UK Working Party on Acute Pancreatitis), although USA 2013 guidelines are substantially similar.

Clinical scenario

Charles Hill, aged 49, is admitted with acute pancreatitis. On arrival, he is in obvious pain, despite having been given 10 mg oromorph an hour previously. The medical team have prescribed an aggressive fluid regime of Hartmann's 500 ml over 1 hour, which has been commenced immediately before transfer. They will review him further within that hour, by when results from serum lipase should be available. He is separated from his wife, and gives his next-of-kin as his daughter, whom he describes as 'close', and who manages a care home 'about 50 miles away'.

1   Using A-B-C-D-E assessment, list immediate priorities of nursing care for Mr Hill. Identify rationales for care.
2   Mr Hill's vital signs are:

> HR 115 regular
> BP 90/60 mmHg
> RR 35 bpm
> temperature 38.5°C

His blood sugar is 24 mmol/litre. He is oliguric, passing 15 ml during the last hour. The medical team have just arrived and are now reviewing Mr Hill. Using A-B-C-D-E assessment, what treatments do you anticipate they will offer Mr Hill? Include rationales for interventions.
3   The medical team's decisions coincide with your expectations. Devise a plan of care for Mr Hill for the next 12 hours, remembering possible complications that may occur. Mr Hill's daughter is expected shortly; include information and support that you will offer her.

Chapter 28

Nutrition

Contents

Fundamental knowledge

- Anatomy and physiology of the gastrointestinal tract

Introduction

Russell and Elia (2009) found 28% of hospital patients are malnourished, with a higher incidence in those aged over 65; Holyday *et al.* (2012) found even higher malnutirion among older patients. Internationally, about 40% of hospitalised patients are malnourished (Barker *et al.*, 2011). Malnutrition causes many complications (see Table 28.1), increases morbidity and mortality (NICE, 2012c), and is widespread (Agarwal *et al.*, 2012). Disease from malnutrition costs the UK £1.3 billion pounds per year (DOH, 2011b).

Table 28.1 Effects of malnutrition

Physical
↓ growth/development
↓ fat and lean body mass
↓ strength and lethargy
↓ ability to cough
↑ pressure sore risk
↓ mobility ↑ falls
↑ risk of respiratory infections

Physiological
impaired immunity
impaired wound healing
↓ gastrointestinal secretions
↑ risk of infection/complications
↑ convalescence
↑ side effects

Psychological
anxiety and depression
↓ quality of life

(DOH, 2011b)

Glucose is normally the preferred energy source for cells, but if diet fails to provide sufficient glucose, the body uses its glycogen stores, then autocannibalises body fat and protein for energy. With catabolic states, 1–2% of muscle is broken down each day (Skipworth *et al.*, 2006). This causes, or predisposes to, most of the complications listed above. Early nutrition reduces mortality (Doig *et al.*, 2009). Most acute hospitals employ dieticians, but good nutrition needs multidisciplinary teamwork (DOH, 2011b). Nurses are core members of this team, usually performing initial assessments (Malone, 2013), co-ordinating referrals and teamwork, and ensuring patients have assistance with eating if needed. Optimising nutrition is a major aspect of nursing care.

Refeeding syndrome

Starvation causes significant metabolic changes:

- reduced insulin release
- increased glucagon release
- protein becomes the main energy source
- protein metabolism causes muscle wasting
- depletion of intracellular phosphate, magnesium and potassium.

(Ormerod *et al.*, 2010)

Very ill/malnourished people who have not eaten for 5 days are at high risk of 'refeeding syndrome'. Suddenly restoring normal supplies of nutrients increases insulin release, transporting sugar, water and micronutrients (potassium, phosphate, magnesium) into cells, causing life-threatening fluid, electrolyte and other imbalances (Mehanna *et al.*, 2008; Fuentebella and Kerner, 2009; Ormerod *et al.*, 2010).

Patients at risk of refeeding syndrome should have feeds (enteral or parenteral) introduced at half estimated requirement for 24–48 hours (NICE, 2006), with electrolyte and micronutrient imbalances restored. Before feeding, vitamin B supplements should be given.

Translocation of gut bacteria

As identified in Chapter 26, lack of enteral nutrition predisposes to translocation of gut bacteria into blood (MacFie, 2013). Blood from the gut flows to the liver, where specialised macrophages destroy pathogens. But ischaemia also compromises liver function (see Chapter 26), exposing the lungs and other organs to infection from gut-derived pathogens. Enteral nutrition prevents gut atrophy (Zarzaur *et al.*, 2000; Fukatsu *et al.*, 2001).

Surgery

Traditional practices of prolonged preoperative fasting have largely been eradicated by admitting many patients on the day of elective surgery, but many patients are malnourished on admission – post-operative mortality is higher among patients with low serum albumin (Palma *et al.*, 2007). When patients are admitted for gut surgery, gut pathology has often contributed to under-nourishment – for example, Crohn's disease.

'Enhanced recovery after surgery' (ERAS) protocols promote preoperative anabolism so that patients can benefit more from post-operative nutrition:

- solid foods up to 6 hours preoperatively;
- 800 ml clear carbohydrate drink before midnight;
- 400 ml carbohydrate drink 2–3 hours preoperatively;
- clear fluids up to 2 hours preoperatively;
- commence oral food 4 hours post-operatively.

(Fearon *et al.*, 2005)

Unless advised otherwise, all drugs should be given preoperatively (RCN, 2005). Enhanced recovery

- reduces preoperative thirst, hunger and anxiety (Fearon *et al.*, 2005);
- reduces post-operative hyperglycaemia and insulin requirements (Fearon *et al.*, 2005);
- improves cardiac output and splanchnic perfusion (Revelley *et al.*, 2001).

Early post-operative feeding is both safe and beneficial, even following gut surgery (Skipworth *et al.*, 2006; Hans-Geurts *et al.*, 2007; Doig *et al.*, 2009), and ERAS is recommended by DOH (2011b).

Absence of bowel sounds is not clinically significant (Baid, 2009), and is not a contra-indication for feeding. Bowel sounds are largely caused by movement of air or gas, so nil-by-mouth patients are unlikely to have sufficient air to cause bowel sounds. While patients with paralytic ileus will not have bowel sounds, patients with no bowel sounds may have absence of peristalsis or absence of air. Nurses should therefore encourage early nutrition whenever possible.

Oral nutrition

Oral nutrition is the safest, simplest and cheapest form of nutrition, provided the patient is able and willing to eat. However, plated food can bring problems of assessing needs/intake, as plated food is generally distributed and cleared away by support staff (Grieve and Finnie, 2002). Nutritional state should therefore be assessed.

NICE (2006) recommends that all hospitals have multidisciplinary nutritional support teams. However, the main barrier to effective nutrition is often that patients are 'not hungry' (Agarwal *et al.*, 2012). Additional strategies to help motivate patients include

- health education about the value of nutrition to help recovery;
- presenting food in appetising ways: small but attractive portions;
- offering supplements between meals;
- protected meal times, giving patients the opportunity to eat food provided (NPSA, 2007d; RCN, 2008b; DOH, 2011b).

Other ways to help improve nutrition include

- 'red trays'– placing meals of patients at risk on a red tray helps identify priorities for observing and helping with oral intake (Leach *et al.*, 2013); support staff should not clear away red trays until a nurse has seen what has been eaten;
- rotas of voluntary workers for meal-time support;
- allowing relatives to help feed patients (Leach *et al.*, 2013).

Any patient with additional or complex nutritional needs, or having an 'at risk' score, should be referred to dieticians.

Enteral nutrition

Where oral diets prove impossible or inadequate, tube feeding into the gut is both the safest and cheapest alternative.

At rest, gastric pH is below 4, providing a hostile environment for any invading micro-organisms. Resting feeds allows gastric acidity to return to normal, although the optimum rest period remains unclear. It should be long enough for the stomach to empty. Resting the gut overnight for 6–8 hours seems physiologically logical – patients taking oral diets would not eat overnight. However, if patients have taken little oral diet in the day, overnight nasogastric supplements may allow time for appetite to develop before main meals the next day.

Tubes

Fine-bore nasogastric tubes (5–8 French gauge) are recommended (NICE, 2006), as they cause less oesophageal erosion/ulceration, and are better tolerated (Best, 2007). The only acceptable tests to confirm initial placement are pH aspirate being 1.0–5.5 or confirmation from a chest X-ray (NHS England, 2013). Check placement before each feed, and each time anything is given through the tube. Patients being treated with antacids are likely to have gastric pH above 5.5. Aspirate is unlikely to be obtained from post-pyloric (jejunostomy) tubes, and should anyway have an alkaline pH. If prolonged tube-feeding is anticipated, a percutaneous gastrostomy (PEG) should be considered.

Total paralytic ileus prevents enteral feeding, but paralysis most often affects the stomach, and least often affects the bowels. As most nutrients are absorbed in the ileum, feeding directly into the small bowel (jejunal tubes) can provide effective nutrition.

Aspirate

Gastric residual volume (aspirate) is the most widely used method to evaluate feed tolerance (Conzalez, 2008). Normal gastric residual volume can be up to 500 ml (Montejo *et al.*, 2009), so current North American guidelines recommend:

- <200 maintain feed;
- 200–500 maintain feed, but careful bedside evaluation;
- >500 withhold feeds and reassess patient's tolerance.

(Conzalez, 2008)

European guidelines are less specific.

Unless excessive, aspirate should be returned, to prevent imbalances from loss of gastric acid, electrolytes and feed (including fluid). If absorption is poor, gut motility can be increased with prokinetic drugs (e.g. metoclopramide, low-dose erythromycin (Booth *et al.*, 2002; Nguyen *et al.*, 2007)).

Blockage

While fine-bore tubes cause less oesophageal irritation than wide-bore ones, they are more likely to block. Risk of blockage can be reduced by

- flushing regularly with water
- flushing tubes after drug administration
- giving drugs in syrup/linctus form rather than crushing tablets.

(Armer and White, 2014)

There are commercial products, made from digestive enzymes, to unblock tubes.

Parenteral nutrition (PN)

Whenever possible, patients should be fed enterally. If the gut cannot be used, parenteral feeding (directly into the bloodstream – sometimes called total parenteral nutrition – TPN) is preferable to starvation. Likely reasons for not using the gut are

- total paralytic ileus (rare);
- following complicated gut surgery it is occasionally necessary to rest the gut to allow healing;
- severe inflammatory bowel/gut conditions.

Disadvantages of parenteral nutrition are

- expense;
- gut atrophy and translocation of gut bacteria from non-use of the gut;
- infection (Turpin *et al.*, 2014);
- (usually) hyperglycaemia/hypertriglyercidaemia (Schloerb, 2004; NICE, 2006);
- thrombophlebitis, from hypertonic glucose in feeds.

Some feeds have to be delivered into central veins, but general practice is that all PN is given centrally. If a central line is inserted, and only needed for feeding, a peripherally inserted central catheter (PICC) is usually chosen. Ideally, parenteral nutrition should be given through a dedicated lumen – a lumen that has not been used for anything else (NCEPOD, 2010). However, while this is preferable to reduce infection risk, as identified in Chapter 16, recent guidance accepts that there are times this may not always be possible.

Parenteral feeds containing fat, protein and glucose are white; those containing only glucose and protein are clear. Feeds also contain other nutrients, each of which should be individually prescribed for each patient, with prescriptions checked against the bag label before administration. Nutrients may be damaged by exposure to light, so bags should be covered.

Large volumes of intravenous glucose may exceed insulin production, so blood sugar should be monitored regularly (initially hourly). Many patients need insulin infusions with parenteral nutrition.

Assessment

Patients are usually seen first and most often by nursing staff, who are therefore best placed to initially assess nutritional needs, and so prevent further muscle wasting. NICE (2006) defines malnourishment as any of

- body mass index (BMI) <18.5 kg/m^2;
- unintentional weight loss >10% in last 3–6 months;
- BMI <20 kg/m^2 and unintentional weight loss >5% within last 3–6 months;

recommending nutritional support for any of these, and anyone who has

- eaten little in last 5 days
- is unlikely to eat little in the next 5 days
- poor absorptive capacity
- high nutrient loss
- increased nutritional needs (e.g. hypercatabolic).

Visual observation may indicate:

- dehydration
- undernourishment
- obesity.

Subcutaneous fat loss (leaving loose skin) often indicates malnutrition. Some muscles, such as biceps, can be felt, indicating muscle wasting. However, muscle and fat wasting may be masked by oedema. Nutritional status should be assessed within 24 hours of admission, to enable early interventions.

Patients and/or relatives should be asked about diet, although problems may be denied. Weight loss may indicate malnutrition, although oedematous patients will gain rather than lose weight. Breathlessness or nausea frequently cause malnourishment in hospitalised patients. Ketonuria indicates catabolism of body tissue. Patients' conditions may also suggest dietary problems. For example, breathless patients are often malnourished because eating exacerbates their breathlessness; alcoholics are often malnourished, because while alcohol supplies carbohydrates (energy), it contains few other nutrients. Seeing what patients eat (e.g. from finished plates) and recording their dietary input is a simple, but often neglected, nursing observation.

Many nutritional screening tools have been developed – Fulbrook *et al.* (2007) found 14 in their pan-European survey, but DOH (2011b) and the British Association for Parenteral and Enteral Nutrition (BAPEN) recommend MUST (Malnutrition Universal Screening Tool – MAG, 2003).

MUST combines scores for body mass index (BMI – kg/m^2), weight loss and disease to identify risk of malnutrition:

- 0 = low risk
- 1 = medium risk
- 2 or more = high risk.

Guidance is included for actions with each score. While MUST is relatively simple, most sicker in-hospital patients score 'high risk', necessitating referral to the nutritional support team (dieticians). Until reviewed by dieticians, nurses should optimise nutritional input.

While effective for most adult patients, the value of MUST for older people has been questioned (Bokorst van der Schueren *et al.*, 2014). The Subjective Global Assessment (SGA – Detsky *et al.*, 1987) is widely used in other countries (Sirodkar and Mohandas, 2005), and can be downloaded from www.hospitalmedicine.org/geriresource/toolbox/subjective_global_assessment.htm.

Implications for nursing

- Many patients admitted to hospital are malnourished.
- Malnourishment often persists and sometimes progresses in hospital.
- Length of stay, morbidity and mortality all increase with malnutrition.
- Nutrition needs multidisciplinary teamwork, but nurses are often central to both initial assessment and co-ordinating care.
- Nutritional status of all patients should be assessed within 24 hours of admission.
- The MUST screening tool is recommended by NICE (2006) and DOH (2011b).
- Red trays (or other means) help identify that 'at risk' patients need priority, and their food intake needs monitoring.
- Patients suffering from or at risk of, malnutrition should be referred to dieticians and other appropriate professionals.

- With refeeding syndrome, feeds should be commenced at low rates, and vitamin supplements prescribed.
- Patients unable to eat an oral diet should be enterally fed whenever possible.
- Before stopping/reducing enteral feeds, consider factors that may reduce gut motility; consider prokinetics.
- Absence of bowel sounds is not a contraindication for enteral/oral diets.
- Nursing care includes assessing and monitoring nutrition and potential complications to minimise risks to patients.

Summary

For decades, major reports continue to raise concerns about malnutrition. Malnutrition adversely affects health, increasing mortality, morbidity and cost. Effective nutrition requires good multidisciplinary teamwork, but ensuring nutritional needs are met is part of the nurse's role (Bloomfield and Pegram, 2012).

Further reading

Many major reports focusing on nutrition include RCN (2008b), NICE (2006, currently being updated), NCEPOD (2010), DOH (2011b) and Health Improvement Scotland (2014). The key text on dietetics is Gandy (2014).

Clinical scenario

Robert Jones, 56 years old, is admitted with an acute exacerbation of chronic obstructive pulmonary disease (COPD). He is being treated with oxygen therapy and drugs, including intravenous antibiotics, steroids and 2 hourly nebulisers. He weighs 62 kg and is 1.7 metres tall; his skin appears dry and loose.

1   How would you assess Mr Jones' nutritional needs? List his risk factors for malnutrition. Using the MUST screening tool, calculate his score (including body mass index – BMI). From reading this chapter, are there any other indicators you might use to identify his risks?
2   Based on your assessment, what actions would you take? Identify the options for nutrition. List the benefits and risks of each.
3   Devise a care plan to minimise the risks identified. Include how to monitor Mr Jones' nutrition to meet any changing needs.

Chapter 29

Infection control

Contents

Introduction

Media 'scares' have given infection, and infection control, high profile that, at least as far as public confidence is concerned, has often been counter-productive. Behind media hype, however, there are justified causes for concern. Approximately one in ten people entering UK hospitals acquires infection (Breathnach, 2005), and of those who do, approximately one in ten die from those infections. Remembering Florence Nightingale's (1859/1960) premise that 'Hospitals should do the sick no harm', infection is therefore a serious concern for all health professionals, and prevention an important duty. This chapter outlines some ways infection can be reduced, and describes some of the more problematic organisms and related nursing care. Specific treatments are not generally discussed, as these should be guided by local microbiologists, and change rapidly with developments of both new drugs and microbial resistance.

People at risk

Falling standards are frequently blamed for infection, yet health services may be victims of their own success. Immunity declines with age, so countries with ageing populations, like the UK, also have increasingly at-risk populations. Many illnesses further compromise immunity, with sicker people being most at risk. Yet sicker people receive more treatments, many of which are invasive. Each invasive treatment/procedure, and exposure to more staff, increases infection risks. Medical advances have enabled people to live to greater ages, further increasing numbers of people at high risk. Preventing all infections is unrealistic, and blame cultures are counter-productive. What realistically can be achieved is reducing infection and mortality rates. Staff who understand implications of infection, especially sepsis, are more likely to reduce risks to their patients. All patients are at risk of healthcare-associated infection, but high risk factors are summarised in Table 29.1

Table 29.1 High risk factors for infection

- sicker patients
- immunocompromise (e.g. low white cell count, chemotherapy, steroids)
- invasive equipment/treatments (especially vascular, and especially central lines)
- very old/young

Colonisation and infection

For each human cell the body has more than 10 bacterial cells (Maczulak, 2010). Some are transient, many are resident. Human bodies are not sterile, and eradicating all body organisms is neither practical nor desirable. As long as bacteria colonise, but do not infect, they are generally harmless (*commensals*), and many are helpful. Infection occurs when organisms cause pathological responses in the host. Most infections are from opportunist pathogens – organisms that cause little harm to healthy people, but which infect the vulnerable.

Infection may be

- *endogenous*, organisms translocating to another part of the body, such as from the gut into blood, or from colonies on indwelling equipment *or*
- *exogenous*, from outside the host.

MICRO-ORGANISMS

Most hospital infections are bacterial. Bacteria are classified as Gram negative or Gram positive, according to whether they retain crystal violet-iodine complex stain. Gram positives include:

- *Staphylococci* (e.g. MRSa)
- *Clostridium*
- *Enterococci*

while Gram negatives include:

- *Pseudomonas*
- *Acinetobacter*

- *Enterobacter*
- *Escherichia coli*
- *Klebsiellae*
- *Proteus*
- *Serratia*
- *Helicobacter pylori.*

Antibiotic resistance rapidly followed introduction of antibiotics: meticillin was marketed in 1960, and six months later resistance was reported (Grundmann, 2006). However, recent exponential increase in microbial resistance ('superbugs') (Larson *et al.*, 2010) raises spectres of antibiotic-resistance epidemics (Cars *et al.*, 2008), prompting promotion of antibiotic stewardship – avoiding unnecessary usage. Emergence of extended spectrum beta-lactamase (ESBL) enables organisms to develop cross-resistance to many antibiotics, making them even more difficult to eliminate. Carbapenems are the 'last resort' anti-biotic (WHO, 2014), so carbapenem-resistant *Enterobactericeae* (CRE, previously called New Delhi Metallo Beta-Lactamase – NDM-1) pose a major threat, which is increasing (CDC, 2013; WHO, 2014).

MRSa

Meticillin-resistant *Staphylococcus aureas* (MRSa) has gained public notoriety. There are many strains of staphylococcus. Resistance varies between strains, with no antibiotics fully effective against all strains. Up to half of the population are colonised by *Staphylococcus* (Lim and Webb, 2005), but even highly resistant strains seldom cause problems to healthy carriers. The UK has 17 epidemic strains of MRSa (EMRSa), of which EMRSa 15 and 16 cause most hospital outbreaks (Barnes and Jinks, 2009).

Most hospitals have policies of screening all patients for MRSa, and for treating MRSa. After patients have washed in antibacterial soap, clean bedding and linen should be provided to prevent recolonisation. Whenever possible, infected patients should be nursed in side rooms (Grundmann, 2006).

Clostridium difficile

Aptly named, *C. difficile* spores are virtually impossible to eliminate (Wren, 2009) and infection difficult to treat. Strain 027 is especially virulent (Shannon-Lowe *et al.*, 2010), causing many high media profile outbreaks and deaths since 1999 (Kelly and LaMont, 2008). About 3% of adults carry *C. difficile* in their gut, incidence rising to over one third in hospitalised patients (Shannon-Lowe *et al.*, 2010). Most people carrying *C. difficile* do not develop infection, but exposure to broad-spectrum antibiotics disrupts normal gut flora, enabling infection (Shannon-Lowe *et al.*, 2010), and potentially fatal pseudomembraneous colitis. Over half of people developing *C. difficile* infection are over eighty-five (Pépin *et al.*, 2005).

C. difficile is the single main cause of healthcare-associated diarrhoea (Voth and Ballard, 2005), which is often profuse, causing life-threatening dehydration. In the 2002 Quebec epidemic, nearly one quarter of those infected died within one month (Pépin *et al.*, 2005). Infection is usually treated with oral metronidazole or vancomycin (Shannon-Lowe *et al.*, 2010).

Toilets/commodes should be cleaned with a chlorine-based disinfectant agent after each use (Hall and Horsley, 2007). *C. difficile* is highly resistant, including to alcohol handrubs, necessitating washing hands with soap and water (Loveday *et al.*, 2014). With most people (staff and visitors) now used to alcohol handrubs, it is probably wise to remove these from the immediate bed area, displaying notices to wash hands instead.

Glycopeptide resistant Enterococci (GRE)

Bowels normally carry more *Entercocci* than any other Gram positive organism (Mascini and Bonten, 2005). *Enterococci*, which cause one third of healthcare-associated infection (Gould, 2008), are usually relatively easily treated, but emergence of strains resistant to most antibiotics poses a major threat. Previously called vancomycin resistant *Enterococci* (VRE), GRE often co-infects with MRSa, to which it can transfer vancomycin-resistance (Zirakzadeh and Patel, 2006). Soap and water handwashes are ineffective against GRE (Lim and Webb, 2005), and it can survive more than a week in the environment (Zirakzadeh and Patel, 2006). Fortunately, linezolid can treat most GREs.

Pseudomonas

Pseudomonas causes one tenth of all healthcare-associated infections (Thuong *et al.*, 2003), more than any other Gram negative organism. It thrives in temperatures between 5 and 45°C and many different environments, especially moist areas, such as baths, washbasins and toilets (Cholley *et al.*, 2008). One quarter of hospital staff carry *Pseudomonas* (Haddadin *et al.*, 2002).

Acinetobacter

Acinetobacter baumannii (Acb) is a common skin surface organism (Grice and Segre, 2011), and also found widely in soil, sewage and water (Pitt, 2007). Recent emergence of multi-resistant strains (Munoz-Price and Weinstein, 2008) poses significant risks for healthcare.

Viruses

Norovirus causes nearly one fifth of cases of acute gastroenteritis (Ahmed *et al.*, 2014), typically during winter, hence its media name of 'winter vomiting virus'. Vomiting is often projectile and watery diarrhoea profuse, potentially causing life-threatening dehydration, so treatment is primarily with fluids and electrolytes (Glass *et al.*, 2009). It is highly contagious, so patients infected should be isolated. Incubation is rapid (10–51 hours) (Glass *et al.*, 2009), so once infection is detected, most people (staff and patients) will have been exposed to it. Preventing spread to other wards is therefore the priority (Hairon, 2008). Norovirus is resistant to alcohol handrubs, necessitating hand washing with soap and water (Loveday *et al.*, 2014).

Influenza ('flu) also typically occurs during winter. Most years bring different strains, usually originating from animals (Stein, 2009). Historically, flu pandemics occur every 10–40 years (Saidi and Brett, 2009); the last one in the UK being in 1968 (Saidi and

Brett, 2009), a flu pandemic is overdue. In popular media, the number classification (e.g. *H5N1*) is usually replaced by the name of the originating species (e.g. bird, swine). Most cases of influenza are mild, but those causing severe illness usually occur in people who have not been vaccinated (Catania *et al.*, 2014).

Fungi

Candida remains the most widespread fungal infection (WHO, 2014). An opportunistic organism, candida typically infects the warm, moist and static areas such as the mouth, skinfolds, and external female genitalia. It remains one of the most common causes of healthcare-associated bacteraemias (CDC, 2013; Loveday *et al.*, 2014). Although still the most prevalent strain, incidence of *Candida albicans* is declining while infections from other, azole-resistant, *Candida* species are increasing (WHO, 2014). Although fairly easily treated, infection is too often missed by failing to assess vulnerable patients. The tongue and skinfolds should therefore be inspected for white coating and rashes.

Controlling infection

All staff should try to prevent infection. Infection occurs only if there is a

■ source
■ means of transmission *and*
■ means of entry.

Removing one link breaks this chain of infection. The source is often within patients themselves – endogenous infection. Although known problem sources should be treated, such as with 'deep cleaning', transmission of micro-organisms from one patient to another is a greater problem. Family and friends rarely move between patients, so although they should be encouraged to use alcohol rubs when entering and leaving wards, they present relatively minor risks. Greater risk of transmission occurs with staff and equipment moving between patients. Hand-hygiene, (see below) and cleaning down equipment, before and after patient contact remains the best way to prevent cross-infection (WHO, 2005b). Readers should ensure they are familiar with hygiene and decontamination local policies.

Even if contact transmission were eradicated, airborne microbes can be transmitted through

■ dust
■ airborne skin scales
■ droplets, such as from coughs.

Close proximity of beds significantly increases risks of airborne infection (Eggimann and Pittet, 2001), often undermining short-term financial savings from closing beds by increasing longer-term costs from cross-infection. Invasive procedures, especially dressing changes, should whenever possible be planned to avoid bed-making, when airborne skin scales are likely to increase. Dirty linen should be carefully folded, and linen skips brought to the bedside. Low staffing levels and high workloads correlate with increased cross-infection (Allen, 2005; Coia *et al.*, 2006; Rogowski *et al.*, 2013), largely because busy staff attempt to cut corners, such as basic hygiene.

Skin generally forms a protective barrier against microbes, but any break in skin, such as wounds or invasive devices, provide microbes with possible means of entry. Two thirds of bloodstream infections occur in patients with intravascular devices (Loveday *et al.*, 2014). Non-sterile gloves should be worn when handling any invasive equipment (Loveday *et al.*, 2014). As identified in Chapter 16, unnecessary cannulae should be removed, and sites inspected at least each shift. Drugs should be given through the least invasive route that will be effective, so prescriptions for intravenous drugs should be reviewed at least daily to assess whether oral, or other, routes are feasible.

Urinary catheters

Nearly one fifth of healthcare associated infections (HCAI) are urinary tract infections, half of which are from urinary catheters (Loveday *et al.*, 2014). Twelve to sixteen per cent of hospitalised patients have catheters (Lo *et al.*, 2014); one fifth of urinary tract infections have negative dipstick results (Nazarko, 2009). Catheters should therefore only be inserted if there is a specific indication, and removed as soon as they are no longer necessary.

Hand hygiene

Since Semmelweis' work, commenced in 1843 and published in 1861, studies have consistently shown hand hygiene to be the single most important way of reducing cross-infection, yet nearly two centuries later, compliance with hand hygiene remains poor (Allegranzi *et al.*, 2013). Alcohol handrubs are usually an effective and easy way to remove transient microbes (Loveday *et al.*, 2014); decontamination is largely caused by drying of the alcohol, so sufficient time should be allowed for drying to occur before touching patients. Efficacy of rubs varies, so readers should check with local guidelines how much rub to use. Hands must be decontaminated immediately

- before each patient-care episode;
- after each patient-care episode;
- after contact with body fluids, mucous membranes and non-intact skin;
- after other activities or contact with objects and equipment in the immediate patient environment which may result in hands becoming contaminated;
- after the removal of gloves.

(Loveday *et al.*, 2014)

Wrist watches and hand jewellery can facilitate microbial colonisation, so should be removed (Loveday *et al.*, 2014).

Implications for practice

- Infection can, and does, kill. Preventing infection is therefore fundamental to preventing harm.
- Invasive techniques and dressings should, when possible, avoid times of dust disturbance.

- Strict asepsis must be observed when breaking any intravenous circuit or treating any open wound.
- Hand hygiene before and after each aspect of care, and before approaching and after leaving each bed area.
- Alcohol handrubs should be available by each bed.
- Invasive devices which are not necessary should be removed as soon as possible.
- Use local resources, such as infection control specialists and link nurses.
- Readers should be familiar with local infection control policies.

Summary

Infection remains, and is likely to remain, a problem in search of solutions. Intense public and media concern about healthcare-associated infections, especially 'superbugs' is generally accompanied by at best limited insight into realities of illness and healthcare.

Health services have faced huge and increasing pressures in recent years, potentially placing targets and short-term financial savings above considerations of preventing harm. Paradoxically, financial costs of treating infections have probably exceeded initial savings. Eradicating all infections is impractical, but many patients admitted to hospital die unnecessarily from healthcare-associated infections. Minimising infection risks is fundamental to everyone's safety. Local infection control teams are a valuable resource for advice, and should be involved whenever infection, or potential sources of infection, cause concern.

Further reading

Readers should be familiar with local and national infection control guidelines – current UK guidelines are Loveday *et al.* (2014). Detailed information about specific organisms can be found in almost any microbiology text. Articles frequently appear in most journals, the *Journal of Hospital Infection* specialising in the topic. Recent nursing texts include Weston (2013). Although there can be differences between different nations, the USA CDC (2013) report makes salutary reading.

Clinical scenario

Mrs Joyce Cantrell is admitted from a residential home, unwell. On examination in A&E she is found to have abdominal cramps, has a dry, coated tongue, and seems to have eaten little since yesterday morning. Vital signs are:

temperature 38.4°C
heart rate 108 beats per minute
blood pressure 103/54 mmHg
respiratory rate 28 breaths per minute

She suffers from mild dementia, and cannot remember whether she took her lisinopril this morning. Her nearest family live many miles away, and seldom visit her. In A&E she is incontinent of urine, and subsequently catheterised. Intravenous compound sodium lactate is commenced at 250 ml/hour.

Following admission to an acute medical ward, where you are looking after her, she develops profuse green diarrhoea, and *C. Diff.* is suspected.

1   List your main concerns from the above history.
2   How can infection risks to Mrs Cantrell, or others, be minimised?
3   Following local protocols, devise a plan of care for Mrs Cantrell.

Part 6

Professional contexts

Chapter 30

Professionalism, accountability, the law and teamwork

Contents

Introduction

Healthcare, and nursing, changed greatly during the twentieth century. In 1900 nurses were not on a professional register, and were not considered professionals. The 'good' nurse was expected to obey the doctor's instructions, without question (Dock, 1917). The register for UK nurses commenced in 1923 (Lloyd Jones, 2012), and during the twentieth century nurses were increasingly recognised as autonomous professionals – nurses regulating themselves (through their professional body) rather than being regulated by others. Autonomy brought responsibility and accountability with it. Henderson's definition of the unique role of the nurse was adopted by the International Council of Nurses in 1960 (Henderson, 1960). Interprofessional collaboration (Zwarenstein *et al.*, 2009) often emphasises the autonomy and independence of nursing practice, yet the number of guidelines from other professions cited, for example, in this book suggest that nursing autonomy is a relative concept.

However, no profession works in a vacuum. Values of individuals, professions and society influence actions. This chapter uses historical perspectives to explore values.

Differing values can be a strength, offering different perspectives and encouraging enquiry. But they can also be a source of conflict and communication breakdown. Communication breakdown causes about 70% of errors in healthcare (Tschannen *et al.*, 2011), and so potentially significantly contributes to avoidable morbidity and mortality.

This chapter includes brief descriptions of UK legal aspects, to give readers insight into what may be expected from them. Any readers directly involved in legal cases should seek professional legal advice.

Collaborative practice

The concept of multidisciplinary teamwork being a collaboration between different, but equally valuable, professions is attractive to many, but contrasts with most of the past. Current professional codes of practice emphasise co-operation (NMC, 2015; HCPC, 2012) and collaboration (GMC, 2013). However, compared with hospitals of 1900, the diversity of professional groups had greatly increased by 2000, some professions having evolved from nursing. This diversity can be both a strength and a challenge. In the busyness of everyday practice, staff may be frustrated by delays in others responding; diversity of roles can cause one professional group not clearly understanding roles of another (Mills *et al.*, 2001), and so not understanding other priorities that may have caused delays. The busyness also limits communication, and time for reflection on practice. Socialisation within nursing encourages many practitioners, and teams, to resort to rituals and routines (Mooney, 2007), which potentially disempowers nurses from giving holistic care (Tonuma and Windbolt, 2001).

Challenges are increased by rapidity of change. The last decade has seen the emergence of the associate practitioner (band 4) role, with often a lack a clarity of what this role involves (RCN Policy Unit, 2009).

Defining nursing

Building on Henderson's (1960) definition, the Royal College of Nursing (RCN 2003) suggest

> Nursing is the use of clinical judgement in the provision of care to enable people to improve, maintain, or recover health, to cope with health problems, and to achieve the best quality of life, whatever their disease or disability, until death. The focus of nursing is the whole person and the human response . . . The purpose is to promote health and healing . . .

More recently, core values of nursing have been identified as 'the six Cs' (Commissioning Board Chief Nursing Officer and DH Chief Nursing Adviser, 2012):

- care
- compassion
- competence
- communication
- courage
- commitment.

Differing values

Multiprofessional teams normally attempt to collaborate. But nurses, patients, doctors and relatives can each differ about what constitutes quality care (Gelling and Provest 1999; Shannon *et al.*, 2002; Florin *et al.* 2005), forming a potential quadrilateral of misunderstanding and conflict. Caring for the person is a core value of nursing (Brown, 2011), while values of medicine have arguably traditionally focused on curing disease. Approaching the same patient from these two different perspectives can cause conflict – for example, whether some treatments are justified.

Coombs (2004) suggests that good multidisciplinary teamwork needs

- respect
- good communication
- working towards the same goals

while avoiding

- traditional power bases
- tribalistic/egoistic behaviour
- empire building.

Accountability

Like everyone else in society, nurses are accountable for their actions and omissions. Dimond (2011) suggests nurses have four 'arenas' of accountability:

- professional
- criminal (statute) law
- civil law
- employer

each of which may act independently of others – actions might be laudable in one and culpable in another.

Each nurse's professional accountability is to the Nursing and Midwifery Council, the regulatory body established by statute law (Act of Parliament) with a primary duty to protect the public (NMC 2015). Expectations of the NMC are published in documents such as the Code of Conduct. Only staff on a professional register have professional accountability, so the widely cited 'responsible but not accountable' description of support staff applies to professional accountability; non-registered staff are accountable in the other arenas.

Breaking statue law (e.g. murder) can result in prosecution by the Crown Prosecution Service, with the state taking the individual to a criminal court. If the case is proven 'beyond reasonable doubt', a criminal conviction may be passed by the court. Relatively few cases of criminal law involve healthcare.

If one person, or group of people, considers another has caused them harm, they can sue in a civil court. If found guilty on the 'balance of probabilities', damages can be awarded to the injured parties. Cases involving healthcare that reach civil court usually involve either assault or negligence (assault can also be a criminal action). For a case of negligence to succeed four elements must be present:

- a duty of care exists;
- there was a breach of that duty of care ('Bolam Test', below);
- there is a causal link between the breach of duty and harm;
- harm was not too remote (reasonably foreseeable).

However, employers have vicarious liability for their staff, so it is usually the employer, rather than the individual, who will be accused. Solicitors representing employers usually attempt to settle out of court if possible, to save the greater costs, and potential adverse publicity, of court cases.

In law, people are accountable for both acts and omissions. Therefore failing to act may be as culpable as doing something that causes harm. If local guidelines lag behind evidence, and perhaps national guidelines, this can create further dilemmas. Recent years have seen a proliferation of guidelines, but many are faulted (Feuerstein *et al.*, 2014); following faulted guidelines arguably conflicts with requirements of professional autonomy, and may not prove a defence in law. Part of professionalism is therefore making decisions and accepting accountability for those decisions.

Each employee has a contract of employment; students and volunteers have honorary contracts. Breach of contract can lead to dismissal through an employment tribunal.

If a number of staff contributed to the harm, accountability may be shared among them. For example, a student nurse may have performed the act, but the supervising registered nurse is accountable for both supervision and delegation. If the harm involves a drug error, the prescribing doctor and ward pharmacist might also share accountability.

There are arguably additional 'moral accountabilities' to oneself, colleagues and the public; public accountability can include anxieties to prevent adverse publicity in the media. While these could not be pursued through any regulatory system, they may influence initial decisions.

Litigation

Until 1991 NHS hospitals had Crown Immunity – like the monarch, they could not be prosecuted. Repealing of Crown Immunity coincided with an increasingly litigious culture. The Clinical Negligence Scheme for Trusts (CNST), a voluntary insurance scheme, was established in 1995 to limit liability by promoting safe and effective practices – some mandatory requirements stem from these requirements. The CNST is now managed by the NHS Litigation Authority, established under the *National Health Service Act 2006* (NHSLA, 2012). Recent UK mandatory requirements for nurses to have professional indemnity may reflect increasing litigiousness.

If possible, civil cases will be settled out of court, which usually incurs less expense. Cases that do reach civil courts may take years to do so – the 2012 NHS Litigation Authority report shows consistent costs being incurred from actions against former Regional Health Authorities, which were abolished in 1996. Think back to what you were doing five years ago today. How accurately can you remember your actions? Imagine yourself being cross-examined in court by a barrister, and attempting to justify those actions. If you were involved in a civil case about your nursing practice, you would probably have to rely heavily on written records made by yourself and your colleagues. How confident are you that your nursing records from your last shift would provide you with sufficient evidence to defend yourself? Remember that opposing lawyers would have had access to the same records. Failure to maintain adequate records is frequently cited in *fitness to practice* cases (NMC, 2011). The NMC posts summaries of fitness to practice cases on its website.

Formal healthcare documentation should be dated, timed, signed and identified as relating to specifically identified patients. However, any written record may be used as evidence. So, for example, reflective journals and case studies could be used, and could be subpoenaed by the Court. Any written records should therefore be documented carefully to ensure accuracy.

If practice is questioned in court, professionals will be judged by the standards of the ordinary competent practitioner (the 'Bolam Test', after case law precedent: Bolam v Friern Hospital Management Committee (1957) 1 WLR 582), not the best possible practice. The standards expected of the ordinary competent nurse are published by the NMC (Code and other publications). If standard practice remained unclear from professional publications, the Court might judge standard practice from statements of expert witnesses.

Rights

Acute illness often makes patients vulnerable. Vulnerable patients have the same rights as others but, if unable to assert them, may need advocates. Advocacy is a fundamental nursing role (Thacker, 2008).

The Mental Capacity Act (Parliament, 2005) established five key principles:

- Presume people have the capacity to make decisions until proved otherwise.
- Support people to make their own decisions using 'all practical means'.
- Do not treat people as lacking capacity to make decisions because their decision is unwise.
- Patients' best interests are paramount.
- Decisions by others must interfere least with the rights and freedom of action of those lacking capacity.

This act promotes the autonomy and rights of people. However, aspects such as proving that people lack capacity, or that 'all practical means' have been used, could be challenging.

Supplementary requirements to the Mental Capacity Act have largely evolved through case law, especially from the European Court of Human Rights. A 2007 amendment to the act established the Deprivation of Liberty Safeguards (DoLS) necessitate authorisation from the Court of Protection for any deprivation of liberty. Traditionally, this was interpreted as lasting more than seven days, but the 'Cheshire West' case defined deprivation of liberty as continuous supervision and control, with the person not being free to leave (Crews *et al.*, 2014). Arguably, many hospitalised patients lacking full consciousness or competence would fit this description.

Three particularly problematic areas for acute healthcare are

- consent
- restraint
- children.

In law, no-one else can decide for another competent adult (DOH, 2009). A deputy appointed by the Court of Protection (established under the Mental Capacity Act) is empowered to make specific decisions – limits of their power will have been identified by the Court – but few patients in acute healthcare are likely to have appointed deputies. The Court of Protection may rule on individual cases, but the unpredictable nature of acute healthcare and acute deterioration often leaves insufficient time to seek advice. At all times, nurses should act in patients' best interests (NMC, 2015), remembering that the Mental Capacity Act requires that actions must interfere least with the rights and freedom of action of those lacking capacity, and that accountability may necessitate nurses being able to prove they acted in patients' best interests. Usually, but not always, the law assumes it is in patients' best interests to be alive rather than dead, so life-saving actions are relatively easy to justify. Actions which prevent harm are usually also easy to justify. However, justifying other actions may prove more problematic.

Maintaining safety is fundamental, and may at times necessitate restraint. However, force used must be proportional to the likelihood and seriousness of harm (Musters, 2010). Restraint may not always involve manual handling. For example, cotsides are potential restraints. Patients who have a one-sided weakness from a stroke may feel safer with cotsides, so consent to their use. But if used to try and keep an agitated patient in bed they may increase the incidence of falls, and from a greater height (Tzeng and Yin, 2012). As identified in Chapter 18, chemical sedation is a form of restraint, so could fall foul of the 'Cheshire West' decision (above). Accountability before the NMC, criminal and civil courts and employer necessitates nurses being able to justify any restraint they use. Restraint without consent, in whatever form, should therefore be a last resort (RCN, 2008c), and only used when no other means to maintain safety are practical.

This book is for nurses caring for acutely ill adults, but some readers may work in departments where children are also admitted. At one time, the law was relatively clear about the ages at which children attained specific rights. In some aspects, such as driving, this remains the case. But since the Gillick Case (originally 1985, resulting in the Fraser Guidelines 1985) and the Children's Act 1989, statute and case law considers the individual competence of each child to make decisions; this might be regardless of parental wishes. A child of eight might be considered competent to make a decision that a 12-year-old might not. If in doubt about decisions when caring for children, it is best to seek advice. Trusts almost invariably have legal departments, employing solicitors who can offer advice. Out-of-hours, concerns may need to be escalated to the administrator on call.

Implications for practice

- As autonomous professionals, nurses are individually accountable for their actions (and omissions).
- The regulating professional body (NMC for nurses) publishes standards it expects of its registrants.

■   All patients have rights; patients unable to assert their rights need advocates.
■   No one else can consent for another competent adult.

Conclusion: The deteriorating patient revisited

Chapter 1 established that the acuity of patients in acute hospitals has increased, and that there is a significant level of avoidable mortality and morbidity. Hospitals and their staff clearly have a duty of care to their patients, and are therefore accountable for their actions. Deterioration is usually accompanied by changes in vital signs. Nurses, and other clinical staff, should therefore assess and monitor their patients.

A key difference between nurses and other healthcare professions is that nurses are continuously present on wards; other professions visit wards to treat identified patients. Nurses are therefore in an ideal position to co-ordinate care, contacting relevant other groups of staff when there are concerns. Henderson's (1960) 'unique function' may now be shared with other groups of staff, but while fundamental aspects of supporting activities of living remain, nursing has since gained greater interventional roles to restore health.

The past has seen many changes to nursing and healthcare. Further change is inevitable. Having now completed reading this book, reflect on your own practice. Questions that can help you develop include

■   What is in the best interests of patients?
■   What do you value about nursing?
■   How can you preserve core values?
■   How far should we extend our own roles?
■   What may be lost by own role expansion?
■   What tasks/aspects should we delegate, and to whom?
■   So what can *you* do in your own ward to develop the practice of yourself and your colleagues?

Further reading

Key further reading is publications by the NMC, especially the professional Code of Conduct (NMC, 2015). Although not a regulatory body, many RCN documents also provide valuable guidance, such as RCN 2008c. DOH guidance on consent (2009) should be followed. Dimond (2011) remains the key text on the law in relation to nursing.

Clinical exercises

Reflecting on your own practice, and material covered in this book, identify:

■   what acutely ill patients need;
■   what you would like if you were acutely ill;
■   how you can help the acutely ill patients in your ward;
■   what relatives value;
■   what makes you feel valued.

Glossary

aerobic in the presence of oxygen

anaerobic in the absence of oxygen

atelectasis collapse of alveoli

bacteraemia bacterial infection in blood

blood–brain barrier capillaries which perfuse the brain (see Chapter 17)

cardioversion restoring normal sinus rhythm – can be chemical (drugs) or electrical (defibrillation)

cirrhosis fibrosis; usually applied to liver disease where scar tissue between cells causes obstruction

cyanocobalamin vitamin B12

deadspace space between where air or gas enters the airway and the alveoli where gas exchange occurs (average physiological adult deadspace = 150 ml)

echocardiogram ultrasound visualisation of the heart, able to measure structures and estimate function

ejection fraction the percentage of blood ejected from the ventricle in relation to total ventricular blood volume. Usually measured by echocardiogram, normal left ventricular ejection fraction is >55% (Jowett and Thompson, 2007)

erythrocyte red blood cell

Glasgow Coma Scale a widely used assessment for level of consciousness (see Chapter 17)

glycocalyx 'slime' coating of cells, helping their function

haemolysis breakdown of red cell

hepatocyte liver cell

hepatomegaly enlarged liver

histamine pro-inflammatory mediator released by mast cells

hypercapnia high (arterial) blood carbon dioxide (>6.0 kPa)

hypertriglyercidaemia high levels of triglycerides in blood (see triglyceeride)

iatrogenic caused by medical treatment

joule measurement of energy: the work involved by one newton moving one metre

kilocalorie (kcal)   measurement of energy: energy needed to warm 1 kilogram of water by 1°C. 1 kcal = 4.184 kJ

leucocyte   white blood cell

leucopenia   lack of leucocytes (white cells) in blood, creating high risk of acquiring infection

metabolic syndrome   a cluster of abnormalities predisposing to cardiovascular disease and diabetes (see Chapters 26 and 27)

mitochondria   the part of the cell where energy (in the form of adenosine triphosphate) is produced

myocyte   muscle cell (including cardiac muscle)

nociceptors   nerve endings that sense pain

oliguria   less than 0.5 ml/kilogram/hour of urine

phlebitis   inflammation of veins (see Chapter 16)

pulse pressure   the difference between arterial systolic and diastolic pressure. High pulse pressure indicates poor vessel compliance (e.g. atherosclerosis), which narrow pulse pressure (e.g. 20) indicates hypovolaemia or poor cardiac output

respiratory failure type 1   failure of oxygen exchange (PaO_2 <8.0, $PaCO_2$ <6.0 kPa)

respiratory failure type 2   failure of oxygen exchange (PaO_2 <8.0, $PaCO_2$ >6.0 kPa)

rhabdomyolysis   acute kidney injury caused by myoglobin, release by extensive muscle damage (e.g. from trauma)

steatorrhoea   fatty stools

stroke volume   amount of blood ejected with each contraction of the left ventricle

thrombocyte   platelet

triglyceride   fatty molecules, which in blood predispose to cardiovascular disease

References

Achike, F.I., To, N.-H. P., Wang, H., Kwan, C.-Y. (2011) Obesity, metabolic syndrome, adipocytes and vascular function: a holistic viewpoint. *Clinical and Experimental Pharmacology and Physiology.* 38 (1): 1–10.

Ackrill, P., France, M.W. (2002) Common electrolyte problems. *Clinical Medicine.* 2 (3): 205–208.

Adam, A., Nicholson, C., Owens, L. (2008) Alcoholic dilated cardiomyopathy. *Nursing Standard.* 22 (38): 42–47.

Adam, S., Odell, M., Welch, J. (2010) *Rapid Assessment of the Acutely Ill Patient.* Oxford. Wiley-Blackwell.

Adam, S.K., Osborne, C. (2005) *Critical Care Nursing: science and practice.* 2nd edn. Oxford. Oxford Medical Publications.

Adler, E.D., Goldfinger, J.Z., Kalman, J., Park, M.E., Meier, D.E. (2009) Palliative care in the treatment of advanced heart failure. *Circulation.* 120 (25): 2597–2006.

Agarwal, E., Ferguson, M., Banks, M., Bauer, J., Capra, S., Isenring, I. (2012) Nutritional status and dietary intake of acute care patients: results from the Nutrition Care Day Survey 2010. *Clinical Nutrition.* 31 (1): 41–47.

Ahern, J., Philpot, P. (2002) Assessing acutely ill patients on general wards. *Nursing Standard.* 16 (47): 47–54.

Ahmed, S., Leurent, B., Sampson, E.L. (2014) Risk factors for incident delirium among older people in acute hospital medical units: a systematic review and meta-analysis. *Age and Ageing.* 43 (3): 326–333.

Ahmed, S.M., Hall, A.J., Robinson, A.E., Verhoef, L., Premkumar, P., Parashar, U.D., Koopmans, M., Lopman, B.A. (2014) Global prevalence of norovirus in cases of gastroenteritis: a systematic review and meta-analysis. *The Lancet Infectious Diseases.* 14 (8): 725–730.

Aiken, L.H., Sloane, D.M., Bruyneel, L., Van den Heede, K., Griffiths, P., Busse, R., Diomidous, M., Kinnunen, J., Kózka, M., Lesaffre, E., McHugh, M.D., Moreno-Casbas, M.T., Rafferty, A.M., Schwendimann, R., Scott, P.A., Tishelman, C., van Achterberg, T., Sermeus, W., RN4CAST consortium. (2014) Nurse staffing and education and hospital mortality in nine European countries: a retrospective observational study. *The Lancet.* 383 (9931): 1824–1830.

Akashi, Y.J., Goldstein, D.S., Barbaro, G., Ueyama, T. (2008) Takotsubo cardiomyopathy: a new form of acute, reversible heart failure. *Circulation.* 118 (25): 2754–2762.

Aksoy, S. (2000) Can the 'quality of life' be used as a criterion in health care services? *Bulletin of Medical Ethics*. 162: 19–22.

Alam, H.B., Rhee, P. (2007) New developments in fluid resuscitation. *Surgical Clinics of North America*. 87 (1): 55–72.

Aldred, H., Gott, M., Gariballa, S. (2005) Advanced heart failure: impact on older patients and informal carers. *Journal of Advanced Nursing*. 49 (2): 116–124.

Allegranzi, B., Gayet-Ageron, A., Damani, N., Bengaly, L., McLaws, M.-L., Moro, M.-L., Memish, Z., Urroz, O., Richet, H., Storr, J., Donaldson, L., Pittet, D. (2013) Global implementation of WHO's multimodal strategy for improvement of hand hygiene: a quasi-experimental study. *The Lancet Infectious Diseases*. 13 (10): 843–851.

Allen, S.J. (2005) Prevention and control of infection in the ICU. *Current Anaesthesia & Critical Care*. 16 (5): 191–199.

Allen, S.J., Martinez, E.G., Gregorio, G.V., Dans, L.F. (2010) Probiotics for treating acute infectious diarrhoea. *Cochrane Database of Systematic Reviews* 2010, Issue 11. Art. No.: CD003048. DOI: 10.1002/14651858.CD003048.pub3

Allen, S.J., Wareham, K., Wang, D., Bradley, C., Hutchings, H., Harris, W., Dhar, A., Brown, H., Foden, A., Gravenor, M.B., Mack, D. (2013) Lactobacilli and bifi dobacteria in the prevention of antibiotic-associated diarrhoea and *Clostridium difficile* diarrhoea in older inpatients (PLACIDE): a randomised, double-blind, placebo-controlled, multicentre trial. *The Lancet*. 382 (9900): 1249–1257.

Allibone, L. (2003) Nursing management of chest drains. *Nursing Standard*. 17 (22): 45–54.

All-Party Parliamentary Group on Sepsis. (2014) *Sepsis and the NHS*. London: HMSO.

Amador, L.F., Goodwin, J.S. (2005) Postoperative delirium in the older patient. *Journal of the American College of Surgeons*. 200 (5): 767–773.

Amathieu, R., Sauvat, S., Reynaud, P., Slavov, V., Luis, D., Dinca, A., Tual, L., Bloc, S., Dhonneur, G. (2012) Influence of the cuff pressure on the swallowing reflex in tracheostomized intensive care unit patients. *British Journal of Anaesthesia*. 108 (4): 578–583.

American Society of Anesthesiologists Task Force on Acute Pain Management. (2012) Practice guidelines for acute pain management in the perioperative setting: an updated report by the American Society of Anesthesiologists Task Force on Acute Pain Management. *Anesthesiology*. 116 (2): 248–273.

American Society of PeriAnesthetic Nurses. (2001) Patient temperature: an introduction to the clinical guideline for the prevention of unplanned perioperative hypothermia. *Journal of PeriAnesthesia Nursing*. 16 (5): 303–304.

Anderson, D. (2005) Preventing delirium in older people. *British Medical Bulletin*. 73 and 74: 25–34.

Andrews, P.J.D., Citero, G., Longhi, L., Polderman, K., Sahuquillo, J., Vajkoczy, P., Neuro-Intensive Care and Emergency Medicine (NICEM) Section of the European Society of Intensive Care Medicine. (2008) Intensive care of aneurismal subarachnoid hemorrhage: an international survey. *Intensive Care Medicine*. 34 (8): 1362–1370.

Anie, K.A., Green, J. (2015) Psychological therapies for sickle cell disease and pain. *Cochrane Database of Systematic Reviews* 2015, Issue 2. Art. No.: CD001916. DOI: 10.1002/14651858.CD001916.pub2.

APPHG. (2014) *Liver Disease: today's complacency, tomorrow's catastrophe*. London: HMSO.

Arbour, R. (2013) Common neurosurgical and neurological disorders. In Morton, P.G., Fontaine, D.K. (eds). *Critical Care Nursing: a holistic approach*. 10th edn. Philadelphia, PA. Lippincott Williams & Wilkins. 762–804.

Argoff, C.E., McCleane, G. (2009) *Pain Management Secrets.* 3rd edn. Philadelphia, PA. Mosby Elsevier.

Armer, S., White, R. (2014) Enteral nutrition. In Gandy, J. (ed). (2014) *Manual of Dietetic Practice.* 5th edn. Oxford. Wiley Blackwell. 344–356.

Asfar, P., Meziani, F., Hamel, J.-F., Grelon, F., Megarbane, B., Anguel, N., Mira, J.-P., Dequin, P.-F., Gergaud, S., Weiss, N., Legay, F., Le Tulzo, Y., Conrad, M., Robert, R., Gonzalez, F., Guitton, C., Tamion, F., Tonnelier, J-M., Guezennec, P., Van Der Linden, T., Vieillard-Baron, A., Mariotte, E., Pradel, G., Lesieur, O., Ricard, J-D., Hervé, F., Du Cheyron, D., Guerin, C., Mercat, A., Teboul, J-L., Radermacher, P., the SEPSISPAM Investigators. (2014) High versus low blood-pressure target in patients with septic shock. *New England Journal of Medicine.* 370 (17): 1583–1593.

Asharani, P.V., Sethu, S., Vadukumpully, S., Zhong, S., Lim, C.T., Hande, M.P., Valiyaveetti, S. (2010) Investigations on the structural damage in human erythrocytes exposed to silver, gold, and platinum nanoparticles. *Advanced Functional Materials.* 20 (8): 1233–1242.

Ataga, K.I., Cappellini, M.D., Rachmilewitz, E.A. (2007) β-Thalassaemia and sickle cell anaemia as paradigms of hypercoagulability. *British Journal of Haematology.* 139 (11): 3–13.

Atherton, J.C. (2003) Acid–base balance: maintenance of plasma pH. *Anaesthesia and Intensive Care Medicine.* 4 (12): 419–422.

AUKUH. (2007) *AUKUH Acuity/Dependency Tool.* London. Critical Care Information Advisory Group. London. Department of Health. The Association of UK University Hospitals.

Azoulay, É., Metnitz, B., Sprung, C.L., Timsit, J.-F., Lemaire, F., Bauer, P., Schlemmer, B., Moreno, R., Metnitz, P., SAPS 3 Investigators. (2009) End-of-life practices in 282 intensive care units: data from the SAPS 3 database. *Intensive Care Medicine.* 35 (4): 623–630.

BACCN (2004) *Position Statement on the Use of Restraint in Adult Critical Care Units.* Newcastle. British Association of Critical Care Nurses.

Baddeley, R.N.B., Skipworth, J.R.A., Pereira, S.P. (2011). Acute pancreatitis. *Medicine.* 39 (2): 108–115.

Bahouth, M.N., Yarbrough, K.L. (2013) Patient management: nervous system. In Morton, P.G., Fontaine, D.K. (eds). *Critical Care Nursing: a holistic approach.* 10th edn. Philadelphia, PA. Lippincott Williams & Wilkins. 744–761.

Baid, H. (2009) A critical review of auscultating bowel sounds. *British Journal of Nursing.* 18 (18): 1125–1129.

Baker, M., Harbottle, L. (2014) Parenteral nutrition. In Gandy, J. (ed). *Manual of Dietetic Practice.* 5th edn. Oxford. Wiley Blackwell. 357–364.

Ball, C.G., Lord, J., Laupland, B.K., Gmora, S., Mulloy, R.H., Ng, A.K., Schieman, C., Kirkpatrick, A.W. (2007) Chest tube complications: How well are we training our residents? *Canadian Journal of Surgery.* 50 (6): 450–458.

Ballantyne, J.C., McKenna, J.M., Ryder, E. (2003) Epidural analgesia – experience of 5628 patients in a large teaching hospital derived through audit. *Acute Pain.* 4 (3–4): 89–97.

Ballard, K., Cheeseman, W., Ripiner, T., Wells, S. (1992) Humidification for ventilated patients. *Intensive & Critical Care Nursing.* 8 (1): 2–9.

Barclay, L. (2013) COPD Linked to cognitive impairment and memory loss. *Mayo Clinic Proceedings.* 88 (12): 1222–1230.

Bar-El, Y., Ross, A., Kablawi, A., Egenburg, S. (2001) Potentially dangerous negative intrapleural pressure generated by ordinary pleural drainage systems. *Chest.* 119 (2): 511–514.

Barker, L.A., Gout, B.S., Crowe, R. (2011) Hospital malnutrition: prevalence, identification and impact on patients and the healthcare system. *International Journal of Environmental Research & Public Health.* 8 (2): 514–527.

Barkun, A.N., Bardou, M., Kulpers, E.J., Sung, J., Hunt, R.H., Martel, M., Sinclair, P., International Consensus Upper Gastrointestinal Bleeding Conference Group. (2010) International consensus recommendations on the management of patients with nonvariceal upper gastrointestinal bleeding. *Annals of Internal Medicine.* 152 (2): 101–113.

Barnes, T.A., Jinks, A. (2009) Meticillin-resistant *Staphylococcus aureus*: the modern-day challenge. *British Journal of Nursing Infection prevention in an evolving healthcare environment.* 4–18.

Barone, J.E. (2009) Fever: fact and fiction. *Journal of Trauma.* 67 (2): 406–409.

Barratt, J. (2007) What to do with patients with abnormal dipstick urinalysis. *Medicine.* 35 (7): 365–367.

Barrett, K.E., Barman, S.M., Boitano, S., Brooks, H.L. (2010) *Ganong's Review of Medical Physiology.* 23rd edn. New York. McGraw Hill Lange.

Basner, M., Babisch, W., Davis, A., Brink, M., Clark, C., Janssen, S., Stansfeld, S. (2014) Auditory and non-auditory effects of noise on health. *The Lancet.* 383 (9925): 1325–1332.

Bateman, D.N. (2007) Poisoning: focus on paracetamol. *Journal of the Royal College of Physicians of Edinburgh.* 37 (4): 332–334.

Bateman, N.T., Leach, R.M. (1998) Acute oxygen therapy. *British Medical Journal.* 317 (7161): 798–801.

Baudouin, S.V. (2002) The pulmonary physician in critical care. 3: Critical care management of community acquired pneumonia. *Thorax.* 57 (3): 267–271.

Bayer, O., Reinhart, K., Sakr, Y., Kabisch, B., Kohl, M., Riedemann, N.C., Bauer, M., Settmacher, U., Hekmat, K., Hartog, C.S. (2011) Renal effects of synthetic colloids and crystalloids in patients with severe sepsis: a prospective sequential comparison. *Critical Care Medicine.* 39 (6): 1335–1342.

Bayer, O., Reinhart, K., Kohl, M., Kabisch, B., Marshall, J., Sakr, Y., Bauer, M., Hartog, C., Schwarzkopf, D., Riedemann, N. (2012) Effects of fluid resuscitation with synthetic colloids or crystalloids alone on shock reversal, fluid balance, and patient outcomes in patients with severe sepsis: a prospective sequential analysis. *Critical Care Medicine.* 40 (9): 2543–2551.

Beach, L., Denehy, L., Lee, A. (2013) The efficacy of minitracheostomy for the management of sputum retention: a systematic review. *Physiotherapy.* 99 (4): 271–277.

Beckett, N.S., Peters, R., Fletcher, A.E., Staessen, J.A., Liu, L., Dumitrascu, D., Stoyanovsky, V., Antikainen, R.L., Nikitin, Y., Anderson, C, Belhani, A, Forette, F, Rajkumar, C, Thijs, L, Banya, W, Bulpitt, C.J., HYVET Study group. (2008) Treatment of hypertension in patients 80 years of age or older. *New England Journal of Medicine.* 358 (18): 1887–1898.

Bell, L., Duffy, A. (2009) Pain assessment and management in surgical nursing: a literature review. *British Journal of Nursing.* 18 (3): 153–156.

Bellot, P., Welker, M.W., Soriano, G., von Schaewen, M., Appenrodt, B., Wiest, R., Whittaker, S., Tzonev, R., Handshiev, S., Verslype, C., Moench, C., Zeuzem, S., Sauerbruch, T., Guarner, C., Schott, E., Johnson, N., Petrov, A., Katzarov, K., Nevens, F., Zapater, P., Such, J. (2013) Automated low flow pump system for the treatment of refractory ascites: A multi-center safety and efficacy study. *Journal of Hepatology.* 58 (5): 922–927.

Benning, A., Ghaleb, M., Suokas, A., Dixon-Woods, M., Dawson, J., Barber, N., Franklin, B.D., Girling, A., Carmalt, M., Rudge, G., Naicker, T., Nwulu, U., Choudhury, S., Lilford, R. (2011) Large scale organisational intervention to improve patient safety in four UK hospitals: mixed method evaluation. *British Medical Journal.* 342:d195 doi:10.1136/British Medical Journal.d195

Bergbom, I., Askwall, A. (2000) The nearest and dearest: a lifeline for ICU patients. *Intensive and Critical Care Nursing.* 16 (6): 384–395.

Bernal, W., Auzinger, G., Dhawan, A., Wendon, J. (2010) Acute liver failure. *The Lancet.* 376 (9736): 190–201.

Bernard, S.A., Buist, M. (2003) Induced hypothermia in critical care medicine: A review. *Critical Care Medicine.* 31 (7): 2041–2051.

Bertuccio, C.A. (2011) Relevance of VEGF and nephrin expression in glomerular diseases. *Journal of Signal Transduction.* doi:10.1155/2011/718609.

Best, C. (2007) Nasogastric tube insertion in adults who require enteral feeding. *Nursing Standard.* 21 (40): 39–43.

Bharucha, A.E., Pemberton, J.H., Locke, G.R. III. (2013) American Gastroenterological Association technical review on constipation. *Gastroenterology.* 144 (1): 218–238.

Bienvenu, O.J., Neufeld, K.J., Needham, D.M. (2012) Treatment of four psychiatric emergencies in the Intensive Care Unit. *Critical Care Medicine.* 40 (9): 2662–2670.

Bishop, L., Dougherty, L., Bodenham, A., Mansi, J., Crowe, P., Kibbler, C., Shannon, M., Treleaven, J. (2007) Guidelines on the insertion and management of central venous access devices in adults. *International Journal of Laboratory Hematology.* 29 (4): 261–278.

Bleeker-Rovers, V., van der Meer, J.W.M., Beechning, N.J. (2009) Fever. *Medicine.* 37 (1): 28–34.

Blich, M., Sebbag, A., Attias, J., Aronson, D., Markiewicz, W. (2008) Cardiac troponin I elevation in hospitalized patients without acute coronary syndromes. *American Journal of Cardiology.* 101 (10): 1384–1388.

Bloomfield, J., Pegram, A. (2012) Improving nutrition and hydration in hospital: the nurse's responsibility. *Nursing Standard.* 26 (34): 52–56.

BNF. (2014) *British National Formulary 68.* London. BMA/Royal Pharmaceutical Society.

Bodenham, A.R., Barry, B.N. (2001) The role of tracheostomy in ICU. *Anaesthesia and Intensive Care Medicine.* 2 (9): 336–339.

Bokorst van der Schueren, M.A.E., Guaitoli, P.R., Jansma, E.P., de Vet, H.C.W. (2014) Nutrition screening tools: does one size fit all? A systematic review of screening tools for the hospital setting. *Clinical Nutrition.* 33 (1): 39–58.

Boldt, J., Suttner, S., Brosch, C., Lehmann, A., Röhm, K., Mengistu, A. (2009) The influence of a balanced volume replacement concept on inflammation, endothelial activation, and kidney integrity in elderly cardiac surgery patients. *Intensive Care Medicine.* 35 (3): 462–470.

Bolliger, D., Steiner, L.A., Kasper, J., Aziz, O.A., Filopovic, M., Seeberger, M.D. (2007) The accuracy of non-invasive carbon dioxide monitoring: a clinical evaluation of two transcutaneous systems. *Anaesthesia.* 62 (4): 394–399.

Bollinger, T., Bollinger, A., Oster, H., Solbach, W. (2010) Sleep, immunity and circadian clocks: a mechanistic model. *Gerontology.* 56 (6): 574–580.

Booth, C., Heyland, D.K., Paterson, W.G. (2002) Gastrointestinal promotility drugs in the critical care setting: A systematic review of the evidence. *Critical Care Medicine.* 30 (7): 1429–1435.

Borthwick, M., Bourne, R., Craig, M., Egan, A., Oxley, J. (2006) *Detection, Prevention and Treatment of Delirium in Critically Ill Patients.* United Kingdom Clinical Pharmacy Association. London.

Bourdages, M., Bigras, J.-L., Farrell, C.A., Hutchison, J.S., Lacroix, J. (2010) Cardiac arrhythmias associated with severe traumatic brain injury and hypothermia therapy. *Pediatric Critical Care Medicine.* 11 (3): 439–441.

Breathnach, A. (2005) Nosocomial infections. *Medicine.* 33 (3): 22–26.

Brochard, L., Abroug, F., Brenner, M., Broccard, A.F., Danner, R.L., Ferrer, M., Laghi, F., Magder, S., Papazian, L., Pelosi, P., Polderman, K.H., TS/ERS/ESICM/SCCM/SRLF Ad Hoc Committee on Acute Renal Failure. (2010) An official ATS/ERS/ESICM/SCCM/SRLF statement: prevention and management of acute renal failure in the ICU patient. *American Journal of Respiratory and Critical Care Medicine.* 181 (10): 1128–1155.

Brown, L.P. (2011) Revisiting our roots: caring in nursing curriculum design. *Nurse Education in Practice.* 11 (6): 360–364.

Brusselle, G.G., Joos, G.F., Bracke, K.R. (2011) New insights into the immunology of chronic obstructive pulmonary disease. *The Lancet.* 378 (9795): 1015–1026.

BTS. (2002) Non-invasive ventilation in acute respiratory failure. *Thorax.* 57 (3): 192–211.

BTS. (2006) *The Burden of Lung Disease.* 2nd edn. London. British Thoracic Society.

BTS. (2008) BTS guideline for emergency oxygen use in adult patients. *Thorax.* 63 (Supplement VI): vi1–vi68.

Buckley, N.H., Hickey, J.V. (2014) Cerebral aneurysms. In Hickey, J.V.(ed). *Neurological and Neurosurgical Nursing.* 7th edn. Philadelphia, PA. Wolters Kluwer Lippincott Williams & Wilkins. 554–591.

Buckman, R. (1988) *I Don't Know What to Say.* London. Pan.

Bunker, J. (2014) Hypertension: diagnosis, assessment and management. *Nursing Standard.* 28 (42): 50–59.

Burke, A.P., Virmani, R. (2007) Pathophysiology of acute myocardial infarction. *Medical Clinics of North America.* 91 (4): 553–572.

Burke, C., Seeley, M.G. (1994) An oncology unit's initiation of bereavement support programme. *Oncology Forum. Nursing.* 21 (10): 1657–1680.

Burns, K.E.A., Adhikari, N.K.J., Keenan, S.P., Meade, M. (2009) Use of non-invasive ventilation to wean critically ill adults off invasive ventilation: meta-analysis and systematic review. *British Medical Journal.* 339 (7706): 1305–1308.

Burt, C.C., Arrowsmith, J.E C. (2009) Respiratory failure. *Surgery.* 27 (11): 475–479.

Cabello, J.B., Burls, A., Emparanza, J.I., Bayliss, S., Quinn, T. (2010) Oxygen therapy for acute myocardial infarction. *Cochrane Database of Systematic Reviews* 2010, Issue 6. Art. No.: CD007160. DOI: 10.1002/14651858.CD007160.pub2.

Camm, A.J., Lip, G.Y.H., De Caterina, R., Savelieva, I., Atar, D., Hohnloser, S.H., Hindricks, G., Kirchhol, P. (2012) 2012 focused update of the ESC Guidelines for the management of atrial fibrillation. *European Heart Journal.* 33: 2719–2747.

Campbell, I. (2003) Physiology of fluid balance. *Anaesthesia and Intensive Care.* 4 (10): 342–344.

Campbell, J., Jackson, A. (2011) Did you know? It takes a minute: check your patient's pulse to see if they are in atrial fibrillation. *Primary Care Nursing.* 8 (1): S3–S5.

Capuzzo, M., Rambaldi, M., Pinelli, G., Campesato, M., Pigna, A., Zanello, M., Barbagallo, M., Girardis, M., Toschi, E. (2012) Hospital staff education on severe sepsis/septic shock and hospital mortality. *BMC Anesthesiology.* 12: 28.

Carron, M., Freo1, U., BaHammam, A.S., Dellweg, D., Guarracino, F., Cosentini, R., Feltracco, P., Vianello, A., Ori1, C., Esquinas, A. (2013) Complications of non-invasive ventilation techniques: a comprehensive qualitative review of randomized trials. *British Journal of Anaesthesia.* 110 (6): 896–914.

Cars, O., Högberg, L.D., Murray, M., Nordberg, O., Sivaraman, S., Lundborg, C.S., So, A.D., Tomson, G. (2008) Meeting the challenge of antibiotic resistance. *British Medical Journal.* 337 (7672): 726–728.

Catania, J., Que, L.G., Govert, J.A., Hollingsworth, J.W., Wolfe, C.R. (2014) High ICU admission rate for 2013–2014 influenza is associated with a low rate of vaccination. *American Journal of Respiratory and Critical Care Medicine.* 189 (4): 485–487.

CDC. (2013) *Antibiotic Resistance Threats in the United States, 2013.* Atlanta, Georgia. Centers for Disease Control and Prevention.

Chadda, K., Louis, B., Benaïssa, L., Annane, D., Gajdos, P., Raphaël, J.C., Lofaso, F. (2002) Physiological effects of decannulation in tracheostomized patients. *Intensive Care Medicine.* 28 (12): 1761–1767.

Chapple, A., Ziebland, S. (2010) Viewing the body after bereavement due to a traumatic death: qualitative study in the UK. *British Medical Journal.* 340 (7754): 1017.

Chesler, M. (2005) Failure and function of intracellular pH regulation in acute hypoxic-ischaemic injury of astrocytes. *Glia.* 50 (4): 398–406.

Chobanian, A.V. (2009) The hypertension paradox – more uncontrolled disease despite improved therapy. *New England Journal of Medicine.* 361 (9): 878–887.

Cholley, P., Thouverez, M., Floret, N., Bertrand, X., Talon, D. (2008) The role of water fittings in intensive care rooms as reservoirs for the colonization of patients with *Pseudomonas aeruginosa. Intensive Care Medicine.* 34 (8): 1428–1433.

Chopra, V., Anand, S., Hickner, A., Buist, M., Rogers, M.A.M., Saint, S., Flanders, S.A. (2013) Risk of venous thromboembolism associated with peripherally inserted central catheters: a systematic review and meta-analysis. *The Lancet.* 382 (9889): 311–325.

Chua, D., Ignaszewski, A. (2009) Clopidogrel in acute coronary syndromes. *British Medical Journal.* 338 (7701): 998–1002.

Chugh, S.S., Havmoeller, R., Narayanan, K., Singh, D., Rienstra, M., Benjamin, E.J., Gillum, R.F., Kim, Y.-H., McAnulty, Jr. J.H., Zheng, Z.-J., Forouzanfar, M.H., Naghavi, M., Mensah, G.A., Ezzati, M., Murray, C.J.L. (2013) Worldwide epidemiology of atrial fibrillation: a global burden of disease 2010 study. *Circulation.* 129 (8): 837–847.

Chumbley, G. (2011) Use of ketamine in uncontrolled acute and procedural pain. *Nursing Standard.* 25 (15–17): 35–37.

Clark, C.E., Taylor, R.S., Shore, A.C., Campbell, J.L. (2012) The difference in blood pressure readings between arms and survival: primary care cohort study. *British Medical Journal.* 344 (7851): 19.

Clark, D., Armstrong, M., Allan, A., Graham, F., Carnon, A., Isles, C. (2014) Imminence of death among hospital inpatients: prevalent cohort study. *Palliative Medicine.* 28 (6): 474–479.

Classen, D.C., Resar, R., Griffin, F., Federico, F., Frankel, T., Kimmel, N., Whittington, J.C., Frankel, A., Seger, A., James, B.C. (2011) 'Global Trigger Tool' shows that adverse events in hospitals may be ten times greater than previously measured. *Health Affairs.* 30 (4): 581–589.

Cnossen, J.S., Vollebregt, K.C., de Vrieze, N., ter Riet, G., Mol, B.W.J., Khan, K.S, van der Post, J.A.M. (2008) Accuracy of mean arterial pressure and blood pressure measurements in predicting pre-eclampsia: systematic review and meta-analysis. *British Medical Journal.* 336 (7653): 1117–1120.

Coca, S.G., Singanamala, S., Parikh, C.R. (2012) Chronic kidney disease after acute kidney injury: a systematic review and meta-analysis. *Kidney International.* 81 (5): 442–448.

Cochrane Injuries Group Albumin Reviewers. (1998) Human albumin in critically ill patients: systematic review of randomised control trials. *British Medical Journal.* 317 (7153): 235–240.

Cohen, A.T., Rapson, V.F., Bergmann, J.-F., Goldhaber, S.Z., Kakkar, A.K., Deslandes, B., Huang, W., Zayaruzny, M., Emery, L., Anderson, F.A. Jr., ENDORSE Investigators. (2008) Venous thromboembolism risk and prophylaxis in the acute hospital care setting (ENDORSE study): a multinational cross-sectional study. *The Lancet.* 371 (9610): 387–394.

Coia, J.E., Duckworth, G.J., Edwards, D.I., Farrington, M., Fry, C., Humphreys, H., Mallaghan, C., Tucker, D.R., Joint Working Party of the British Society of Antimicrobial Chemotherapy, the Hospital Infection Society, and the Infection Control Nurses Association. (2006) Guidelines for the control and prevention of meticillin-resistant *Staphylococcus aureus* (*MRSa*) in healthcare facilities. *Journal of Hospital Infections.* 63S: S1–S44.

Commission on Human Medicines. (2012) Paracetamol overdose: new guidance on use of intravenous acetylcysteine (letter, dated 3rd September). Secretary of Commission, S. Singh, www.mhra.gov.uk/Safetyinformation/Safetywarningsalertsandrecalls/Safetywarningsand messagesformedicines/CON178225 (last accessed 8 January 2014).

Commissioning Board Chief Nursing Officer and DH Chief Nursing Adviser. (2012) *Compassion in Practice*. London. Department of Health.

Conti, C.R. (2011) Is hyperoxic ventilation important to treat acute coronary syndromes such as myocardial infarction? *Clinical Cardiology*. 34 (3): 132–133.

Conzalez, J.C.M. (2008) Gastric residuals – are they important in the management of enteral nutrition. *Clinical Nutrition Highlights*. 4 (1): 2–8.

Cook, S., Windecker, S. (2008) Percutaneous ventricular assist devices for cardiogenic shock. *Current Heart Failure Reports*. 5 (3): 163–169

Coolican, M.B. (1994) Families facing the sudden death of a loved one. *Critical Care Clinics of North America*. 6 (3): 607–612.

Coombs, M. (2004) *Breaking the Inner Circle*. London. Routledge.

Cooper, N., Forrest, K., Cramp, P. (2006) *Essential Guide to Acute Care*. London. 2nd edn. British Medical Journal Books.

Coppen, R., Friele, R.D., Marquet, R.L., Gevers, S.K. (2006) Opting-out systems: no guarantee for higher donation rates. *Transplant International*. 18 (11): 1275–1279.

Corley, A., Caruana, L., Barnett, A., Tronstad, O., Fraser, J. (2011) Oxygen delivery through high-flow nasal cannulae increases end-expiratory volume and reduces respiratory rate in post-cardiac surgical patients. *British Journal of Anaesthesia*. 107 (6): 998–1004.

Cox, M., Kemp, R., Anwar, S., Athey, V., Aung, T., Moloney, E.D. (2006) Non-invasive monitoring of CO_2 levels in patients using NIV for AECOPD. *Thorax* 61 (4):363–364.

Craig, J.J.O., McClelland, D.B.L., Watson, H.G. (2010) Blood disease. In Colledge, N.R., Walker, B.R., Ralston, S.H. (eds) *Davidson's Principles and Practice of Medicine*. 21st edn. Edinburgh. Churchill Livingstone Elsevier. 985–1051.

Crawford, D., Greene, N., Wentworth, S. (2005) *Thermometer Review: UK market survey. Medicines and Healthcare products Regulatory Agency Evaluation 04144*. London. Department of Health.

Cretikos, M.A., Bellomo, R., Hillman, K., Chen, J., Finfer, S., Flabouris, A. (2008) Respiratory rate: the neglected vital sign. *Medical Journal of America*. 188 (11): 657–659.

Crews, M., Garry, D., Phillips, C., Wong, A., Troke, B., Ruck Keene, A., Danbury, C. (2014) Deprivation of liberty in intensive care. *Journal of the Intensive Care Society*. 15 (4): 320–324.

Crombie, I.K., Davies, H.T.O., Macrae, W.A. (1998) Cut and thrust: antecedent surgery and trauma among patients attending a chronic pain clinic. *Pain*. 76 (1–2): 167–172.

Cunningham, C., McWilliam, K. (2006) Caring for people with dementia in A&E. *Emergency Nurse*. 14 (6): 12–16.

Curtis, R.L. (2009) Catheter-related bloodstream infection in the intensive care unit. *Journal of the Intensive Care Society*. 10 (2): 102–108.

Czura, C.J. (2011) 'Merinoff Symposium 2010: Sepsis'– speaking with one voice. *Molecular Medicine*. 17 (1–2): 2–3.

Daneshmandi, M., Neiseh, F., SadeghiShermeh, M., Ebadi, A. (2012) Effect of eye mask on sleep quality in patients with acute coronary syndrome. *Journal of Caring Sciences*. 1 (3), 135–143.

Danis, M. (1998) Improving end-of-life care in the intensive care unit: what's to be learned from outcomes research? *New Horizons*. 6 (1): 110–118.

Darouiche, R. (2006) Spinal epidural abscess. *New England Journal of Medicine*. 355 (19): 2012–2020.

Davenport, A., Stevens, P. (2008) *Clinical Practice Guidelines: Acute Kidney Injury*. 4th edn. London. UK Renal Association.

Davidhizer, R., Giger, J.N. (1997) When touch in not the best approach. *Journal of Clinical Nursing*. 6 (3): 203–206.

Davidson., K.W., Rieckmann, N., Schwartz, J.E., Shimbo, D., Medina, V., Albanese, G., Kronish, I., Hegel, M., Burg, M.M. (2010) Enhanced depression care for patients with acute coronary syndrome and persistent depressive symptoms. *Archives of Internal Medicine*. 170 (7): 600–608.

Davies, H.E., Davies, R.J.O., Davies, C.W.H., BTS Pleural Disease Guideline Group. (2010) Management of pleural infection in adults: British Thoracic Society pleural disease guideline 2010. *Thorax*. 65 (Supplement 2): ii41–ii53.

De, D. (2008) Acute nursing care and management of patients with sickle cell. *British Journal of Nursing*. 17 (13): 818–823.

De Keulenaer, B.L., De Waele, J.J., Powell, B., Malbrain, M.L.N.G. (2009) What is normal intra-abdominal pressure and how is it affected by positioning, body mass and positive end-expiratory pressure? *Intensive Care Medicine*. 35 (6): 969–976.

Dellinger, R.P., Carlet, J.M., Masur, H., Gerlach, H., Calandra, T., Cohen, J., Gea-Banacloche, J., Keh, D., Marshall, J.C., Parker, M.M., Ramsay, G., Zimmerman, J.L., Vincent, J.-L., Levy, M.M. (2004) Surviving sepsis campaign guidelines for management of severe sepsis and septic shock. *Intensive Care Medicine*. 30 (3): 536–555.

Dellinger, R.P., Levy, M.M., Rhodes, A., Annane, D., Gerlach, H., Opal, S.M., Sevransky, J.E., Sprung, C.L., Douglas, I.S., Jaeschke, R., Osborn, T.M., Nunnally, M.E., Townsend, S.R., Reinhart, K., Kleinpell, R.M., Angus, D.C., Deutschman, C.S., Machado, F.R., Rubenfeld, D.G., Webb, S.A., Beale, R.J., Vincent, J.-L., Moreno, R., Surviving Sepsis Campaign Guidelines Committee including the Pediatric Subgroup. (2013) Surviving Sepsis Campaign: international guidelines for management of severe sepsis and septic shock. *Critical Care Medicine*. 4 (2): 580–637.

Deroy, R. (2000) Crystalloids or colloids for fluid resuscitation – is that the question? *Current Anaesthesia and Critical Care*. 11 (1): 20–26.

Detsky, A.S., McLaughlin, J.R., Baker, J.P., Johnston, N., Whittaker, S., Mendelson, R.A., Jeejeebhoy, K.N. (1987) What is subjective global assessment? *Journal of Parenteral Nutrition*. 11 (1): 8–13.

Dezfulian, C., Shiva, S., Alekseyenko, A., Pendyal, A., Besiser, D.G., Munasinghe, J.P., Anderson, S.A., Chesley, C.F., Hoek, V., Gladwin, M.T. (2009) Nitrite therapy after cardiac arrest reduces reactive oxygen species generation, improves cardiac and neurological function, and enhances survival via reversible inhibition of mitochondrial complex I. *Circulation*. 120 (10): 897–905.

Dickson, R.P., Erb-Downward, J.R., Huffnagle, G.B. (2014) Towards an ecology of the lung: new conceptual models of pulmonary microbiology and pneumonia pathogenesis. *The Lancet Respiratory Medicine*. 2: 238–246.

Dimond, B. (2011) *Legal Aspects of Nursing*. 6th edn. Harlow. Pearson.

Docherty, B., Bench, S. (2002) Tracheostomy management for patients in general ward settings. *Professional Nurse*. 18 (2): 100–104.

Dock, S.1917. The relationship of the nurse to the doctor and the doctor to the nurse. *American Journal of Nursing*.17 (5): 394–396.

DOH. (2000) *Comprehensive Critical Care*. London. Department of Health.

DOH. (2007) *High Impact Intervention 1: Central Venous Care Bundle*. London. Department of Health.

DOH. (2008a) *National Infarct Angioplasty Project (NIAP)*. London. Department of Health.

DOH. (2008b) *Organs for Transplants*. London. Department of Health.

DOH. (2009) *Reference Guide to Consent for Examination or Treatment*. 2nd edn. London. Department of Health.

DOH. (2011a) *An Outcome Strategy for People with Chronic Obstructive Pulmonary Disease (COPD) and Asthma in England.* London. Department of Health.

DOH. (2011b) (updated 2012) *Promoting Good Nutrition.* London. Department of Health.

DOH. (2013) *In-Patient Care. Health Building Note 04-01: Adult In-Patient Facilities.* London. Department of Health.

Doherty, M., Buggy, D.J. (2012) Intraoperative fluids: how much is too much? *British Journal of Anaesthesia.* 109 (1): 69–79.

Doig, G.S., Heighes, P.T., Simpson, F., Sweetman, E.A., Davies, A.R. (2009) Early Enteral nutrition, provided within 24 h of injury or intensive care unit admission, significantly reduces mortality in critically ill patients: a meta-analysis of randomised controlled trials. *Intensive Care Medicine.* 35 (12): 2018–2027.

Dougherty, L., Lamb, J. (2008) *Intravenous Therapy in Nursing Practice.* 2nd edn. Oxford. Blackwell Publishing.

Dougherty, L., Lister, S. (eds). (2011) *The Royal Marsden Hospital Manual of Clinical Nursing Procedures.* 8th edn. Oxford. Wiley-Blackwell.

Dumas, F., Bougouin, W., Geri, G., Lamhaut, L., Bougle, A., Daviaud, F., Morichau-Beauchant, T., Rosencher, J., Marijon, E., Carli, P., Jouven, X., Rea, T.D., Cariou, A. (2014) Is epinephrine during cardiac arrest associated with worse outcomes in resuscitated patients? *Journal of the American College of Cardiology.* 64 (22): 2360–2367.

Durai, R., Hoque, H., Davies, T.W. (2010) Managing a chest tube and drainage system. *AORN.* 91 (2): 275–280.

Dutta, R., Baha, S., Al-Shaikh, B. (2006) Humidification, humidifiers and nebulizers. *CPD Anaesthesia.* 8 (2): 78–82.

EASL. (2010) EASL clinical practice guidelines on the management of ascites, spontaneous bacterial peritonitis, and hepatorenal syndrome in cirrhosis. *Journal of Hepatology.* 53 (4): 397–417.

EASL. (2014) Hepatic Encephalopathy in Chronic Liver Disease: 2014 Practice Guideline by the European Association for the Study of the Liver and the American Association for the Study of Liver Diseases. *Journal of Hepatology.* http://dx.doi.org/10.1016/j.jhep.2014.05.042 (last acessed 4 January 2015).

Eastland, J. (2001) A framework for nursing the dying patient in ICU. *Nursing Times.* 97 (3): 36–39.

Eckardt, K.-U., Coresh, J., Devuyst, O., Johnson, R.J., Köttgen, A., Levey, A.S., Levin, A. (2013) Evolving importance of kidney disease: from subspecialty to global health burden. *The Lancet.* 382 (9887): 158–169.

Edmunds, S., Graham, C., Hollis, V., Lamb, J., Todd J. (2011) Observations. In Dougherty, L., Lister, S. (eds). (2008) *The Royal Marsden Hospital Manual of Clinical Nursing Procedures.* 8th edn. Oxford. Wiley-Blackwell. 746–827.

Eeles, E.M.P., Hubbard, R.E., White, S.V., O'Mahony, M.S., Savva, G.M., Bayer, A.J. (2010) Hospital use, institutionalisation and mortality associated with delirium. *Age & Ageing.* 39 (4): 470–475.

Eggimann, P., Pittet, D. (2001) Infection control in the ICU. *Chest.* 120 (6): 2059–2093.

Ehlenbach, W.J., Hough, C.L., Crane, P.K., Haneuse, S.J.P.A., Carson, S.S., Curtis, J.R., Larson, E.B. (2010) Association between acute care and critical illness hospitalization and cognitive function in older adults. *Journal of the American Medical Association.* 303 (8): 763–770.

Ellershaw, J., Ward, C. (2003) Care of the dying patient: The last hours or days of life. *British Medical Journal.* 326 (30): 30–34.

Elliot, P., Anderson, B., Arburstini, E., Bilinska, Z., Cecchi, F., Charron, P., Dubourg, O., Kühl, B., McKenna, W.J., Monseettat, L., Pankuweit, S., Rapezzzi, C., Seferovic, P.,

Tavazzzi, L., Kerem, A. (2008) Classification of the cardiomyopathies: a position statement from the European Society of Cardiology working group on myocardial and pericardial disease. *European Heart Journal.* 29 (2): 270–276.

Ellis, J.J., Eagle, K.A., Kline-Rogers, E.M., Erickson, S.R. (2005) Depressive symptoms and treatment after acute coronary syndrome. *International Journal of Cardiology.* 99 (3): 443–447.

Ellison, G. (1992) A private disaster. *Nursing Times.* 88 (52): 52–53.

El-Sharkawy, A.M., Sahota, O., Maughan, R.J., Lobo, D.N. (2014) The pathophysiology of fluid and electrolyte balance in the older adult surgical patient. *Clinical Nutrition.* 33 (1): 6–13.

Emmanuel, E.J., Fairclough, D.L., Emanuel, L.L. (2000) Attitudes and desires related to euthanasia and physician-assisted suicide among terminally ill patients and their caregivers. *Journal of the American Medical Association.* 284 (19): 2460–2468.

Esteban, A., Frutos-Vivar, F., Ferguson, N.D., Arabi, Y., Apeztegufa, C., González, M., Epstein, S.K., Hill, N.S., Nava, S., Soares, M.-A., D'Empaire, G., Alía, I., Anzueto, A. (2004) Noninvasive positive pressure ventilation for respiratory failure after extubation. *New England Journal of Medicine.* 350 (24): 2452–2460.

Ewens, J.P. (2001) Assessment of a breathless patient. *Nursing Standard.* 15 (16): 48–53.

Ewins, D., Bryant, J. (1992) Relative comfort. *Nursing Times.* 88 (52): 61–63.

Eyers, I., Young, E., Luff, R., Arber, S. (2012) Striking the balance: night care versus the facilitation of good sleep. *British Journal of Nursing.* 21 (5): 303–307.

Farrell, M. (1999) The challenge of breaking bad news. *Intensive and Critical Care Nursing.* 15 (2): 101–110.

Faulds, M., Meekings, T. (2013) Temperature management in critically ill patients. *Continuing Education in Anaesthesia, Critical Care & Pain.* 13 (3): 75–79.

Fazel, S., Wolf, A., Pillas, D., Lichtenstein, P., Långström, N. (2014) Suicide, fatal injuries, and other causes of premature mortality in patients with traumatic brain injury. A 41-year Swedish population study. *Journal of the American Medical Association Psychiatry.* 71 (3): 326–333.

Fearon, K.C.H., Ljunqvist, O., von Meyenfeldt, M., Revhaug, A., Dejong., C.H.C., Lassen, K., Nygren, J., Hausel, J., Soop, M., Andersen, J., Kehlet, H. (2005) Enhanced recovery after surgery: a consensus review of clinical care for patients undergoing colonic resection. *Clinical Nutrition.* 24 (3); 466–477.

Ferer, M., Esquinas, A., Leon, M., Gonzalez, G., Alarcon, A., Torres, A. (2003) Noninvasive ventilation in severe hypoxemic respiratory failure. *American Journal of Respiratory and Critical Care Medicine.* 168 (12): 1438–1444.

Feuerstein, J.D., Akbari, M., Gifford, A.E., Hurley, C.M., Leffler, D.A., Sheth, S.G., Cheifetz, A.S. (2014) Systematic analysis underlying the quality of the scientific evidence and conflicts of interest in interventional medicine subspecialty guidelines. *Mayo Clinic Proceedings.* 89 (1): 16–24.

Finlay, I., Dallimore, D. (1991) Your child is dead. *British Medical Journal.* 302 (6791): 1524–1525.

Finney, A., Rushton, C. (2007) Recognition and management of patients with anaphylaxis. *Nursing Standard.* 21 (37): 50–57.

Fisher, L., Macnaughton, P. (2006) Electrolyte and metabolic disturbances in the critically ill. *Anaesthesia and Intensive Care Medicine.* 7 (5): 151–154.

Florin, J., Ehrenberg, A., Ehnfors, M. (2005) Patients' and nurses' perceptions of nursing problems in an acute care setting. *Journal of Advanced Nursing.* 51 (2): 140–149.

Fontana, R.J. (2008) Acute liver failure including acetaminophen overdose. *Medical Clinics of North America.* 92 (4): 761–794.

Ford, H. (2013) Use of statins to reduce the risk of cardiovascular disease in adults. *Nursing Standard*. 27 (39): 48–56.

Forsyth, R.J., Wolny, S., Rodrigues, B. (2010) Routine intracranial pressure monitoring in acute coma. *Cochrane Database of Systematic Reviews* 2010, Issue 2. Art. No.: CD002043. DOI: 10.1002/14651858.CD002043.pub2.

Foxall, F. (2008) *Arterial Blood Gas Analysis*. Keswick. M&K Update.

Francis, R. (2013) *Report of the Mid Staffordshire NHS Foundation Trust Public Inquiry*. London. The Stationery Office Limited.

Fuentebella, J., Kerner, J.A. (2009) Refeeding syndrome. *Pediatric Clinics of North America*. 56 (5): 1201–1210.

Fukatsu, K., Zarzaur, B.L., Johnson, C.D., Lundberg, A.H., Wilcox, H.G., Kudsk, K.A. (2001) Enteral nutrition prevents remote organ injury and death after a gut ischaemia insult. *Annals of Surgery*. 233 (5): 660–668.

Fulbrook, P., Bonkers, A., Albarran, J.W. (2007) A European survey of adult intensive care nurses' practice in relation to nutritional assessment. *Journal of Clinical Nursing*. 16 (11): 2132–2141.

Fysh, E.T.H., Smith, N.A., Lee, Y.C.G. (2010) Optimal chest drain size: the rise of the small-bore pleural catheter. *Seminars in Respiratory Critical Care Medicine*. 31 (6): 760–768.

Galbois, A., Meurisse, Z.S., Kernéis, S., Margetis, D., Alves, M., Ait-Oufella, M., Baudel, J.-L., Offenstadt, G., Maury, E., Guidet, B. (2012) Outcome of spontaneous and iatrogenic pneumothoraces managed with small-bore chest tubes. *Acta Anaesthesiologica Scandinavica*. 56 (4): 507–512.

Gallagher, A., Wainwright, P. (2007) Terminal sedation: promoting ethical nursing practice. *Nursing Standard*. 21 (34): 42–46.

Galley, H.F. (2011) Oxidative stress and mitochondrial dysfunction in sepsis. *British Journal of Anaesthesia*. 107 (1): 57–64.

Gandy, J. (ed). (2014) *Manual of Dietetic Practice*. 5th edn. Oxford. Wiley Blackwell.

Gardner, K., Bell, C., Bartram, J.L., Allman, M., Awogbade, M., Reed, D.C., Ervine, M., Thein, S.L. (2010) Outcome of adults with sickle cell disease admitted to critical care of a single institution in the UK. *British Journal of Haematology*. 151 (5): 610–613.

Garry, P., Garry, D., Kapila, A. (2010) Surviving sepsis – the physiology behind why we should intervene early. *Care of the Critically Ill*. 25 (2): 36–39.

Gelinas, C., Puntillo, K.A., Joffe, A.M., Barr, J. (2013) A validated approach to evaluating psychometric properties of pain assessment tools for use in nonverbal critically ill adults. *Seminars in Respiratory and Critical Care Medicine*. 34 (2): 153–168.

Gelling, L., Provest, T. (1999) The needs of relatives of critically ill patients admitted to a neuroscience critical care unit: a comparison of the perceptions of relatives, nurses and doctors. *Care of the Critically Ill*. 15 (2): 53–58.

Gerich, J.E. (2010) Role of the kidney in normal glucose homeostasis and in the hyperglycaemia of diabetes mellitus: therapeutic implications. *Diabetic Medicine*. 27 (2): 136–142.

Gianni, M., Dentali, F., Grandi, A.M., Sumner, G., Hiralal, R., Lonn, E. (2006) Apical ballooning syndrome or takotsubo cardiomyopathy: a systematic review. *European Heart Journal*. 27 (13): 1523–1529.

Gibbison, B., Sheikh, A., McShane, P., Haddow, C., Soar, J. (2012) Anaphylaxis admissions to UK critical care units between 2005 and 2009. *Anaesthesia*. 67 (8): 833–838.

Gines, P., Cardenas, A. (2008) The management of ascites and hyponatremia in cirrhosis. *Seminars in Liver Disease. Complications of Cirrhosis*. 28 (1):43–58.

Glass., R.I., Parashar, U.D., Estes, M.K. (2009) Norovirus gastroenteritis. *New England Journal of Medicine*. 361 (18): 1776–1785.

Global Initiative for Asthma. (2012) Global Strategy for Asthma Management and Prevention. www.ginasthma.org/local/uploads/files/GINA_Report_2012Feb13.pdf (last accessed 19 April 2015).

Glossop, A.J., Shepherd, N., Bryden, D., Mills, G.H. (2012) Non-invasive ventilation for weaning, avoiding reintubation after extubation and in the postoperative period: a meta-analysis. *British Journal of Anaesthesia.* 108 (3): 305–314.

GMC. (2010) *Treatment and care towards the end of life: good practice in decision making.* London. General Medical Council.

GMC. (2013) *Good Medical Practice.* London. General Medical Council.

GOLD. (2013) Global strategy for the diagnosis, management, and prevention of chronic obstructive pulmonary disease. Updated 2013. Global initiative for chronic Obstructive Lung Disease. Available from: http://www.goldcopd.org/ (last accessed 21 August 2014).

Goldhill, D., McNarry, A. (2003) Physiological abnormalities are associated with increased mortality – appendix 2. In *National Outreach Forum. Critical Care Outreach 2003: Progress in Developing Services.* London. Department of Health Modernisation Agency.

Golembiewski, J.A., O'Brien, D. (2002) A systematic approach to the management of postoperative nausea and vomiting. *Journal of Perianesthesia Nursing.* 17 (6): 364–376.

Gould, D. (2008) Enterococcal infection. *Nursing Standard.* 22 (27): 40–43.

Gray, A., Goodacre, S., Newby, D.E., Masson, M., Sampson, F., Nicholl, J., 3CPO Triallists. (2008) Noninvasive ventilation in acute cardiogenic pulmonary edema. *New England Journal of Medicine.* 359 (2): 142–151.

Gray, E. (2001) Pain management for patients with chest drains. *Nursing Standard.* 14 (23): 40–44.

Grech, E.D., Jackson, M.J., Ramsdale, D.R. (1995) Reperfusion injury after acute myocardial infarction. *British Medical Journal.* 310 (6978): 477–478.

Green, S.M. (2011) Cheerio, Laddie! Bidding farewell to the Glasgow Coma Scale. *Annals of Emergency Medicine.* 58 (5): 427–430.

Greenlee, M., Wingo, C.S., McDonough, A.A., Youn, J.-H., Kone, B.C. (2009) Narrative review: evolving concepts in potassium homeostasis and hypokalaemia. *Annals of Internal Medicine.* 150 (9): 619–625.

Grice, E.A., Segre, J.A. (2011) The skin microbiome. *Nature Reviews Microbiology.* 9 (4): 244–253.

Grieve, R.J., Finnie, A. (2002) Nutritional care: implications and recommendations for nursing. *British Journal of Nursing.* 11 (7): 432–437.

Grundmann, H. (2006) Emergence and resurgence of meticillin-resistant *Staphylococcus aureus* as a public-health threat. *The Lancet.* 368 (9538): 874–885.

Guly, H.R., Bouramra, O., Lecky, F.E. (2008) The incidence of neurogenic shock in patients with isolated spinal cord injury in the emergency department. *Resuscitation.* 76 (1): 57–62.

Gumbley, E., Pearson, J. (2006) Tissue donation: benefits, legal issues and the nurse's role. *Nursing Standard.* 21 (1): 51–56.

Güneş, Ü.Y., Zaybak, A. (2008) Does the body temperature change in older people? *Journal of Clinical Nursing.* 17 (17): 2284–2287.

Gunning, K. (2009) Hepatic failure. *Anaesthesia and Intensive Care Medicine.* 10 (3): 124–126.

Gupta, R.K., Nikkar-Esfahani, A., Jamjoom, D.Z.A. (2010) Spontaneous intracerebral haemorrhage: a clinical review. *British Journal of Hospital Medicine.* 71 (9): 499–506.

Hackett, M.L., Köhler, S., O'Brien, J.T., Mead, G.E. (2014) Neuropsychiatric outcomes of stroke. *The Lancet Neurology.* 13 (5): 525–534.

Haddad, S.H., Arabi, Y.M. (2012) Critical care management of severe traumatic brain injury in adults. *Scandinavian Journal of Trauma, Resuscitation and Emergency Medicine.* 20:12. www.sjtrem.com/content/20/1/12 (last accessed 22 July 2014).

Haddadin, A.S., Fappiano, S.A., Lipsett, P.A. (2002) Meticillin resistant *Staphylococcus aureus* (*MRSa*) in the intensive care unit. *Postgraduate Medical Journal.* 78 (921): 385–392.

Hadingham, J. (1997) Talking about tissue donation. *Professional Nurse.* 12 (7): 473.

Haines, L., Wan, K.C., Lynn, R., Barrett, T.G., Shield, J.P.H. (2007) Rising incidence of type 2 diabetes in children in the UK. *Diabetes Care.* 30 (5): 1097–1011.

Hairon, N. (2008) Action to prevent the spread of norovirus infection. *Nursing Times.* 104 (2): 27–28.

Hale, A.S., Moseley, M.J., Warner, S.C. (2000). Treating pancreatitis in the acute care setting. *Dimensions of Critical Care Nursing.* 19 (4): 15–21.

Hall, A.P., Henry, J.A. (2006) Acute toxic effects of 'Ecstasy' (MDMA) and related compounds: overview of pathophysiology and clinical management. *British Journal of Anaesthesia.* 96 (6): 678–685.

Hall, B., Hall, D.A. (1994) Learning from the experience of loss: people bereaved during intensive care. *Intensive and Critical Care Nursing.* 10 (4): 265–1709.

Hall, J., Horsley, M. (2007) Diagnosis and management of patients with *Clostridium-difficile*-associated diarrhoea. *Nursing Standard.* 21 (46): 49–56.

Hall, J.E. (2011) *Guyton and Hall. Textbook of Medical Physiology.* 12th edn. Philadelphia, PA. Saunders Elsevier.

Hampton, J.R. (2013a) *The ECG Made Easy.* 8th edn. Edinburgh. Churchill Livingstone Elsevier.

Hampton, J.R. (2013b) *150 ECG Problems.* 4th edn. Edinburgh. Churchill Livingstone Elsevier.

Hans-Geurts, I.J.M., Hop, W.C.J., Kok, N.F.M., Lim, A., Brouwer, K.J., Jeekel, J. (2007) Randomized clinical trial of the impact of early enteral feeding on postoperative ileus and recovery. *British Journal of Surgery.* 94 (5): 555–561.

Hare, M., McGowan, S., Wynaden, D., Speed, G., Landsborough, I. (2008) Nurses' descriptions of changes in cognitive function in the acute care setting. *Australian Journal of Advanced Nursing.* 26 (1), 21–25.

Hartog, C.S., Rothaug, J., Goettermann, A., Zimmer, A., Meissner, W. (2010) Room for improvement: nurses' and physicians' views of a post-operative pain management program. *Acta Anaesthesiologica Scandinavica.* 54 (5): 277–283.

Hartog, C.S., Bauer, M., Reinhart, K. (2011) The efficacy and safety of colloid resuscitation in the critically ill. *Anesthesia & Analgesia.* 112 (1):156–164.

Harvey, L. 2008. *Management of Spinal Cord Injuries.* Edinburgh. Churchill Livingstone.

Havelock, T., Teoh, R., Laws, D., Gleeson, F., BTS Pleural Disease Guideline Group. (2010) Pleural procedures and thoracic ultrasound: British Thoracic Society pleural disease guideline 2010. *Thorax.* 65 (Supplement 2): ii61-ii76.

Hayden, P., Wyncoll, D. (2008) Severe acute pancreatitis. *Current Anaesthesia & Critical Care.* 19 (1) 1–7.

Hayes, C., Browne, S., Lantry, G., Burstal, R. (2002) Neuropathic pain in the acute pain service: a prospective survey. *Acute Pain.* 4 (2): 45–48.

HCPC (2012) *Standards of Conduct, Performance and Ethics.* London. Health & Care Professions Council.

Health Improvement Scotland. (2014) *Food, Fluid and Nutritional Care.* Edinburgh. Health Improvement Scotland.

Heart Protection Study Collaborative Group. (2012) Effects on 11-year mortality and morbidity of lowering LDL cholesterol with simvastatin for about 5 years in 20536 high-risk individuals: a randomised controlled trial. *The Lancet.* 378 (9808): 2013–2020.

Hebert, P.C., Wells, G., Blajchman, M.A., Marshall, J., Martin, C., Pagliarello, G., Tweeddale, M., Schweitzer, I., Yetisir, E., Transfusion Requirements Investigators for the Canadian

Critical Care Trials Group. (1999) A multicenter randomized, controlled clinical trial of transfusion requirements in critical care. *New England Journal of Medicine.* 340 (6): 409–417.

Heidbuchel, H., Verhamme, P., Alings, M., Antz, M., Hacke, W., Oldgren, J., Sinnaeve, P., Camm, A.J., Kirchhof, P. (2013) European Heart Rhythm Association practical guide on the use of new oral anticoagulants in patients with non-valvular atrial fibrillation. *Europace.* 15 (5): 625–651.

Henderson, V. (1960) *Basic Principles of Nursing Care.* Geneva. International Council of Nurses.

Hennessey, I.A.M., Japp, A.G. (2007) *Arterial Blood Gases Made Easy.* Edinburgh. Churchill Livingstone.

Henricson, M., Berglund, A.-L., Määttä, S., Ekman, R., Segesten, K. (2008) The outcome of tactile touch on oxytocin in intensive care patients: a randomised controlled trial. *Journal of Clinical Nursing.* 17 (19): 2624–2633.

Hernandez, A.F., Hammill, B.G., O'Connor, C.M., Schulman, K.A., Curtis, L.H., Fonarow, G.C. (2009) Clinical effectiveness of beta-blockers in heart failure. *Journal of the American College of Cardiology.* 53 (2): 184–192.

Herrod, P.J.J., Awad, S., Redfern, A., Morgan, L., Lobo, N.H. (2010) Hypo- and hypernatraemia in surgical patients: is there room for improvement? *World Journal of Surgery.* 34 (3): 495–499.

Hex, N., Bartlett, C., Wright, D., Taylor, M., Varley, D. (2012) Estimating the current and future costs of Type 1 and Type 2 diabetes in the UK, including direct health costs. *Diabetic Medicine.* 29 (7): 855–862.

Hickey, J.V. (ed). (2014) *Neurological and Neurosurgical Nursing.* 7th edn. Philadelphia, PA. Wolters Kluwer Lippincott Williams & Wilkins.

Hickey, J.C., Kanusky, J.T. (2014) Overview of neuroanatomy and neurophysiology. In Hickey, J.V. (ed). *Neurological and Neurosurgical Nursing.* 7th edn. Philadelphia, PA. Wolters Kluwer Lippincott Williams & Wilkins. 48–93.

Higgins, C. (2008) Low platelet count and spontaneous bleeding. *The Biomedical Scientist.* 65 (4): 673–675.

Higgins, C. (2013) *Understanding Laboratory Investigations.* 3rd edn. Oxford. Wiley-Blackwell.

Hilmer, S., Gnjidic, D. (2013) Statins in older adults. *Australian Prescriber.* 36 (3): 79–82.

Hinds, C.J., Watson, D. (2008) *Intensive Care: a concise textbook.* 3rd edn. Edinburgh. Saunders Elsevier.

Hinkelbein, J., Genzwuerker, H.V. (2008) Fingernail polish does not influence pulse oximetry to a clinically relevant dimension. *Intensive & Critical Care Nursing.* 24 (1): 4–5.

Hoffman, J.J., Hausman, K.A. (2013) Spinal cord injury. In Morton, P.G., Fontaine, D.K.(eds). *Critical Care Nursing: a holistic approach.* 10th edn. Philadelphia, PA. Lippincott Williams & Wilkins. 824–850.

Holyday, M., Daniells, S., Bare, M., Caplan, G.A., Petocz, T., Bolin, P. (2012) Malnutrition screening and early nutrition intervention in hospitalised patients in acute aged care: a randomised controlled trial. *The Journal of Nutrition Health & Aging.* 16 (6): 562–568.

Horeczko, T., Green, J.P., Panacek, E.A. (2014). Epidemiology of the systemic inflammatory response syndrome (SIRS) in the emergency department. *Western Journal of Emergency Medicine.* 15 (3): 329–336.

Hou, W., Sanyal, A.J. (2009) Ascites: diagnosis and management. *Medical Clinics of North America.* 93 (4): 801–807.

Hough, A. (2001) *Physiotherapy in Respiratory Care.* 3rd edn. Cheltenham. Nelson Thornes.

Houghton, A.R., Gray, D. (2014) *Making Sense of the ECG*. 4th edn. London. Hodder Education.

Howard, L.S. (2009) Oxygen therapy. *Clinical Medicine*. 9 (2): 156–159.

Hughes, E. (2004) Understanding the care of patients with acute pancreatitis. *Nursing Standard*. 18 (18): 45–52.

Hussein, H.K., Lewington, A.J.P., Kanagasundaram, S. (2009) General management of acute kidney injury. *British Journal of Hospital Medicine*. 70 (7): M104-M107.

Hyers, T.M. (2003) Management of venous thromboembolism. *Archives of Internal Medicine*. 163 (7): 759–768.

ICS (2002) *Levels of Critical Care for Adult Patients*. London. Intensive Care Society.

ICS (2007) *Investigation of Suspected Infection in Critically Ill Patients*. London. Intensive Care Society.

ICS (2009) *Levels of Critical Care for Adult Patients*. London. Intensive Care Society.

ICS (2014) *Standards for the Care of Adult Patients with a Temporary Tracheostomy*. London. Intensive Care Society.

International Association for the Study of Pain. (1986) *Classification of Chronic Pain*. 2nd edn. Seattle. International Association for the Study of Pain.

Isaac, R., Taylor, B.L. (2003) Fever in ICU patients. *Anaesthesia and Intensive Care*. 4 (5): 153–155.

IST-3 Collaborative Group. (2012) The benefits and harms of intravenous thrombolysis with recombinant tissue plasminogen activator within 6h of acute ischaemic stroke (the third international stroke trial [IST-3]): a randomised controlled trial. *The Lancet*. 379 (9834): 2352–2363.

Jackson, T., Hallam, C., Corner, T., Hill, S. (2013) Right line, right patient, right time: every choice matters. *British Journal of Nursing*. 22 (supplement 5).

Jackson, I. (1996) Critical care nurses' perception of a bereavement follow-up service. *Intensive and Critical Care Nursing*. 12 (1): 2–11.

Jackson, I. (1998) A study of bereavement in an intensive care unit. *Nursing in Critical Care*. 3 (3): 141–150.

Jacques, T., Harrison, G.A., McLaws, M.-L., Kilborn, G. (2006) Signs of critical conditions and emergency responses (SOCCER): a model for predicting adverse events in the inpatient setting. *Resuscitation*. 69: 175–183.

Jain, S., Bellingan, G. (2007) Basic science of acute lung injury. *Surgery*. 25 (3): 112–116.

Jarvis, H. (2006) Exploring the evidence base of the use of non-invasive ventilation. *British Journal of Nursing*. 15 (14): 756–759.

JBDS (2010) *Guidance on Management of Hyperosmolar Hyperglcaemic State (HHS) in Adults*. London. Joint British Diabetes Societies.

JBDS (2013) *The Management of Diabetic Ketoacidosis in Adults*. 2nd edn. London. Joint British Diabetes Societies.

Jensen, L.O., Thayssen, P., Pedersen, K.E., Stender, S., Torben, H. (2004) Regression of coronary atherosclerosis by Simvastatin. *Circulation*. 110 (3): 265–270.

Jevon, P. (2007) Respiratory procedures part 1 – use of a non-rebreathe oxygen mask. *Nursing Times*. 103 (32): 26–27.

Jevon, P. (2009) *Clinical Examination Skills*. Chichester. Wiley-Blackwell.

Jevon, P., Ewens, B. (2012) *Monitoring the Critically Ill Patient*. 3rd edn. Chichester. Blackwell Publishing Ltd.

Joffe, A.M., Hallman, M., Gélinas, C., Herr, D.L., Puntillo, K. (2013) Evaluation and treatment of pain in critically ill adults. *Seminars in Respiratory and Critical Care Medicine*. 34 (2): 189–200.

Jolliet, P., Abajo, B., Pasquina, P., Chevrolet, J.-C. (2001) Non-invasive pressure support ventilation in severe community-acquired pneumonia. *Intensive Care Medicine.* 27 (5): 812–821.

Jones, S.K.B. (2011) *Chest Tube Dressings: A Comparison of Different Methods.* PhD Thesis. University of Oklahoma/Proquest. Ann Arbor, Michigan.

Jowett, N.I., Thompson, D.R. (2007) *Comprehensive Coronary Care.* 4th edn. London. Baillière Tindall.

Kalanuria, A., Nyquist, P., Ling, G. (2012) The prevention and regression of atherosclerotic plaques: emerging treatments. *Vascular Health and Risk Management.* 8: 549–561.

Kamel, H., Navi, B.B., Nakagawa, K., Hemphill, J.C. III, Ko, N.U. (2011) Hypertonic saline versus mannitol for the treatment of elevated intracranial pressure: A meta-analysis of randomized clinical trials. *Critical Care Medicine.* 39 (3): 554–559.

KDIGO (2012) Clinical Practice Guideline for Acute Kidney Injury. *Kidney International.* 2 (Supplement 1): 1–138.

Keays, R. (2014) Diabetic emergencies. In Bersten, A.D., Soni, N. (eds) *Intensive Care Manual.* 7th edn. Edinburgh. Butterworth-Heinemann. 629–636.

Kee, J.L. (2009) *Handbook of Laboratory & Diagnostic Tests.* New Jersey. Prentice Hall Health.

Keeling, D., Baglin, T., Tait, C., Watson, H., Perry, D., Baglin, C., Kitchen, S., Makris, S., British Committee for Standards in Haematology (2011) Guidelines on oral anticoagulation with warfarin – fourth edn. *British Journal of Haematology.* 154 (3): 311–324.

Kelly, C.P., LaMont, J.T. (2008) *Clostridium difficile* – more difficult than ever. *New England Journal of Medicine.* 359 (18): 1932–1940.

Kemper, M.J., Harps, E., Muller-Wiefel, D.E. (1996) Hyperkalaemia: therapeutic options in acute and chronic renal failure. *Clinical Nephrology.* 46 (1): 67–69.

Kent, H., McDowell, J. (2004) Sudden bereavement in acute care settings. *Nursing Standard.* 19 (6): 38–42.

Kesieme, E.B., Dongo, A., Ezemba, N., Irekpita, E., Jebbin, N., Kesieme, C. (2012) Tube thoracostomy: complications and its management. *Pulmonary Medicine.* Article ID 256878.

Kim, S.M., Han, H.-R. (2013) Evidence-based strategies to reduce readmission in patients with heart failure. *Journal for Nurse Practitioners.* 9 (4): 224–232.

Kingsnorth, A., O'Reilly, D. (2006) Acute pancreatitis. *British Medical Journal.* 332 (7549): 1072–1076.

Kitwood, T. (1997) *Dementia Reconsidered.* Buckingham. Open University Press.

Klein, A.M., Howell, K., Vogler, J., Grill, E., Straube, A., Bender, A. (2013) Rehabilitation outcome of unconscious traumatic brain injury patients. *Journal of Neurotrauma.* 30 (17): 1476–1483.

Knight, A.R., Fry, L.E., Clancy, R.L., Pierce, J.D. (2011) Understanding the effects of oxygen administration in haemorrhagic shock. *Nursing in Critical* Care.16 (1): 28–33.

Kolmodin, L., Sekhon, M.S., Henderson, W.R., Turgeon, A.F., Griesdale, D.E.G. (2013) Hypernatremia in patients with severe traumatic brain injury: a systematic review. *Annals of Intensive Care.* 3: 35.

Kramer, C.K., Zinman, B., Retnakaran, R. (2013) Are metabolically healthy overweight and obesity benign conditions?: a systematic review and meta-analysis. *Annals of Internal Medicine.* 159 (11): 758–769.

Krinsley, J.S., Keegan, M.T. (2010) Hypoglycemia in the critically ill: how low is too low? *Mayo Clinic Proceedings.* 85 (3): 217–224.

Krum, H., Abraham, W.T. (2009) Heart failure. *The Lancet.* 373 (9667): 941–955.

Kubler-Ross, E. (1970) *On Death and Dying.* London. Routledge.

Kubler-Ross, E. (1991) *On Life after Death.* California. Celestial Arts.

Kuffler, D.P. (2012) Maximizing neuroprotection: where do we stand? *Therapeutics and Clinical Risk Management.* 8 (1): 185–194.

Kyriacou, C. (2012) Identifying Takotsubo Cardiomyopathy. *e-journal of the ESC Council for Cardiology Practice.* Volume 10.

LaBrecque, D.R., Abbas, Z., Anania, F., Ferenci, P., Khan, A.G., Goh, K.-L., Hamid, S.S., Isakov, V., Lizarzabal, M., Peñaranda, M.M., Ramos, J.F.R., Sarin, S., Stimac, D., Thomson, A.B.R., Umar, M., Krabshuis, J., LeMair, A. (2014) World gastroenterology organisation global guidelines nonalcoholic fatty liver disease and nonalcoholic steatohepatitis. *Journal of Clinical Gastroenterology.* 48 (6): 467–473.

Lackland, D.T., Roccella, E.J., Deutsch, A.F., Fornage, M., George, M.G., Howard, G., Kissela, B.M., Kittner, S.J., Lichtman, J.H., Lisabeth, L.D., Schwamm, L.H., Smith, E.E., Towfighi, A. (2013) Factors influencing the decline in stroke mortality. A statement from the American Heart Association/American Stroke Association. *Stroke.* 45 (1): 315–353.

Lakasing, E., Francis, H. (2006) Diagnosis and management of heart failure. *Primary Health Care.* 16 (5): 36–39.

Lambert, P., Bingley, P.J. (2002) What is type 1 diabetes? *Medicine.* 30 (1): 1–5.

Landis, E.M. (1930) Micro-injection studies of capillary blood pressure in human skin. *Heart.* V15: 209–228.

Langhorne, P., Bernhardt, J., Kwakkel, G. (2011) Stroke rehabilitation. *The Lancet.* 377 (9778): 1693–1702.

Larson, E.L., Cohen, B., Ross, B., Behta, M. (2010) Isolation precautions for methicillin-resistant staphylococcus aureus: electronic surveillance to monitor adherence. *American Journal of Critical Care.* 19 (1): 16–26.

Law, M.R., Morris, J.K., Wald, N.J. (2009) Use of blood pressure lowering drugs in the prevention of cardiovascular disease: meta-analysis of 147 randomised trials in the context of expectations from prospective epidemiological studies. *British Medical Journal.* 338 (7705): 1245–1253.

Leach, R. (2010) Fluid management on hospital medical wards. *Clinical Medicine.* 10 (6): 611–615.

Leach, R.M., Brotherton, A., Stroud, M. (2013) Nutrition and fluid balance must be taken seriously. *British Medical Journal.* 346 (7895): 22–24.

Leadership Alliance for the Care of Dying People. (2014) *One Chance to Get It Right.* London. NHS England.

Lebeaux, D., Fernández-Hidalgo, N., Chauhan, A., Lee, S., Ghigo, J.-M., Almirante, B., Beloin, C. (2014) Management of infections related to totally implantable venous-access ports: challenges and perspectives. *The Lancet Infectious Diseases.* 14 (2): 146–159.

Lee, J.-H., Bahk, J.-H., Jung, C.-W., Jeon, Y. (2009) Comparison of the bedside central venous catheter placement techniques: landmark vs electrocardiogram guidance. *British Journal of Anaesthesia.* 102 (5): 662–666.

Lefor, A.T. (2002) *Critical Care on Call.* New York. Lange/McGraw-Hill. 238–240.

Lewis, T., Oliver, G. (2005) Improving tracheostomy care for ward patients. *Nursing Standard.* 19 (19): 33–37.

Lichtman, J.H., Froelicher, E.S., Blumenthal, J.A., Carney, R.M., Doering, L.V., Frasure-Smith., N., Freedland, K.E., Jaffe, A.S., Leifheit-Limson, E.C., Sheps, D.S., Vaccarino, V., Wulsin, L., the American Heart Association Statistics Committee of the Council on Epidemiology and Prevention and the Council on Cardiovascular and Stroke Nursing. (2014) Depression as a risk factor for poor prognosis among patients with acute coronary syndrome: systematic review and recommendations a scientific statement from the American Heart Association. *Circulation.* 129 (12): 1350–1369.

Light, R.W., Lee, Y.C.G. (2010) Pneumothorax, chylothorax, hemothorax and fibrothorax. In Mason, R.J., Broaddus, V.C., Martin, T.R., King, E.T. Jr., Schraufnagel, D.E., Murray, J.F., Nadel, J.A. (eds) *Murray & Nadel's Textbook of Respiratory Diseases.* 5th edn. Philadelphia, PA. Saunders Elsevier. 1764–1791.

Light, R.W. (2011) Pleural controversy: optimal chest tube size for drainage. *Respirology.* 16 (2): 244–248.

Lim, S.-M., Webb, S.A. (2005) Nosocomial bacterial infections in Intensive Care Units. I: Organisms and mechanisms of antibiotic resistance. *Anaesthesia.* 60 (9): 887–902.

Lima, A., Bakker, J. (2005) Noninvasive monitoring of peripheral perfusion. *Intensive Care Medicine.* 31 (10): 1316–1326.

Lindermann, E. (1994) Symptomatology and management of acute grief. *American Journal of Psychiatry.* 151 (6): 155–160.

Ling, J.M., Klimaj, S., Toulouse, T., Mayer, A.R. (2013) A prospective study of gray matter injuries in mild traumatic brain injury. *Neurology.* 81 (24): 2121–2127.

Lip, G.Y.H., Beevers, D.G. (2007) Hypertension and vascular risk. In Beevers, D.G., Lip, G.Y.H., O'Brien, E. (eds). *ABC of Hypertension.* 5th edn. London. British Medical Journal Books. 7–11.

Lip, G.Y.H. (2003) *Clinical Hypertension in Practice.* RSM Press. London.

Lloyd, D.G., Ma, D., Vizcaychipi, M.P. (2012) Cognitive decline after anaesthesia and critical care. *Continuing Education in Anaesthesia, Critical Care & Pain.* 12 (3): 105–109.

Lloyd Jones, M. (2012) A brief history of the registration of nurses. *British Journal of Healthcare Assistants.* 6 (1): 41–44.

Lo, E., Nicolle, L.E., Coffin, S.E., Gould, C., Maragakis, L.L., Meddings, J., Pegues, D.A., Pettis, A.M., Saint, S., Yokoe, D.S. (2014) Strategies to prevent catheter-associated urinary tract infections in acute care hospitals. *Infection Control and Hospital Epidemiology.* 35 (5): 464–479.

Lobo, S.M.A., Lobo, F.R.M., Bota, D.P., Lopes-Ferreira, F., Soliman, H.M., Mélot, C., Vincent, J.L. (2003) C-reactive protein levels correlate with mortality and organ failure in critically ill patients. *Chest.* 123 (6): 2043–2049.

Lough, M.E. (2008) Cardiovascular assessment and diagnostic procedures. In Urden, L.D., Stacy, K.M., Lough, M.E. (eds). *Priorities in Critical Care Nursing.* 5th edn. St Louis. Mosby. 121–173.

Loveday, H.P., Wilson, J.A., Pratt, R.J., Golsorkhi, M., Tingle, A., Bak, A., Browne, J., Prieto, J., Wilcox, M. (2014) epic3: National Evidence-Based Guidelines for Preventing Healthcare-Associated Infections in NHS Hospitals in England. *Journal of Hospital Infection.* 86 (supplement 1): S1–S70.

Low, P.A. (2008) Prevalence of orthostatic hypotension. *Clinical Autonomic Research.* 18 (Supplement 1): 8–13.

Lowe, M.E., Sevilla, W.A. (2012) Nutritional advice for prevention of acute pancreatitis: review of current opinion. *Nutrition and Dietary Supplements.* 4: 71–81.

Lower, J. (2003) Using pain to assess neurologic response. *Nursing2003.* 33 (6): 56–57.

Lumb, A.B. (2010) *Nunn's Applied Respiratory Physiology.* 7th edn. Edinburgh. Churchill Livingstone Elsevier.

Maben, J. (2009) Splendid isolation? The pros and cons of single rooms for the NHS. *Nursing Management.* 16 (2): 18–19.

McCusker, J., Cole, M.G., Voyer, P., Monette, J., Champoux, H., Clampi, A., Vu, M., Belzile, E. (2011) Prevalence and incidence of delirium in long-term care. *International Journal of Geriatric Psychology.* 26 (11): 1152–1161.

McDonough, M. (2009) Managing atrial fibrillation. *Nursing2009.* 39 (11): 59–63.

MacDuff, A., Arnold, A., Harvey, J., BTS Pleural Disease Guideline Group. (2010) Management of spontaneous pneumothorax: British Thoracic Society pleural disease guideline 2010. *Thorax.* 65 (Supplement 2): ii18-ii31.

MacFie, J. (2013) Surgical sepsis. *British Journal of Surgery.* 100 (S6): S36–S39.

McHugh, M.D., Chenjuan, M. (2013) Hospital nursing and 30-day readmissions among Medicare patients with heart failure, acute myocardial infarction, and pneumonia. *Medical Care.* 51 (1): 52–59.

McHugh, M.D., Berez, J., Small, D.S. (2013) Hospitals with higher nurse staffing had lower odds of readmissions penalties than hospitals with lower staffing. *Health Affairs.* October.

Macintyre, P., Schug, S.S. (2007) *Acute Pain Management: A Practical Guide.* 3rd edn. Saunders Elsevier. Edinburgh.

Mackintosh, C. (2007) Assessment and management of patients with post-operative pain. *Nursing Standard.* 22 (5): 49–55.

McLellan, S.A., McClelland, D.B.L., Walsh, T.S. (2003) Anaemia and red blood cell transfusion in the critically ill patient. *Blood Reviews.* 17 (4): 195–208.

McLenachen, J.M., Machin, S., Marley, C. (2010) National roll-out of Primary PCI for patients with ST segment elevation myocardial infarction: an interim report. Leicester. Improvement NHS.

McMahon, S.B., Koltzenburg, M., Tracey, I., Turk, D.C. (eds) (2013) *Wall and Melzack's Textbook of Pain.* 6th edn. Elsevier Saunders. Philadelphia PA.

McMillan, A., Bratton, D.J., Faria, R., Laskawiec-Szkonter, M., Griffin, S., Davies, R.J., Nunn, A.J., Stradling, J.R., Riha, R.L., Morrell, M.J., PREDICT Investigators. (2014) Continuous positive airway pressure in older people with obstructive sleep apnoea syndrome (PREDICT): a 12-month, multicentre, randomised trial. *The Lancet.* 2 (10): 804 – 812.

McNicholas, M.J., Rowley, D.I., McGurty, D., Adalberth, T., Abdon, P., Lindstrand, A., Lohmander, L.S. (2000) Total meniscectomy in adolescence: a thirty-year follow-up. *Journal of Bone and Joint Surgery.* 82-B (2): 217–221.

McQuay, H., Moore, A. (1998) *An Evidence-Based Resource for Pain Relief.* Oxford. Oxford Medical.

McQuillan, P., Pilkington, S., Allan, A., Taylor, B., Short, A., Morgan, G., Nielsen, M., Barrett, D., Smith, G. (1998) Confidential inquiry into quality of care before admission to intensive care. *British Medical Journal.* 316 (7148): 1853–1858.

Maczulak, A. (2010) *Allies and Enemies: How the World Depends on Bacteria.* Upper Saddle River, New Jersey. FT Press. Pearson Education Ltd.

MAG. (2003) *Malnutrition Universal Screening Tool.* Worcestershire. Malnutrition Advisory Group, BAPEN.

Maggiore, S.M., Idone, F.A., Vaschetto, R., Festa, R., Cataldo, A., Antonicelli, F., Montini, L., De Gaetano, A., Navalesi, R., Antonelli, M. (2014) Nasal High-Flow versus Venturi mask oxygen therapy after extubation. Effects on oxygenation, comfort, and clinical outcome. *American Journal of Respiratory Critical Care Medicine.* 190 (3): 282–288.

Magraph, H.P., Boulstridge, L.J. (2005) Tissue donation after death in the accident and emergency department: an opportunity wasted? *Journal of Accident and Emergency Medicine.* 16 (2): 117–119.

Maitland, K., Kiguli, S., Opoka, R.O., Engoru, C., Olupot-Olupot, P., Akech, S.O., Nyeko, R., Mtove, G., Reyburn, H., Lang, T., Brent, B., Evans, J.A., Tibenderana, J.K., Crawley, J., Russell, E.C., Levin, M., Babiker, A.G., Gibb, D.M., FEAST Trial Group. (2011). Mortality after fluid bolus in African children with severe infection. *New England Journal of Medicine.* 364 (26): 2483–2495.

Mak, S., Newton, G.E. (2001) The oxidative stress hypothesis of congestive heart failure. *Chest.* 120 (6): 2035–2046.

Mäkitalo, O., Liikanen, E. (2013) Improving quality at the preanalytical phase of blood sampling: literature review. *International Journal of Biomedical Laboratory Science.* 2 (1): 7–16.

Malaise, O., Bruyere, O., Reginster, J.-Y. (2007) Intravenous paracetamol: a review of efficacy and safety in therapeutic use. *Future Neurology.* 2 (6): 673–688

Malangoni, M.A., Martin, A.S. (2005) Outcome of severe acute pancreatitis. *American Journal of Surgery.* 189 (3): 273–77.

Malbrain., M.L.N.G. Chiumello, D., Pelosi, P., Bihari, D., Innes, R., Ranieri, V.M., del Turco, M., Wilmer, A., Brienza, N., Malcangi, V., Cohen, J., Japiassu, A., de Keulenaer, B.L., Daelemans, R., Jacquet, L., Laterre, P.-F., Frank, G., de Souza, P., Cesana, B., Gattinoni, L. (2005) Incidence and prognosis of intraabdominal hypertension in a mixed population of critically ill patients: a multiple-center epidemiological study. *Critical Care Medicine.* 33 (2): 315–332.

Malone, A. (2013) Addressing hospital malnutrition – the time is now! *Journal of Parenteral & Enteral Nutrition.* 37 (4): 439–440.

Manning, L., Hirakawa, Y., Arima, H., Wang, X., Chalmers, J., Wang, J., Lindley, R., Heeley, E., Delcourt, C., Neal, B., Lavados, P., Davis, S.M., Tzourio, C., Huang, Y., Stapf, C., Woodward, M., Rothwell, P.M., Robinson, T.G., Anderson, C.S., for the INTERACT2 investigators. (2014) Blood pressure variability and outcome after acute intracerebral haemorrhage: a post-hoc analysis of INTERACT2, a randomised controlled trial. *The Lancet.* 13 (4): 364–373.

March, K.S., Hickey, J.V. (2014a) Intracranial hypertension: theory and management of increased intracranial pressure. In Hickey, J.V. (ed). *Neurological and Neurosurgical Nursing.* 7th edn. Philadelphia, PA. Wolters Kluwer Lippincott Williams & Wilkins. 266–299.

March, K.S., Hickey, J.V. (2014b) Craniocerebral injuries. In Hickey, J.V. (ed). *Neurological and Neurosurgical Nursing.* 7th edn. Philadelphia, PA. Wolters Kluwer Lippincott Williams & Wilkins. 343–381.

Marieb, E.N., Hoehn, K. (2013) *Human Anatomy and Physiology.* 9th edn. Boston. Pearson.

Marik, P.E. (2000) Fever in the ICU. *Chest.* 117 (3): 859–869.

Marik, P.E., Lemson, J. (2014) Fluid responsiveness: an evolution of our understanding. *British Journal of Anaesthesia.* 112 (4): 617–620.

Marques, P., Sousa, P., Silva, A. (2014) Acute confusion and advanced nursing practice. *American Journal of Nursing Research.* 2 (2): 17–19.

Marret, E., Remy, C., Bonnet, F., Postoperative Pain Forum Group. (2007) Meta-analysis of epidural analgesia versus parenteral opioid analgesia after colorectal surgery. *British Journal of Surgery.* 94 (6): 665–673.

Martinez, F.J., Donohue, J.F., Rennard, S.I. (2011) The future of chronic obstructive pulmonary disease treatment – difficulties of and barriers to drug development. *The Lancet.* 378 (9795): 1027–1037.

Martinson, B.C., O'Connor, P.J., Pronk, N.P. (2001) Physical inactivity and short-term all-cause mortality in adults with chronic disease. *Archives of Internal Medicine.* 161 (9): 1173–1180.

Mascini, E.M., Bonten, M.J.M. (2005) Vancomycin-resistant *enterococci*: consequences for therapy and infection control. *Clinical Microbiology and Infection.* 11 (supplement 4), 43–56.

Massey, D., Aitken, L.M., Chaboyer, W. (2010) Literature review: do rapid response systems reduce the incidence of major adverse events in the deteriorating ward patient? *Journal of Clinical Nursing.* 19 (23–24): 3260–3273.

Maund, E., McDaid, C., Rice, S., Wright, K., Jenkins, B., Woolacott, N. (2011) Paracetamol and selective and non-selective non-steroidal anti-inflammatory drugs for the reduction in morphine-related side-effects after major surgery. *British Journal of Anaesthesia.* 106 (3): 292–297.

May, K. (2009) The pathophysiology and causes of raised intracranial pressure. *British Journal of Nursing.* 18 (15): 911–914.

Medford, A., Maskell, N. (2005) Pleural effusion. *Postgraduate Medical Journal.* 81 (961): 702–710.

Mehanna, H.M., Moledina, J., Travis, J. (2008) Refeeding syndrome: what it is, and how to prevent and treat it. *British Medical Journal.* 336 (7659): 1495–1498.

Mehta, P.A., Cowie, M.R. (2006) Epidemiology and pathophysiology of heart failure. *Medicine.* 34 (6): 210–214.

Mehta, R.L., Paascual, M.T., Soroko S, Chertow GM, PICARD Study Group. (2002) Diuretics, mortality, and nonrecovery of renal function in acute renal failure. *Journal of the American Medical Association.* 188 (19): 2547–2553.

Meier, R., Ockenga, J., Pertkiewicz, M., Pap, A., Milinic, N., MacFie, J., Löser, C., Keim, V. (2006) ESPEN guidelines on enteral nutrition: pancreas. *Clinical Nutrition.* 25 (2): 275–284.

Melzack, R., Wall, P. (1988) *The Challenge of Pain.* 2nd edn. London. Penguin.

Messer, P.B., Sweenie, A.C., Whittle, R.J., McEleavy, I.M. (2012) The effect of repeated audit on the quality of transfer of brain-injured patients into a regional neurosciences centre. *Journal of the Intensive Care Society.* 13 (1): 39–42.

Meyer, G., Roy, P.-M. Gilberg, S., Perrier, A. (2010) Pulmonary embolism. *British Medical Journal.* 340 (7753): 974–976.

MHRA. (2009) *One Liners 67.* Medicines and Healthcare Products Regulatory Agency. London.

Mickiewicz, P., Binkowski, M., Bursig, H., Wróbel, Z. (2013) Preservation and sterilization methods of the meniscal allografts: literature review. *Cell and Tissue Banking.* 15 (3): 307–317.

Mills, N., Scullion, P., Gopee, N. (2001) Understanding nursing roles to facilitate collaboration. *British Journal of Therapy and Rehabilitation.* 8 (1): 6–11.

Mishriky, B.M., Waldron, N.H., Habib, A.S. (2015) Impact of pregabalin on acute and persistent postoperative pain: a systematic review and meta-analysis. *British Journal of Anaesthesia.* 114 (1): 10–31.

Mitchell, R.M.S., Byrne, M.F., Baillie, J. (2003) Pancreatitis. *The Lancet.* 361 (9367): 1447–1455.

Molyneux, A.J., Birks, J., Clarke, A., Sneade, M., Kerr, F.S.C. (2014) The durability of endo-vascular coiling versus neurosurgical clipping of ruptured cerebral aneurysms: 18 year follow-up of the UK cohort of the International Subarachnoid Aneurysm Trial (ISAT). *The Lancet,* Early Online Publication, 28 October 2014 DOI:10.1016/S0140–6736(14)60975–2.

Montague, B.T., Ouellette, J.R., Buller, G.K. (2008) Retrospective review of the frequency of ECG changes in hyperkalemia. *Clinical Journal of the American Society of Nephrolology.* 3 (2): 324–330.

Montejo, J.C., Miñambres., E., Bordejé, L., Masejo, A., Acosta, J., Heras, A., Ferré, M., Fernandez-Ortega, F., Vasquizo, C.I., Manzanedo, R. (2009) Gastric residual volume during enteral nutrition in ICU patients: the REGANE study. *Intensive Care Medicine.* 36 (8): 1386–1393.

Moody, W.E., Edwards, N.C., Chue, C.D., Ferro, C.F., Townend, J.N. (2013) Arterial disease in chronic kidney disease. *Heart.* 99 (6): 365- 372.

Mooney, M. (2007) Professional socialisation: the key to survival as a newly qualified nurse. *International Journal of Nursing Practice.* 13 (2): 75–80.

Moore, A. (2009) Minimising pain during intravenous cannulation. *British Medical Journal.* 338: a2993.

Moore, C., Dobson, A., Kinago, M., Dillon, B. (2008) Comparison of blood pressure measure at the arm, ankle and calf. *Anaesthesia.* 63 (12): 1327–1331.

Morley, R. (2002) Respiratory physiotherapy. *Nursing Times.* 98 (12): 58–60.

Morris, W. (2011) Complications. In Philips, S., Collins, M., Dougherty, L.(eds). *Venepuncture and Cannulation.* Oxford. Wiley Blackwell. 175–222.

Morton, P.G., Rempher, K.J. (2013) Patient management: respiratory system. In Morton, P.G., Fontaine, D.K.(eds). *Critical Care Nursing: a holistic approach.* 10th edn. Philadelphia, PA. Lippincott Williams & Wilkins. 485–505.

Mourvillier, B., Tubach, F., van de Beek, D., Garot, D., Pichon, N., Georges, H., Lefevre, L.M., Bollaert, P.-E., Boulain, T., Luis, D., Cariou, A., Girardie, P., Chelha, R., Megarbane, B., Delahaye, A., Chalumeau-Lemoine, L., Legriel, S., Beuret, P., Brivet, F., Bruel, C., Camou, F., Chatellier, D., Chillet, P., Clair, B., Constantin, J-M., Duguet, A., Galliot, R., Bayle, F., Hyvernat, H., Ouchenir, K., Plantefeve, G., Quenot, J.-P., Richecoeur, J., Schwebel, C., Sirodot, M., Esposito-Farèse, M., Le Tulzo, Y., Wolff, M. (2013) Induced hypothermia in severe bacterial meningitis. *Journal of the American Medical Association.* 310 (20): 2174–2183.

Mukhopadhyay, D., Mohanaruban, K. (2002) Iron deficiency anaemia in older people: investigation, management and treatment. *Age and Ageing.* 31 (2): 87–91.

Munoz-Price, L.S., Weinstein, R.A. (2008) Acinetobacter infection. *New England Journal of Medicine.* 358 (12): 1271–1281.

Murdoch, J., Larsen, D. (2004) Assessing pain in cognitively impaired older adults. *Nursing Standard.* 18 (38): 33–39.

Murphy, T., Robinson, S. (2006) Renal failure and its treatment. *Anaesthesia and Intensive Care Medicine.* 7 (7): 247–252.

Musters, C. (2010) Managing patients without their consent: a guide to recent legislation. *British Journal of Hospital Medicine.* 71 (2): 87–90.

Nag, S., Kapadia, A., Stewart, D.J. (2011) Review: Molecular pathogenesis of blood–brain barrier breakdown in acute brain injury. *Neuropathology and Applied Neurobiology.* 37 (1) 3–23.

Nash, K.L., Bentley, I., Hirschfield, G.M. (2009) Managing hepatitis C virus infection. *British Medical Journal.* 339 (7711): 37–42.

Nathens, A.B., Curtis, J.R., Beale, R.J., Cook, D.J., Moreno, R.P., Romand, J.-A., Skerrett, S.J., Stapleton, R.D., Ware, L.B., Waldmann, C.S. (2004). Management of the critically ill patient with severe acute pancreatitis. *Critical Care Medicine.* 32 (12): 2524–2536.

National Collaborating Centre for Women's and Children's Health. (2013) *Feverish illness in children: Assessment and initial management in children younger than 5 years.* 2nd edn. London. Royal College of Obstetricians and Gynaecologists.

Nava, S., Hill, N. (2009) Non-invasive ventilation in acute respiratory failure. *The Lancet.* 374 (9685): 250–259.

Nava, S., Grassi, M., Fanfulla, M., Domenighetti, G., Carlucci, A., Perren, A., Dell'orso, D., Vitacca, M., Ceriana, P., Karakurt, Z., Clini, E. (2011) Non-invasive ventilation in elderly patients with acute hypercapnic respiratory failure: a randomised controlled trial. *Age and Ageing.* 40 (4): 444–450.

Nazarko, L. (2009) Urinary tract infection: diagnosis, treatment and prevention. *British Journal of Nursing.* 18 (19): 1170–1174.

NCEPOD. (2008) *A Sickle Crisis?* London. National Confidential Enquiry into Patient Outcome and Death.

NCEPOD. (2009a) *Caring to the End?* London. National Confidential Enquiry into Patient Outcome and Death.

NCEPOD. (2009b) *Adding Insult to Injury.* London. National Confidential Enquiry into Patient Outcome and Death.

NCEPOD. (2010) *A Mixed Bag.* London. National Confidential Enquiry into Patient Outcomes and Death.

NCEPOD. (2013) *Managing the flow? A review of the care received by patients who were diagnosed with an aneurysmal subarachnoid haemorrhage.* London. National Confidential Enquiry into Patient Outcome and Death.

NCEPOD. (2014) "On the Right Trach?" London. National Confidential Enquiry into Patient Outcome and Death.

Needleman, J. (2013) Increasing acuity, increasing technology, and the changing demands on nurses. *Nursing Economics.* 31 (4): 200–202.

Needleman, J., Buerhaus, P., Pankratz, S., Leibson, C.L., Stevens, S.R., Harris, M. (2011) Nurse staffing and inpatient hospital mortality. *New England Journal of Medicine.* 364 (11): 1037–1045.

Nelson, R.A., Yu, H., Ziegler, M.G., Mills, P.J., Clausen, J.L., Dinsdale, J.E. (2001) Continuous positive airway pressure normalizes cardiac autonomic and hemodynamic responses to a laboratory stressor in apneic patients. *Chest.* 119 (4): 1092–1101.

Neubauer, S. (2007) The failing heart – an engine out of fuel. *New England Journal of Medicine.* 356 (11): 1140–1151.

Nguyen, N.Q., Chapman, M.J., Fraser, R.J., Bryant, L.K., Holloway, R.H. (2007) Erythromycin is more effective than metoclopramide in the treatment of feed intolerance in critical illness. *Critical Care Medicine.* 35 (2): 483–489.

NHS Choices. (2013) at www.nhs/uk/Conditions/Cholesterol/Pages/Diagnosis.aspx (last accessed 19 April 2015).

NHS England. (2013) *Placement devices for nasogastric tube insertion DO NOT replace initial position checks.* www.england.nhs.uk/patientsafety Publications Gateway Reference 00876. (last accessed 19 April 2015).

NHS England. (2014) Safer Staffing: *A Guide to Care Contact Time.* Leeds. NHS England. Available at: /www.england.nhs.uk/wp-content/uploads/2014/11/safer-staffing-guide-care-contact-time.pdf (last accessed 19 April 2015).

NHS Quality Improvement Scotland. (2007) *Caring for the Patient with a Tracheostomy.* NHS Quality Improvement Scotland. Edinburgh.

NHSLA. (2012) *Report and Accounts for 2011–2012.* Norwich. The Stationery Office.

NICE. (2006) *Nutrition Support in Adults.* London. National Institute for Clinical Excellence.

NICE. (2007) *Clinical Guideline 50. Acutely Ill Patients in Hospital: Recognition of and Response to Acute Illness in Adults in Hospital.* London. National Institute for Clinical Excellence.

NICE. (2010a) *Chronic Obstructive Pulmonary Disease. Management of Chronic Obstructive Pulmonary Disease in Adults in Primary and Secondary Care (Partial Update). Clinical Guideline 101.* London. National Institute for Clinical Evidence.

NICE. (2010b) *Chronic Heart Failure: Management of Chronic Heart Failure in Adults in Primary and Secondary Care. Clinical Guideline 108.* London. National Institute for Clinical Excellence.

NICE. (2010c) *Chest Pain of Recent Onset. Clinical Guideline 95.* National Institute for Clinical Excellence. London.

NICE. (2010d) *Delirium. Diagnosis, Prevention and Management. NICE clinical guideline 103.* London. National Institute for Clinical Excellence.

NICE. (2011a) *Hypertension. Clinical Guideline 127.* London. National Institute for Clinical Excellence.

NICE. (2011b) *Therapeutic hypothermia following cardiac arrest.* Interventional procedure guidance 386. London. National Institute for Clinical Excellence.

NICE/National Collaborating Centre for Cancer. (2012a) *Neutropenic Sepsis: prevention and management of neutropenic sepsis in cancer patients.* London. National Institute for Health and Clinical Excellence.

NICE. (2012b) *Venous Thromboembolic diseases: the management of venous thromboembolic diseases and the role of thrombophilia testing. CG144.* London. National Institute for Health and Care Excellence

NICE. (2012c) *Quality standard for nutrition support in adults. QS24.* London. National Institute for Clinical Excellence.

NICE. (2013a) *Acute kidney injury. Prevention, detection and management of acute kidney injury up to the point of renal replacement therapy.* NICE clinical guideline 169. London. National Institute for Clinical Excellence.

NICE. (2013b) *Intravenous fluid therapy in adults in hospital. NICE clinical guideline 174.* London. National Institute for Clinical Excellence.

NICE. (2014a) *Acute heart failure: diagnosing and managing acute heart failure in adults. Clinical guideline 187.* London. National Institute for Clinical Excellence.

NICE. (2014b) Head Injury: Triage, assessment, investigation and early management of head injury in children, young people and adults. London. National Institute for Clinical Excellence.

NICE-SUGAR Study investigators. (2009) Intensive versus conventional glucose control in critically ill patients. *New England Journal of Medicine.* 360 (130): 1283–1297.

Nielsen, N., Wetterslev, J., Cronberg, T., Erlinge, D., Gasche, Y., Hassager, C., Horn, J., Hovdenes, J., Kjaergaard, J., Kuiper, M., Pellis, T., Stammet, P., Wanscher, M., Wise, M.P., Åneman, A., Al-Subaie, N., Boesgaard, S., Bro-Jeppesen, J., Brunetti, I., Bugge, J.F., Hingston, C.D., Juffermans, N.P., Koopmans, M., Køber, L., Langørgen, J., Lilja, G., Møller, JE., Rundgren, M., Rylander, C., Smid, O., Werer, C., Winkel, P., Friberg, H., for the TTM Trial Investigators. (2013) Targeted temperature management at 33°C versus 36°C after cardiac arrest. *New England Journal of Medicine.* 369 (23): 2197–2206.

Nightingale, F. (1859/1980) *Notes on Nursing: what it is, and what it is not.* Edinburgh. Churchill Livingstone.

Nilles, K.M., Subramanian, R.M. (2012) Intensive care management of patients prior to liver transplantation. In Abdeldayem, H. (ed) *Liver Transplantation – Basic Issues.* Rijeka, Croatia. InTech. 321–331.

NMC. (2007) *Standards for Medicines Management.* London. Nursing and Midwifery Council.

NMC. (2015) *The Code: professional standards of practice and behaviour for nurses and midwives.* London. Nursing and Midwifery Council.

NMC. (2011) *Annual Fitness to Practice Report: 2010–2011.* London. Nursing and Midwifery Council.

Nolan, J.P., Kelley, F.E. (2011) Airway challenges in critical care. *Anaesthesia.* 66 (supplement 2): 81–92.

Norberg, A., Brauer, K.I., Prough, D.S., Gabrielsson, J., Hahn, R.G., Uchida, T., Traber, D.L., Svensén, C.H. (2005) Volume turnover kinetics of fluid shifts after hemorrhage, fluid infusion, and the combination of hemorrhage and fluid infusion in sheep. *Anesthesiology.* 109 (5): 985–994.

Northfield, T.C. (1971) Oxygen therapy for spontaneous pneumothorax. *British Medical Journal.* 4 (5779): 86–88.

NPSA. (2007a) *Safer Care for the Acutely Ill Patient: Learning from Serious Incidents*. London. National Patient Safety Agency.

NPSA. (2007b) *Patient Safety Alert 21: Safer Practice with Epidural Injections and Infusions.* London. National Patient Safety Agency.

NPSA. (2007c) *Patient Safety Alert 22: Reducing the Risk of Hyponatraemia when Administering Intravenous Infusions to Children*. London. National Patient Safety Agency.

NPSA. (2007d) *Protected Mealtimes*. (ref0367). London. National Patient Safety Agency.

NPSA. (2008) *Rapid Response Report: Risks of Chest Drain Insertion*. NPSA/2008/RRR03. London. National Patient Safety Agency.

NPSA. (2009) *Rapid Response Report: Oxygen Safety in Hospitals. NPSA/ 2009/RRR006:* London. National Patient Safety Agency.

Nunnally, M.E., Jaeschke, R., Bellingan, G.J., Lacroix, J., Mourvillier, B., Rodriguez-Vega, G.M., Rubertsson, S., Vassilakopoulos, T., Craig, W. (2011) Targeted temperature management in critical care. A report and recommendations from five professional societies. *Critical Care Medicine.* 39 (5): 1113–1125.

Nyirenda, M., Tang, J.I., Padfield, P.L., Seckl, J.R. (2009) Hyperkalaemia. *British Medical Journal.* 339 (7728): 1019–1024.

O'Brien, E., Parati, G., Stergiou, G., Asmar, R., Beilin, L., Bilo, G., Clement, D., de la Sierra, A., de Leeuw, P., Dolan, E., Fagard, R., Graves, J., Head, G.A., Imai, Y., Kario, K., Lurbe, E., Mallion, J.-M., Mancia, G., Mengden, T., Myers, M., Ogedegbe, G., Ohkubo, T., Omboni, S., Palatini, P., Redon, J., Ruilope, L.M., Shennan, A., Staessen, J.A., van Montfrans, G., Verdecchia, P., Waeber, B., Wang, J., Zanchetti, A., Zhang, Y., on behalf of the European Society of Hypertension Working Group on Blood Pressure Monitoring. (2013) European Society of Hypertension position paper on ambulatory blood pressure monitoring. *Journal of Hypertension.* 31 (8):1731–1768.

Ochola, J., Venkatesh, B. (2009) Rational approach to fluid therapy in acute diabetic ketoacidosis. In Vincent, J.-L. (ed). *2009 Yearbook of Intensive Care and Emergency Medicine.* 254–262.

O'Grady, N.P., Alexander, M., Burns, L.A., Dellinger, E.P., Garland, J., Heard, S.O., Lipsett, P.A., Masur, H., Mermel, L.A., Pearson, M.L., Raad, I.I., Randolph, A., Rupp, M.E., Saint, S., the Healthcare Infection Control Practices Advisory Committee (HICPAC). (2011) Guidelines for the prevention of intravascular catheter-related infections, 2011. *Clinical Infectious Diseases.* 52 (9): e162-e193.

Olin, K., Eriksdotter-Jönhagen, M., Jansson, A., Herrington, M.K., Kristiansson, M., Permert, J. (2005) Postoperative delirium in elderly patients after major abdominal surgery. *British Journal of Surgery.* 92 (12): 1559–1564.

Ormerod, C., Farrer, K., Lal, S. (2010) Refeeding syndrome: a clinical review. *British Journal of Hospital Medicine.* 71 (12): 686–690.

Osanai, T., Kuroda, S., Sugiyama, T., Kawabori, M., Ito, M., Shichinoheb, H., Kuge, Y., Houkin, K., Tamaki, N., Iwasaki, Y. (2012) Therapeutic effects of intra-arterial delivery of bone marrow stromal cells in traumatic brain injury of rats – in vivo cell tracking study by near-infrared fluorescence imaging. *Neurosurgery.* 70 (2): 435–444.

O'Shea, P. (1997) Altered consciousness and stroke. In Goldhill, D.R., Withington, P.S. (eds) *Textbook of Intensive Care.* London. Chapman & Hall. 495–502.

O'Shea, R.S., Dasarathy, S., McCullough, A.J., the Practice Guideline Committee of the American Association for the Study of Liver Diseases and the Practice Parameters Committee of the American College of Gastroenterology. (2010) Alcoholic liver disease. *Hepatology.* 53 (3): 307–328.

Ouldred, E., Bryant, C. (2011) Delirium: prevention, clinical features and management. *Nursing Standard.* 25 (28): 47–56.

Overgaard-Steensen, C. (2010) Initial approach to the hyponatremic patient. *Acta Anaesthesiologica Scandinavica.* 55 (2): 139–148.

Owen, J.A., Punt, J., Stranford, S.A., Jones, P.P. (2013) *Kuby Immunology.* 7th edn. New York. WH Freeman and Company.

Page, V.J., Ely, E.W., Gates, S., Zhao, X.B., Alce, T., Shintani, A., Jackson, J., Perkins, G.D., McAuley, D.F. (2013) Effect of intravenous haloperidol on the duration of delirium and coma in critically ill patients (Hope-ICU): a randomised, double-blind, placebo-controlled trial. *The Lancet Respiratory Medicine.* 1 (7): 515–523.

Palma, S., Cosano, A., Mariscal, M., Martinez-Gallego, G., Medina-Cuadros, M., Delgado-Rodriguez, M. (2007) Cholesterol and serum albumin as risk factors for death in patients undergoing general surgery. *British Journal of Surgery.* 94 (3): 369–375.

Pandharipande, P.P., Girard, T.D., Jackson, J.C., Morandi, A., Thompson, J.L., Pun, B.T., Brummel, N.E., Hughes, C.G., Vasilevskis, E.E., Shintani, A.K., Moons, K.G., Geevarghese, S.K., Canonico, A., Hopkins, R.O., Bernard, G.R., Dittus, R.S., Ely, E.W., for the BRAIN-ICU Study Investigators. (2013) Long-term cognitive impairment after critical illness. *New England Journal of Medicine.* 369 (14): 1306–1316.

Papiris, S., Kotanidou, A., Malagari, K., Roussos, C. (2002) Clinical review: severe asthma. *Critical Care.* 6: 30–44.

Papiris, S.A., Roussos, C. (2004) Pleural disease in the intensive care unit. In Bouros, D. (ed) *Pleural Disease (Lung Biology in Health and Disease).* New York. Marcel Dekker. 771–777.

Parikh, M., Webb, S.T. (2012) Cations: potassium, calcium, and magnesium. *Continuing Education in Anaesthesia, Critical Care & Pain.* 12 (4): 195–198.

Parkes, C. (1996) *Bereavement: studies of grief in adult life.* London. Penguin.

Parliament. (2000) *Adults with Incapacity (Scotland) Act.* London. Stationery Office.

Parliament. (2005) *Mental Capacity Act.* London. Stationery Office.

Parliamentary and Health Service Ombudsman. (2013) *Time To Act: Severe sepsis: rapid diagnosis and treatment saves lives.* London. Parliamentary and Health Service Ombudsman.

Parola, D., Romani, S., Petroianni, A., Locorriere, L., Terzano, C. (2012) Treatment of acute exacerbations with non-invasive ventilation in chronic hypercapnic COPD patients with pulmonary hypertension. *European Review of Medical and Pharmacological Science.* 16 (2): 183–191.

Parsons, T. (1951) *The Social System.* Free Press. New York.

Parsons, C.L., Sole, M.L., Byers, J.F. (2000) Noninvasive positive-pressure ventilation: averting intubation of the heart failure patient. *Dimensions of Critical Care Nursing.* 19 (6): 18–24.

Pasero, C., McCaffery, M. (2011) *Pain assessment and pharmacologic management.* St. Louis. Mosby Elsevier.

Pasero, C., Stannard, D. (2012) The role of intravenous acetaminophen in acute pain management: a case-illustrated review. *Pain Management Nursing.* 13 (2): 107–124.

Patel, A.S., Burnard, K.G. (2009) Cardiovascular haemodynamics and shock. *Surgery.* 27 (11): 459–464.

Patel, S.R., White, D.P., Malhotra, A., Stanchina, M.L., Ayas, N.T. (2003) Continuous Positive Airway Pressure therapy for treating sleepiness in a diverse population with obstructive sleep apnea. *Archives of Internal Medicine.* 163 (5): 565–571.

Pathology Harmony. (2011) *Harmonisation of Reference Intervals.* www.pathology harmony.co.uk/ . . . /Pathology%Harmony%201120%f (last accessed 19 April 2015).

Patil, B.B., Dowd, T.C. (2000) Physiological functions of the eye. *Current Anaesthesia and Critical Care.* 11 (6): 291–298.

Patton, H., Misel, M., Gish, R.G. (2012) Acute liver failure in adults: an evidence-based management protocol for clinicians. *Gastroenterology & Hepatology.* 8 (3): 161–212.

Pépin, J., Valiquette, L., Cossette, B. (2005) Mortality attributable to nosocomial *Clostridium difficile*–associated disease during an epidemic caused by a hypervirulent strain in Quebec. *Canadian Medical Association Journal.* 173 (9): 1037– 042.

Perazella, M.A. (2012) Drug use and nephrotoxicity in the Intensive Care Unit. *Kidney International.* 81 (12): 1172–1178.

Perel, P., Roberts, I., Ker, K. (2013) Colloids versus crystalloids for fluid resuscitation in critically ill patients. *Cochrane Database of Systematic Reviews* 2013, Issue 2. Art. No.: CD000567. DOI: 10.1002/14651858.CD000567.pub6.

Peris, A., Zagli, G., Bonizzoli, M., Cianchi, G., Ciapetti, M., Spina, R., Anichini, V., Lapi, F., Batacchi, S. (2010) Implantation of 3951 long-term central venous catheters: performances, risk analysis, and patient comfort after ultrasound-guidance introduction. *Anesthesia & Analgesia.* 111 (5): 1194–201

Peters, M., Heijboer, H., Smiers, F., Goprado, P.C. (2012) Diagnosis and management of thalassaemia. *British Medical Journal.* 344 (7841): 40–44.

Philips, S., Collins, M., Dougherty, L. (2011) *Venepuncture and Cannulation.* Oxford. Wiley Blackwell.

Pierce, J.D., Cackler, A.B., Arnett, M.G. (2004) Why should you care about free radicals? *American Journal of Nursing.* 67 (1): 38–42.

Pilwer, A., Åkeson, A., Lindgren, S. (2012) Complications associated with peripheral or central routes for central venous cannulation. *Anaesthesia.* 67 (1): 65–71.

Pitt, T. (2007) Management of antimicrobial-resistant Acinitobacter in hospitals. *Nursing Standard.* 21 (35): 51–56.

Poponcik, J.M., Renston, J.P., Bennett, R.P., Emerman, C.L. (1999) Use of a ventilatory support system (BiPAP) for acute respiratory failure in the emergency department. *Chest.* 116 (1): 166–171.

Porter, J.B. (2009) Optimizing iron chelation strategies in beta-thalassaemia major. *Blood Reviews.* 23 (supplement 1): S3–S7.

Powell-Tuck, J., Gosling, P., Lobo, D.N., Allison, S.P., Carlson, G.L., Gore, M., Lewington, A.J., Pearse, R.M., Mythen, M.G. (2008/2011) *British Consensus Guidelines on Intravenous Fluid Therapy for Adult Surgical Patients. GIFTASUP.* London. BAPEN, Association for Clinical Biochemistry, Association of Surgeons of Great Britain and Ireland, Society of Academic and Research Surgery, Renal Association, Intensive Care Society.

Power, B. (2014) Acute cardiac syndromes, investigations and interventions. In Bersten, A.D., Soni, N. (eds) *Intensive Care Manual.* 7th edn. Edinburgh. Butterworth-Heinemann. 167–190.

Preise, J.-C., Devos, P., Ruiz-Santana, S., Mélot, C., Annane, D., Groeneveld, J., Iapichino, G., Leverve, X., Nitenberg, G., Singer, P., Wernerman, J., Joannidis, M., Stecher, A., Chioléro, R. (2009) A prospective randomised multi-centre controlled trial on tight glycaemic control by intensive insulin therapy in adult intensive care units: the Glucontrol study. *Intensive Care Medicine.* 35 (10): 1738–1748.

Price, A.M., Plowright, C., Makowski, A., Misztal, B. (2008) Using a high-flow respiratory system (Vapotherm) within a high dependency setting. *Nursing in Critical Care.*13 (6): 298–303.

Priestley J. (1775) *Philosophical transactions.* London. Royal Society.

Pritchard, M.J. (2009) Identifying and assessing anxiety in pre-operative patients. *Nursing Standard.* 23 (51): 35–40.

Pruss, A., Caspari, G., Krüger, D.H., Blümel, J., Nübling, C.M., Gürtler, L., Gerlich, W.H. (2010) Tissue donation and virus safety: more nucleic acid amplification testing is needed. *Transplant Infectious Disease.* 15 (5): 375–386.

Pryor, J.A., Prasad, S.A. (2008) *Physiotherapy for Respiratory and Cardiac Problems.* 4th edn. Edinburgh. Churchill Livingstone Elsevier.

Prytherch, D.R., Smith, G.B., Schmidt, P.A., Featherstone, P.I. (2010) ViEWS – Towards a national early warning score for detecting adult inpatient deterioration. *Resuscitation.* 81 (8): 932–937.

Puntillo, K.A., Max, A., Timsit, J.F., Vignoud, L., Chanques, G., Robleda, G., Roche-Campo, F., Mancebo, J., Divatia, J.V., Soares, M., Ionescu, D.C., Grintescu, I.M., Vasiliu, I.L., Maggiore, S.M., Rusinova, K., Owczuk, R., Egerod, I., Papathanassoglou, E.D.E., Kyranou, M., Joynt, G.M., Burghi, G., Freebairn, R.C., Ho, K.K., Kaarlola, A., Gerritsen, R.T., Kesecioglu, J., Sulaj, M.M.S., Norrenberg, M., Benoit, D.D., Seha, M.S.G., Hennein, A., Periera, F.J., Benbenishty, J.S., Abroug, F., Aquilina, A., Monte, J.R.C., An, Y., Azoulay, E. (2014) Determinants of procedural pain intensity in the intensive care unit. The Europain® study. *American Journal of Respiratory and Critical Care Medicine.* 189 (1): 39–47.

Putaala, J., Metso, T.M., Metso, A.J., Mäkelä, E., Haapaniemi, E., Salonen, O., Kaste, M., Tatisumak, T. (2009) Thrombolysis in young adults with ischaemic stroke. *Stroke.* 40 (6): 2085–2091.

Rahman, T.M., Treacher, D. (2002) Management of acute renal failure on the intensive care unit. *Clinical Medicine.* 2 (2): 108–113.

Raithatha, A., Pratt, G., Rash, A. (2013) Developments in the management of acute ischaemic stroke implications for anaesthetic and critical care management. *Continuing Education in Anaesthesia, Critical Care & Pain.* 13 (3): 80–86.

Randhawa., G. (2012) Death and organ donation: meeting the needs of multiethnic and multifaith populations. *British Journal of Anaesthesia.* 108 (supplement 1): i88–i91.

Rashid, M., Goldin, R., Wright, M. (2004) Drugs and the liver. *Hospital Medicine.* 65 (8): 456–461.

Ratcliffe, A.T., Pepper, C. (2008) Thrombolysis or primary angioplasty? Reperfusion therapy for myocardial infarction in the UK. *Postgraduate Medical Journal.* 84 (988): 73–77.

Ravenscroft, A.J., Bell, M.D.D. (2000) 'End-of-life' decision making within intensive care – objective, consistent, defensible? *Journal of Medical Ethics.* 26 (6): 435–440.

RCN. (2003) *Defining Nursing.* London. Royal College of Nursing.

RCN. (2005) *Clinical Practice Guidelines: Perioperative Fasting in Adults and Children.* London. Royal College of Nursing.

RCN. (2008a) *Bowel Care, Including Digital Rectal Examination and Removal of Faeces.* London. Royal College of Nursing.

RCN. (2008b) *Enhancing Nutritional Care.* London. Royal College of Nursing.

RCN. (2008c) *Let's Talk about Restraint Revisited.* London. Royal College of Nursing.

RCN. Policy Unit. (2009) *The Assistant Practitioner Role. A Policy Discussion Paper. Policy Brief 06/2009.* London. Royal College of Nursing.

RCN. (2010) *Standards for Infusion Therapy.* London. Royal College of Nursing.

RCN. (2012) *Mandatory Nurse Staffing Levels.* London. Royal College of Nursing.

RCP. (2011) *Standardising the Assessment of Acute Illness Severity in the NHS.* London. Royal College of Physicians.

RCP. (2012a) *National Early Warning Score (NEWS): Standardising the assessment of acute illness severity in the NHS. Report of a working party.* London. Royal College of Physicians. (revision scheduled 2015)

RCP. (2012b) *National Clinical Guideline for Stroke.* 4th edn. London. Royal College of Physicians.

RCP/BTS/ICS. (2008) *Chronic Obstructive Pulmonary Disease: Non-invasive Ventilation with Bi-phasic Positive Airways Pressure in the Management of Patients with Acute Type 2 Respiratory Failure.* London. Royal College of Physicians, British Thoracic Society, Intensive Care Society.

Reding, M.T., Cooper, D.L. (2012) Barriers to effective diagnosis and management of a bleeding patient with undiagnosed bleeding disorder across multiple specialties: results of a quantitative case-based survey. *Journal of Multidisciplinary Healthcare.* 5: 277–287.

Redón, J., Bartolin, V., Giner, V., Lurbe, E. (2001) Assessment of blood pressure: early morning rise. *Blood Pressure Monitoring.* 6 (4): 207–210.

Rees, D.C., Williams, T.N., Gladwin, M.T. (2010) Sickle-cell disease. *The Lancet.* 376 (9757): 2018–2031.

Reitsma, S., Slaaf, D.W., Vink, H., van Zandvoort, M.A.M.J., oude Egbrink, M.G.A. (2007) The endothelial glycocalyx: composition, functions, and visualization. *European Journal of Physiology.* 454 (3): 345–359.

Resuscitation Council (UK). (2008) *Emergency treatment of anaphylactic reactions. Guidelines for healthcare providers.* London. Resuscitation Council (UK).

Resuscitation Council. (2010) *Resuscitation Guidelines.* London. Resuscitation Council.

Revelley, J.P., Tappy, L., Berger, M.M., Gerbach, P., Cayeux, C., Chiolero, R. (2001) Early metabolic and splanchnic responses to enteral nutrition in postoperative cardiac surgery patients with circulatory compromise. *Intensive Care Medicine.* 27 (3): 540–547.

Reynolds, R.M., Padfield, P.L., Seckl, J.R. (2006) Disorders of sodium balance. *British Medical Journal.* 332 (7543): 702–705.Rutherford IA. (1996) Haemostasis and disseminated intravascular coagulation. *Intensive and Critical Care Nursing.* 12 (3): 161–167.

Richardson, A., Allsop, M., Coghill, E., Turnock, C. (2007) Earplugs and eye masks: do they improve critical care patients' sleep? *Nursing in Critical Care.* 12 (6): 278–286.

Richardson, C. (2008) Nursing aspects of phantom limb pain following amputation. *British Journal of Nursing.* 17 (7): 422–426.

Rickes, S., Uhle, C. (2009) Advances in the diagnosis of acute pancreatitis. *Postgraduate Medical Journal.* 85 (2002): 208–212.

Riley, B., de Beer, T. (2014) Acute cerebrovascular complications. In Bersten, A.D., Soni, N. (eds) *Intensive Care Manual.* 7th edn. Edinburgh. Butterworth-Heinemann Elsevier. 568–579.

Roberts, I., Shakur, H., Ker, K., Coats, T, on behalf of the CRASH-2 Trial collaborators. (2011) *Antifibrinolytic drugs for acute traumatic injury.* Cochrane Database of Systematic Reviews, Issue 1. Art. No.: CD004896. DOI: 10.1002/14651858.CD004896.pub3.

Roberts, M.E., Neville, E., Berrisford, R.G., Antunes, G., Ali, N.J., BTS Pleural Disease Guideline Group. (2010) Management of a malignant pleural effusion: British Thoracic Society pleural disease guideline 2010. *Thorax.* 65 (Supplement 2): ii32-ii40.

Robinson, J. (2009) Information on practical procedures following death. *Nursing Standard.* 23 (19): 42–46.

Rodden, A.M., Spicer, L., Diaz, V.A., Steyer, T.E. (2007) Does fingernail polish affect pulse oximeters readings? *Intensive and Critical Care Nursing.* 23 (1): 51–55.

Rodríguez-Villar, C., Paredes, D., Ruiz, A., Alberola, M., Montilla, C., Vilardell, J., Manyalich, M., Miranda, B. (2009) Attitude of health professionals toward cadaveric tissue donation. *Transplantation Proceedings.* 41 (6): 2064–2066.

Rogowski, J.A., Staiger, D., Patrick, T., Horbar, J., Kenny, M., Lake, E.T. (2013) Nurse staffing and NICU infection rates. *Journal of the American Medical Association Pediatrics.* 167 (5): 444–450.

Romero, C.M., Marambio, A., Larrondo, J., Walker, K., Lira, M.-T., Tobar, E., Cornejo, R., Ruiz, M. (2010) Swallowing dysfunction in nonneurologic critically ill patients who require percutaneous dilational tracheostomy. *Chest. 137* (6): 1278–1282.

Roper, N., Logan, W., Tierney, A. (1996) *The Elements of Nursing.* 4th edn. Edinburgh. Churchill Livingstone.

Roskelly, L., Smith, A.P. (2011) Respiratory Care. In Dougherty, L., Lister, S (eds). *The Royal Marsden Hospital Manual of Clinical Nursing Procedures.* 8th edn. Oxford. Wiley-Blackwell. 534–614.

Rotondi, F., Manganelli, F. (2013) Takotsubo cardiomyopathy and arrhythmic risk: the dark side of the moon. *European Review for Medical and Pharmacological Sciences.* 17 (1): 105–111.

Runcimann, W.B., Ludbrook, G.L. (1996) The measurement of systemic arterial blood pressure. In Prys-Roberts, C., Brown, B.R. Jr. (eds) *International Practice of Anaesthesia.* Oxford. Butterworth Heinemann. 2/154/1–11.

Russell, C.A., Elia, M. (2009) *Nutrition Screening Survey in the UK in 2008.* London. British Association for Parenteral and Enteral Nutrition (BAPEN).

Rutledge, T., Reis, V.A., Linke, S.E., Greenberg, B.H., Millis, P.I. (2006) Depression in heart failure. A meta-analytic review of prevalence, interaction effects, and associations with clinical outcomes. *Journal of the American College of Cardiology.* 48 (8): 1527–1537.

Ruxton, C. (2012) Promoting and maintaining healthy hydration in patients. *Nursing Standard.* 26 (31): 50–56.

Ryan, K., Bain, B.J., Worthington, D., James, J., Plews, D., Mason, A., Roper, D., Rees, D.C., de la Salle, B., Streetly, A., British Committee for Standards in Haematology. (2010) Significant haemoglobinopathies: guidelines for screening and diagnosis. *British Journal of Haematology.* 149 (1): 35–49.

Safar, M.E., Levy, B.I., Struijker-Boudier, H. (2003) Current perspectives on arterial stiffness and pulse pressure in hypertension and cardiovascular diseases. *Circulation.* 107 (22): 2864–2869.

Sahin, T., Celikyurt, U., Geyik, B., Oner, G., Kilic, T., Bildirici, U., Kozdag, G., Ural, D. (2012) Relationship between endothelial functions and acetylsalicylic acid resistance in newly diagnosed hypertensive patients. *Clinical Cardiology.* 35 (12): 755–763.

Saidi, M., Brett, S. (2009) Pandemic influenza: clinical epidemiology. In Ridley, S. (ed) *Critical Care Focus 16: Infection.* London. Intensive Care Society. 117–134.

Saliba, W., Wazni, O.M. (2011) Sinus rhythm restoration and treatment success: insight from recent clinical trials. *Clinical Cardiology.* 34 (1): 12–22.

Sargent, S. (2005) The aetiology, management and complications of alcoholic hepatitis. *British Journal of Nursing.* 14 (10): 556–562.

Sargent, S. (2007) Pathophysiology and management of hepatic encephalopathy. *British Journal of Nursing.* 16 (6): 335–339.

Saw, M.M., Chandler, B., Ho, K.M. (2012) Benefits and risks of using gelatin solution as a plasma expander for perioperative and critically ill patients: a meta-analysis. *Anaesthesia & Intensive Care.* 40 (1): 17–32

Sawhney, N.S., Feld, G.K. (2008) Diagnosis and management of typical atrial flutter. *Medical Clinics of America.* 92 (1): 65–85.

SBAR. www.institute.nhs.uk/quality_and_service_improvement_tools/quality_and_service_improvement_tools/sbar_-_situation_-_background_-_assessment_-_recommendation.html (last accessed 29 June 2015)

Schalk, B.W.M., Deeg, D.J.H., Penninx, B.W.J.H., Bouter, L.M., Visser, M. (2005) Serum albumin and muscle strength: a longitudinal study in older men and women. *Journal of the American Geriatrics Society.* 53 (8): 1331–1338.

Scheer, F.A.J.L., Shea, S.A. (2014) Human circadian system causes a morning peak in prothrombotic plasminogen activator inhibitor-1 (PAI-1) independent of the sleep/wake cycle. *Blood.* 123 (4): 590–593.

Schloerb, P.R. (2004) Glucose in parenteral nutrition: a survey of US medical centres. *Journal of Parenteral & Enteral Nutrition.* 28 (6): 447–452.

Scrase, W., Tranter, S. (2011) Improving evidence-based care for patients with pyrexia. *Nursing Standard*. 25 (29): 37–41.

Sego, S. (2007) Pathophysiology of diabetic nephropathy. *Nephrology Nursing Journal*. 34 (6): 631–633.

Seligman, M.E.P. (1975) *Helplessness: on depression, development and death*. New York. W. H. Freeman.

Sendelbach, S., Guthrie, P. (2009) Acute confusion/delirium: identification, assessment, treatment, and prevention. *Journal of Gerontological Nursing*. 35 (11): 11–18.

Sessler, D.I. (2008) Temperature monitoring and perioperative thermoregulation *Anesthesiology*. 109 (2): 318–338.

Shannon, S.A., Mitchell, P.H., Cain, K.C. (2002) Patients, nurses, and physicians have differing views of quality of critical care. *Journal of Nursing Scholarship*. 34 (2): 173–179.

Shannon-Lowe, J., Matheson, N.J., Cooke, F.J., Aliyu, S.H. (2010) Prevention and medical management of *Clostridium difficile* infection. *British Medical Journal*. 340 (7747): 605–662.

Sickle Cell Society. (2008) *Standards for the Clinical Care of Adults with Sickle Cell Disease in the UK*. London. Sickle Cell Society.

Siddiqi, N., House, A.O., Holmes, J.D. (2006) Occurrence and outcome of delirium in medical in-patients: a systematic literature review. *Age & Ageing*. 35 (4): 350–364.

SIGN/BTS. (2012) *British Guideline on the Management of Asthma*. Edinburgh/London.

Simons, F.E.R., Ardusso, L.R.F., Bilò, M.B., El-Gamal, Y.M., Ledford, D.K., Ring, J., Sanchez-Borges, M., Senna, G.E., Sheikh, A., Thong, B.Y., World Allergy Organization. (2011) World Allergy Organization guidelines for the assessment and management of anaphylaxis. *WAO Journal*. 4 (1):13–37.

Sin, D.D., Logan, A.G., Fitzgerald, F.S., Liu, P.P., Bradley, T.D. (2000) Effects of continuous positive airway pressure on cardiovascular outcomes in heart failure patients and without cheyne-stokes respiration. *Circulation*. 102 (1): 61–66.

Singh, S., Trikha, S.P., Lewis, J. (2004) Acute compartment syndrome. *Current Orthopaedics*. 18 (6): 468–476.

Sirodkar, M., Mohandas, K.M. (2005) Subjective global assessment: a simple and reliable screening tool for malnutrition among Indians. *Indian Journal of Gasterenterology*. 24 (6): 246–250.

Skipworth, R.J.E., Stewart, G.D., Ross, J.A., Guttridge, D.C., Fearon, K.C.H. (2006) The molecular mechanisms of skeletal muscle wasting: implications for therapy. *The Surgeon*. 4 (5): 273–283.

Smith, D.H. (2007) Managing acute acetaminophen toxicity. *Nursing (2007)* 37 (1): 58–63.

Smith, K.A., Bigham, M. (2013) Cardiogenic shock. *The Open Pediatric Medicine Journal*. 7 (supplement 1: M5): 19–27.

Smorenberg, A., Ince, C., Groeneveld, A.B.J. (2013) Dose and type of crystalloid fluid therapy in adult hospitalized patients. *Perioperative Medicine*. 2 (1): 17.

Somauroo, J.D., Wilkinson, M., White, V.J., Rodrigues, E., Connelly, D.T., Calverley, P.M.A., Angus, R.M. (2000) Effect of nasal bilevel positive airway pressure (BiPAP) and continuous positive airway pressure (CPAP) ventilation on cardiac haemodynamics in patients with congestive heart failure. *Heart*. 83 (supplement II): A20.

Soo, L.H., Gray, D., Young, T., Hampton, J.R. (2000) Circadian variation in witnessed out of hospital cardiac arrest. *Heart*. 84 (4): 370–376.

Spasovski, G., Vanholder, R., Allolio, B., Annane, D., Ball, S., Bichet, D., Decaux, G., Fenske, W., Hoorn, E.J., Ichai, C., Joannidis, M., Soupart, A., Zietse, R., Haller, M., van der Veer, S., Van Biesen, W., Nagler, E., on behalf of the Hyponatraemia Guideline Development Group. (2014) Clinical practice guideline on diagnosis and treatment of hyponatraemia. *European Journal of Endocrinology*. 170: G1–G47.

Spirito, P., Autore, C. (2006) Management of hypertrophic cardiomyopathy. *British Medical Journal*. 332 (7552): 1251–1255.

Spodick, D.H. (2003) Acute cardiac tamponade. *New England Journal of Medicine*. 349 (7): 684–690.

Sque, M., Long, T., Payne, S., Allardyce, D. (2008) Why relatives do not donate organs for transplants: 'sacrifice' or 'gift of life'? *Journal of Advanced Nursing*. 61 (2): 134–144.

Sridhar, S., Botbol, Y., Macian, F., Cuervo1, A.M. (2012) Autophagy and disease: always two sides to a problem. *Journal of Pathology*. 226 (1): 255–273.

St George's Healthcare Trust. (2006) *Guidelines for the Care of Patients with Tracheostomy Tubes*. London. Smiths-Medical.

Starling, E. (1896) On the absorption of fluid from the connective tissue spaces. *Journal of Physiology*. 19 (4): 312–326.

Steggall, M.J. (2007) Urine samples and urinalysis. *Nursing Standard*. 22 (14–16): 42–45.

Stein, P.D., Woodward, P.K., Weg, J.G., Wakefield, T., Tapson, V., Sostman, H., Sos, T., Quinn, K., Leaper, K. Jr., Hull, R. (2006) Diagnostic pathways in acute pulmonary embolism: recommendations of the PIOPED II investigators. *American Journal of Medicine*. 119 (12): 1048–1055.

Stein, R.A. (2009) Lessons from outbreaks of H1N1 influenza. *Annals of Internal Medicine*. 151 (1): 59–62.

Stevens, K.R. (2013) The impact of evidence-based practice in nursing and the next big ideas. *OJIN: The Online Journal of Issues in Nursing*. 18 (2).

Stevens, P. (2007) Assessment of patients presenting with acute renal failure (acute kidney injury). *Medicine*. 35 (8): 429–433.

Straus, S.M.J.M., Kors, J.A., de Bruin, M.L., van der Hooft, C.S., Hofman, A., Heeringa, J., Deckers, J.W., Kingma, J.H., Sturkenboom, M.C.J.M., Stricker, B.M.C., Witteman, J.C.M. (2006) Prolonged QTc interval and risk of sudden cardiac death in a population of older adults. *Journal of the American College of Cardiology*. 47 (2): 362–367.

Strickler, J. (2010) Traumatic hypovolaemic shock. *Nursing 2010*. 40 (10): 34–40.

Stringer, S. (2007) Quality of death: humanisation versus medicalisation. *Cancer Nursing Practice*. 6 (3): 23–28.

Sturgess, D.J. (2014) Haemodynamic monitoring. In Bersten, A.D., Soni, N. (eds) *Intensive Care Manual*. 7th edn. Edinburgh. Butterworth-Heinemann Elsevier. 122–137.

Sullivan, B. (2008) Nursing management of patients with a chest drain. *British Journal of Nursing*. 17 (6): 388–393.

Swift, C., Calcutawalla, S., Elliot, R. (2007) Nursing attitudes towards recording of religious and spiritual data. *British Journal of Nursing*. 16 (20): 1279–1282.

Taher, A.T., Musallam, K.M., Cappellini, M.D., Weatherall, D.J. (2011) Optimal management of beta-thalassaemia intermedia. *British Journal of Haematology*. 152 (5): 512–523.

Tanaka, A., Kawarabayashi, T., Fukuda, D., Nishibori, Y., Sakamoto, T., Nishida, Y., Shimada, K., Yashikawa, J. (2004) Circadian variation of plaque rupture in acute myocardial infarction. *American Journal of Cardiology*. 93 (1): 1–5.

Tarassenk, L., Hann, A., Young, D. (2006) Integrated monitoring and analysis for early warning of patient deterioration. *British Journal of Anaesthesia*. 97 (1): 64–68.

Task Force for the management of acute coronary syndromes (ACS) in patients presenting without persistent ST-segment elevation of the European Society of Cardiology (ESC). (2011) ESC Guidelines for the management of acute coronary syndromes in patients presenting without persistent ST-segment elevation. *European Heart Journal*. 32 (23): 2999–3054.

Task Force for the Management of Arterial Hypertension of the European Society of Hypertension (ESH) and of the European Society of Cardiology (ESC). (2013) 2013

ESH/ESC Guidelines for the management of arterial hypertension. *European Heart Journal.* 34 (28): 2159–2219.

Task Force for the Management of Atrial Fibrillation of the European Society of Cardiology (ESC). (2010a) Guidelines for the management of atrial fibrillation. *European Heart Journal.* 31 (19): 2369–2429.

Task Force on Myocardial Revascularization of the European Society of Cardiology (ESC) and the European Association for Cardio-Thoracic Surgery (EACTS). (2010b) Guidelines on myocardial revascularization. *European Heart Journal.* 31 (20): 2501–2555.

Taylor, F., Ward, K., Moore, T.H.M., Burke, M., Davey Smith, G., Casas, J.P., Ebrahim, S. (2011) Statins for the primary prevention of cardiovascular disease. *Cochrane Database of Systematic Reviews* 2011, Issue 1. Art. No.: CD004816. DOI: 10.1002/14651858. CD004816.pub4.

Taylor, S.A. (2010) Safety and satisfaction provided by patient-controlled analgesia. *Dimensions of Critical Care Nursing.* 29 (4): 163–166.

Taylor, V., Ashelford, S. (2008) Understanding depression in palliative and end-of-life care. *Nursing Standard.* 23 (12): 48–57.

Teasdale, G., Jennett, B. (1974) Assessment of coma and impaired consciousness. *The Lancet.* ii (7872): 81–83.

Telfer, M., Lewin, A., Jenkins, P. (2007) Assisted ventilation in acute exacerbation of chronic obstructive pulmonary disease. *Journal of the Royal College of Physicians of Edinburgh.* 37 (1): 44–48.

Tenner, S., Baillie, J., DeWitt, J., Vege, S.S. (2013) American College of Gastroenterology Guideline: Management of Acute Pancreatitis. *American Journal of Gastroenterology.* 108 (9): 1400–1415.

Teoh, L.S.G., Gowardman, J.R., Larsen, P.D., Green, R., Galletly, D.C. (2000) Glasgow Coma Scale: variation in mortality among permutations of specific total scores. *Intensive Care Medicine.* 26 (2): 157–161.

Terrio, H., Brenner, L.A., Irvins, B., Cho, J.M., Helmick, K., Schwab, K., Scally K, Bretthauer R, Warden D. (2009) Preliminary findings regarding prevalence and sequelae in a US Army brigade combat team. *Journal of Head Trauma & Rehabilitation.* 24 (1): 14–23.

Thacker, K. (2008) Nurses' advocacy behaviors in end-of-life nursing care. *Nursing Ethics.* 15 (2): 174–185.

The IST-3 Collaborative Group. (2012) The benefits and harms of intravenous thrombolysis with recombinant tissue plasminogen activator within 6h of acute ischaemic stroke (the third international stroke trial [IST-3]): a randomised controlled trial. *The Lancet.* 379 (9834): 2352–2363.

Thiele, H., Zeymer, U., Neumann, F-J., Ferenc, M., Olbrich, H-G., Hausleiter, J., Richardt, G., Hennersdorf, M., Empen, K., Fuernau, G., Desch, S., Eitel, I., Hambrecht, R., Fuhrmann, J., Böhm, M., Ebelt, H., Schneider, S., Schuler, G., Werden, K., IABP-SHOCK II Trail Investigators. (2012) Intraaortic balloon support for myocardial infarction with cardiogenic shock. *New England Journal of Medicine.* 367 (14): 1287–1296.

Thomas, C., Lumb, A.B. (2012) Physiology of haemoglobin. *Continuing Education in Anaesthesia, Critical Care & Pain.* 12 (5): 251–256.

Thomas, D.R., Cote, T.R., Lawhorne, L., Levenson, S.A., Rubenstein, L.Z., Smith, D.A., Stefanacci, R.G., Tangalos, E.G., Morley, J.E., The Dehydration Council. (2008) Understanding clinical dehydration and its treatment. *Journal of the American Medical Directors Association.* 9 (5): 292–301.

Thomas, N (ed). (2014) *Renal Nursing.* 4th edn. Oxford. Wiley-Blackwell.

Thuong, M., Arvaniti, K., Ruimy, R., de la Salmonière, P., Scanvic-Hameg, A., Lucet, J.C., Régnier, B. (2003) Epidemiology of *Pseudomonas aeruginosa* and risk factors for carriage acquisition in an intensive care unit. *Journal of Hospital Infection.* 53 (4): 274–282.

Thygesen, K., Alpert, J.S., Jaffe, A.S., Simoons, M.L., Chaitman, B.R., White, H.D., Writing Group on behalf of the Joint ESC/ACCF/AHA/WHF Task Force for the Universal Definition of Myocardial. Infarction. (2012) Third universal definition of myocardial infarction. *European Heart Journal.* 33 (20): 2551–2567.

To, T., Stanojevic, S., Moores, G., Gershon, A.S., Bateman, E.D., Cruz, A.A., Boulet, L.-P. (2012) Global asthma prevalence in adults: findings from the cross-sectional world health survey. *BMC Public Health.* 12. 204.

Tocci, G., Ferrucci, A., Guida, P., Avogaro, A., Comaschi, C., Corsini, A., Cortese, C., Giorda, C.B., Manzato, E., Medea, G., Mureddu, G.F., Riccardi, G., Titta, G., Ventriglia, G., Zito, G.B., Volpe, M., EFFECTUS Steering Committee. (2011) Impact of diabetes mellitus on the clinical management of global cardiovascular risk: analysis of the results of the evaluation of final feasible effect of control training and ultra sensitization (EFFECTUS) educational program. *Clinical Cardiology.* 34 (9): 560–566.

Todaro, J.F., Shen, B.J., Niaura, R., Spiro, A. III, Ward, K.D. (2003) Effect of negative emotions on frequency of coronary heart disease (The Normative Aging Study). *American Journal of Cardiology.* 92 (8): 901–906.

Tonuma, M., Windbolt, M. (2001) From rituals to reason: creating an environment that allows nurses to nurse. *International Journal of Nursing Practice.* 6 (4): 214–218.

Toubia, N., Sanyal, A.J. (2008) Portal hypertension and variceal hemorrhage. *Medical Clinics of North America.* 92 (3): 551–574.

Townsend, N., Wickramasinghe, K., Bhatnagar, P., Smolina, K., Nichols, M., Leal, J., Luengo-Fernandez, R., Rayner, M. (2012) *Coronary Heart Disease Statistics 2012 edn.* London. British Heart Foundation.

Treadwell, L., Mendelow, D., Head Injury Audit Team. (1994) Audit of head injury management in the northern region. *British Journal of Nursing.* 3 (3): 136–140.

Treger, R., Pirouz, S., Kamangar, N., Corry, D. (2010) Agreement between central venous and arterial blood gas measurements in the Intensive Care Unit. *Clinical Journal of the American Society of Nephrologists.* 5 (3): 390–394.

Treleaven, J., Meller, S.T. (2000) Acute leukaemia. *Medicine.* 28 (3): 58–62.

Tschannen, D., Keenan, G., Aebersold, M., Kocan, M.J., Lundy, F., Averhart, V. (2011) Implications of nurse-physician relations: report of a successful intervention. *Nursing Economics.* 29 (3):127–135.

Turnbull, B. (2008) High-flow humidified oxygen therapy used to alleviate respiratory distress. *British Journal of Nursing.* 17 (19): 1226–1230.

Turpin, R.S., Solem, C., Pontes-Arruda, A., Sanon, M., Mehta, S., Liu, F.X., Botteman, M. (2014) The impact of parenteral nutrition preparation on bloodstream, infection risk and costs. *European Journal of Clinical Nutrition.* 68 (8): 953–958.

Tveit, A., Flonaes, B., Aaser, E., Korneliussen, K., Froland, G., Gullestad, L., Grundtvig, M. (2011) No impact of atrial fibrillation on mortality risk in optimally treated heart failure patients. *Clinical Cardiology.* 34 (9): 537–542.

Twigg, D.E., Duffield, C.M., Thompson, P., Rapley, P. (2010) The impact of nurses on patient morbidity and mortality – the need for a policy change in response to the nursing shortage. *Australian Health Review.* 34 (3), 312–316.

Tzeng, H.-M., Yin, C.-Y. (2012) Physical restraint use rate and total fall and injurious fall rates: an exploratory study in two US acute care hospitals. *Open Journal of Nursing.* 2: 170–175.

UK Working Party on Acute Pancreatitis. (2005) UK guidelines for the management of acute pancreatitis. *Gut.* 54: iii1–iii9.

United Kingdom Thalassaemia Society. (2008) Standards for the Clinical Care of Children and Adults with Thalassaemia in the UK. London. United Kingdom Thalassaemia Society.

Ünsal, A., Demir, G. (2012) Evaluation of sleep quality and fatigue in hospitalized patients. *International Journal of Caring Sciences.* 5 (3): 311–319.

Unverzagt, S., Wachsmuth, L., Hirsch, K., Thiele, H., Buerke, M., Haerting, J., Werdan, K., Prondzinsky, R. (2014) Inotropic agents and vasodilator strategies for acute myocardial infarction complicated by cardiogenic shock or low cardiac output syndrome. *Cochrane Database of Systematic Reviews* 2014, Issue 1. Art. No.: CD009669. DOI: 10.1002/14651858.CD009669.pub2.

Valiee, S., Negarandeh, R., Naueri, N.D. (2012) Exploration of Iranian intensive care nurses' experience of end-of-life care: a qualitative study. *Nursing in Critical Care.* 17 (6): 309–315.

Varghese, G,M., Trowbridgem P., Dohertym T. (2010) Investigating and managing pyrexia of unknown origin in adults. *British Medical Journal.* 341 (October): 878–881.

Venkatesh, B. (2014) Disorders of consciousness. In Bersten, A.D., Soni, N. (eds) *Intensive Care Manual.* 7th edn. Edinburgh. Butterworth-Heinemann Elsevier. 549–559.

Viles-Gonzalez, J.F., Fuster, V., Halperin, J., Calkins, H., Reddy, V.Y. (2011) Rhythm control for management of patients with atrial fibrillation: balancing the use of antiarrhythmic drugs and catheter ablation. *Clinical Cardiology.* 34 (1): 23–29.

Vinson, G.P., Coghlan, J.P. (2010) Expanding view of aldosterone action, with an emphasis on rapid action. *Clinical and Experimental Pharmacology and Physiology.* 37 (4): 410–416.

Viscusi, E.R., Siccardi, M., Damaraju, C.V., Hewitt, D.J., Kershaw, P. (2007) The safety and efficacy of fentanyl iontrophoretic transdermal system compared with morphine intravenous patient-controlled analgesia for postoperative pain management: an analysis of pooled data from three randomized, active-controlled clinical studies. *Anesthesia & Analgesia.* 105 (5): 1428–1436.

Visser, E., Schug, S.A. (2006) The role of ketamine in pain management. *Biomedicine & Pharmacology.* 60 (7): 341–348.

von Klemperer, K., Bunce, N.H. (2007) Chronic heart failure. *Care of the Critically Ill.* 23 95): 134–144.

Von Rueden, K.T., Des Champs, E.S., Johnson, K.L. (2013) Shock, systemic inflammatory response syndrome, and multiple organ dysfunction. In Morton, P.G., Fontaine, D.K.(eds). *Critical Care Nursing: a holistic approach.* 10th edn. Philadelphia, PA. Lippincott Williams and Wilkins. 1209–1233.

Voth, D.E., Ballard, J.D. (2005) *Clostridium difficile* toxins: mechanism of action and role in disease. *Clinical Microbiology Reviews.* 18 (2): 2247–2263.

Wakefield, B.J., Mentes, J., Holman, J.E., Culp, K. (2009) Postadmission dehydration: risk factors, indicators and outcomes. *Rehabilitation Nursing.* 34 (5): 209–216.

Waldmann, C., Barnes, R. (2004) Cannulation of central veins. *Anaesthesia and Intensive Care Medicine.* 5 (1): 6–9.

Walltmahmed, M. (2006) Insulin therapy in the management of type 1 and type 2 diabetes. *Nursing Standard.* 21 (6): 50–56.

Walsh, S.B., Tang, T., Wijewardena, C., Yarham, S.I., Boyle, J.R., Gaunt, M.E. (2007) Postoperative arrhythmias in general surgical patients. *Annals of the Royal College of Surgeons of England.* 89 (2): 91–95.

Walthour, A., Dassow, P. (2014) How should a positive urine urobilinogen dipstick test be evaluated? Family Physicians Inquiries Network. *Evidence Based Practice.* 17(12): E-1. URI: https://hdl.handle.net/10355/44601 (last accessed 4 January 2015).

Wang, J., Xu, E., Xiao, Y. (2014) Isotonic versus hypotonic maintenance IV fluids in hospitalized children: a meta-analysis. *Pediatrics.* 133 (1): 105–113.

Waterhouse, C. (2005) The Glasgow Coma Scale and other neurological observations. *Nursing Standard.* 19 (33): 56–64.

Waterhouse, J., Campbell, I. (2002) Respiration: gas transfer. *Anaesthesia & Critical Care.* 3 (9): 340–343.

Watkins, P.J. (2003) Retinopathy. *British Medical Journal.* 326 (7395): 924–926

Weatherall, D.J. 2010. The inherited diseases of hemoglobin are an emerging global health burden. *Blood.* DOI 10.1182/blood-2010-01-251348.

Weaver, L.K., Churchill, S.K., Deru, K., Cooney, D. (2013) False positive rate of carbon monoxide saturation by pulse oximetry of Emergency Department patients. *Respiratory Care.* 58 (2): 232–242.

Weetman, C., Allison, W. (2006) Use of epidural analgesia in post-operative pain management. *Nursing Standard.* 20 (44): 54–64.

Welch, J. (2000) Using assessment to identify and prevent critical illness. *Nursing Times.* 96 (20): 3–4.

Weng, C.-L., Zhao, Y.-T., Liu, Q.-H., Fu, C.-J., Sun F, Ma, Y.-L., Chen, Y.-W., He, Q.-Y. (2010) Meta-analysis: noninvasive ventilation in acute cardiogenic pulmonary edema. *Annals of Internal Medicine.* 152 (9): 590–600.

West, E., Barron, D.N., Reeves, R. (2005) Overcoming the barriers to patient-centred care: time, tools and training. *Journal of Clinical Nursing.* 14 (4): 435–443.

Weston, D. (2013) *Fundamentals of Infection Prevention and Control: Theory and Practice.* 2nd edn. Chichester. John Wiley & Sons.

White, D. (2002) Cardiogenic Shock: a more aggressive approach is now warranted. *European Heart Journal.* 21 (23): 1897–1901.

WHO (1968) *Nutritional Anaemias*: Report of a WHO Group of Experts. 1968. Geneva. World Health Organization.

WHO (1996) *Cancer Pain Relief.* 2nd edn. Geneva. World Health Organization.

WHO (2005a) *World Alliance for Patient Safety. WHO Draft Guidelines for Adverse Event Reporting and Learning Systems.* Geneva. World Health Organization.

WHO (2005b) *Global Patient Safety Challenge*: 2005–2006. Geneva. World Health Organization.

WHO (2014) *Antimicrobial Resistance. Global Report on Surveillance.* Geneva. World Health Organization.

Wigfull, J., Welchew, E. (2001) Survey of 1057 patients receiving postoperative patient-controlled epidural analgesia. *Anaesthesia.* 56 (1): 70–75.

Willard, C., Luker, K. (2006) Challenges to end of life care in the acute hospital setting. *Palliative Medicine.* 20 (6): 611–615.

Williams, A.M., Irurita, V.F. (2004) Therapeutic and non-therapeutic interpersonal interactions: the patient's perspective. *Journal of Clinical Nursing.* 13 (7): 806–815.

Williams, J.M.L., Williamson, RCN (2010) Alcohol and the pancreas. *British Journal of Hospital Medicine.* 71 (10): 556–561.

Williams, R., Aspinall, R., Bellis, M., Camps-Walsh, G., Cramp, M., Dhawan, A., Ferguson, J., Forton, D., Foster, G., Gilmore, I., Hickman, M., Hudson, M., Kelly, D., Langford, A., Lombard, M., Longworth, L., Martin, N., Moriarty, K., Newsome, P., O'Grady, J., Pryke, R., Rutter, H., Ryder, S., Sheron, N., Smith, T. (2014) Addressing liver disease in the UK: a blueprint for attaining excellence in health care and reducing premature mortality from lifestyle issues of excess consumption of alcohol, obesity, and viral hepatitis. *The Lancet.* 384 (9958): 1953–1997.

Wilson, L.A. (2005) Urinalysis. *Nursing Standard.* 19 (35): 51–54.

Winslow, E.H., Jacobson, A.F. (1998) Dispelling the petroleum jelly myth. *American Journal of Nursing.* 98 (11): 16.

Witlox, J., Eurelings, L.S.M., de Jonghe, J.F.M., Kalisvaart, K.J., Eikelenboom, P., van Gool, W.A. (2010) Patients and the risk of postdischarge mortality, institutionalization, and dementia: a meta-analysis. *Journal of the American Medical Association.* 304 (4): 443–451.

Wong, C.-K., Gao, W., Refel, C., French, J.K., Stewart, R.A., White, H.D., HERO-2 Investigators. (2006) Initial Q waves accompanying ST-segment elevation at presentation of acute myocardial infarction and 30-day mortality in patients given streptokinase therapy: an analysis from HERO-2. *The Lancet.* 367 (9528): 2061–2067.

Woodcock, T.E., Woodcock, T.M. (2012) Revised Starling equation and the glycocalyx model of transvacular fluid exchange: an improved paradigm for prescribing intravenous fluid therapy. *British Journal of Anaesthesia.* 108 (3): 384–394.

Woodford, H. (2010) *Essential Geriatrics.* Oxford. Radcliffe Publishing.

Woodward, S, Waterhouse C. (2009) *Oxford Handbook of Neuroscience Nursing.* Oxford. Oxford University Press.

Wren, M. (2009) *Clostridium difficile*: How big? How bad? In Ridley, S. (ed) *Critical Care Focus 16: Infection.* London. Intensive Care Society. 46–55.

Wright, B. (1991) *Sudden Death. Intervention skills for the caring professionals.* Edinburgh. Churchill Livingstone.

Wright, B. (1996) *Sudden Death. A research base for practice.* 2nd edn. Edinburgh. Churchill Livingstone.

Wu, C.L., Raja, S.N. (2011) Treatment of acute postoperative pain. *The Lancet.* 377 (9784): 2215–2225.

Yagihashi, S., Mizukami, H., Sugimoto, K. (2011) Mechanism of diabetic neuropathy: Where are we now and where to go? *Journal of Diabetes Investigation.* 2 (1): 18–32.

Yates, D.W., Elison, G., McGuiness, S. (1990) Care of the suddenly bereaved. *British Medical Journal.* 301 (6742): 29–31.

Yawn, B.P., Buchanan, G.R., Afenyi-Annan, A.N., Ballas, S.K., Hassell, K.L., James, A.H., Jordan, L., Lanzkron, S.M., Lottenberg, R., Savage, W.J., Tanabe, P.J., Ware, R.E., Murad, M.H., GoldSmith, J.C., Ortiz, E., Fulwood, R., Horton, A., John-Sowah, J. (2014) Management of sickle cell disease. Summary of the 2014 evidence-based report by expert panel members. *Journal of the American Medical Association.* 312 (10): 1033–1048.

Yellon, D.M., Hausenloy, D.J. (2007) Myocardial reperfusion injury. *New England Journal of Medicine.* 357 (11): 1121–1135.

Yin, A.T., Bradley, T.D., Liu, P.P. (2001) The role of continuous positive airway pressure in the treatment of congestive heart failure. *Chest.* 120 (5): 1675–1685.

Yip, P.D., Hannam, J.A., Cameron, A.J.D., Campbell, D. (2010) Incidence of residual neuromuscular blockade in a post-anesthetic care unit. *Anesthesia and Intensive Care.* 38 (1): 91–95.

Yki-Järvinen, H. (2014) Non-alcoholic fatty liver disease as a cause and a consequence of metabolic syndrome. *The Lancet Diabetes & Endocrinology.* 2 (11): 901–910.

Ympa, Y.P., Sakr, Y., Reinhart, K., Vincent, J.-L. (2005) Has mortality from acute renal failure decreased? A systematic review of the literature. *American Journal of Medicine.* 118 (8): 827–832.

Yoon, P.W., Bastian, B., Anderson, R.N., Collins, J.L., Jaffe, H.W. (2014) Potentially preventable deaths from the five leading causes of death – United States, 2008–2010. *Morbidity and Mortality Weekly Report.* 63 (17): 369–374.

Young, J., Stiffleet, J., Nikoletti, S., Shaw, T. (2006) Use of a behavioural pain scale to assess pain in ventilated, unconscious and/or sedated patients. *Intensive & Critical Care Nursing.* 22 (1): 32–39.

Yunos, N.M., Bellomo, R., Hegarty, C., Story, D., Ho, L., Bailey, M. (2012) Association between a chloride-liberal vs chloride-restrictive intravenous fluid administration strategy and kidney injury in critically ill adults. *Journal of the American Medical Association.* 308 (15): 1566–1572.

Zamani, M., Soleimani, M., Golab, F., Mohamadzadeh, F., Mehdizadeh, M., Katebi, M. (2013) Neuroprotective effects of adenosine receptor agonist coadministration with ascorbic acid on CA1 hippocampus in a mouse model of ischemia reperfusion injury. *Metabolic Brain Disease.* 28 (3): 367–374.

Zandieh, S., Katz, E.S. (2010) Retrograde lacrimal duct airflow during nasal positive pressure ventilation. *Journal of Clinical Sleep Medicine.* 6 (6): 603–604.

Zarzaur, B.L., Fukatsu, K., Kudsk, K.A. (2000) The influence of nutrition on mucosal immunology and endothelial cell adhesion molecules. In Vincent, J.-L. (ed) *Yearbook of Intensive Care and Emergency Medicine.* Berlin. Springer. 63–71.

Zhang, J., Ho, K.-Y., Wang, Y. (2011) Efficacy of pregablin in acute postoperative pain: a meta-analysis. *British Journal of Anaesthesia.*106 (4): 454–462.

Zilberstein, J., McCurdy, M.T., Winters, M.E. (2014) Anaphylaxis. *The Journal of Emergency Medicine.* 47 (2): 182–187.

Zirakzadeh, A., Patel, R. (2006) Vancomycin-resistant enterococci: colonization, infection, detection, and treatment. *Mayo Clinical Proceedings.* 81 (4): 529–536.

Zwarenstein, M., Goldman, J., Reeves, S. (2009) Interprofessional collaboration: effects of practice-based interventions on professional practice and healthcare outcomes. *Cochrane Database of Systematic Reviews* 2009, Issue 3. Art. No.: CD000072. DOI: 10.1002/14651858.CD000072.pub2.

Index